The Burden of Musculoskeletal Diseases

in the United States

Prevalence,

Societal

and Economic Cost

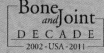

The Burden of Musculoskeletal Diseases in the United States is a joint project of the **American Academy of Orthopaedic Surgeons, American Academy of Physical Medicine and Rehabilitation, American College of Rheumatology, American Society for Bone and Mineral Research, Arthritis Foundation, National University of Health Sciences, Orthopaedic Research Society, Scoliosis Research Society, and the United States Bone and Joint Decade.**

Management Oversight Team and Major Contributing Organizations

Joshua J. Jacobs, MD
> Chair, Management Oversight Team, *The Burden of Musculoskeletal Diseases in the United States*

Gunnar B. J. Andersson, MD, PhD
John-Erik Bell, MD
Stuart L. Weinstein, MD
American Academy of Orthopaedic Surgeons (AAOS)

John P. Dormans, MD
Scoliosis Research Society (SRS)

Steve M. Gnatz, MD, MHA
American Academy of Physical Medicine and Rehabilitation (AAPM&R)

Nancy Lane, MD
United States Bone and Joint Decade (USBJD)

J. Edward Puzas, PhD
Orthopaedic Research Society (ORS)
President, United States Bone and Joint Decade (USBJD)

E. William St. Clair, MD
Edward H. Yelin, PhD
American College of Rheumatology (ACR)

Additional Contributing Organizations

American Society for Bone and Mineral Research (ASBMR)
Arthritis Foundation
National University of Health Sciences

Project Coordinator
Sylvia I. Watkins-Castillo, PhD

Staff
Robert H. Haralson, III, MD, MBA, Medical Director, AAOS
Toby R.W. King, CAE, Executive Director, USBJD
Amy Miller, Senior Director, Research, Training and Quality, ACR
Thomas E. Stautzenbach, MA, MBA, CAE, Executive Director, AAPM&R
Charles M. Turkelson, PhD, Director, Research and Scientific Affairs, AAOS
Marilyn Fox, PhD, Director, Publications, AAOS
Mary Steermann Bishop, Senior Manager, Production & Archives, AAOS
Courtney Astle, Assistant Production Manager, AAOS

Cover Design
Rick Cosaro, Cosaro & Associates, Ltd.

The Burden of Musculoskeletal Diseases in the United States
6300 N. River Road
Rosemont, IL 60018
United States of America
1-800-626-6726

Visit **www.boneandjointburden.org** for upcoming new chapters and an electronic version of this publication.

Authors and Reviewers

Gunnar B. J. Andersson, MD, PhD

Jeannette Bouchard

Kevin J. Bozic, MD, MBA

Robert M. Campbell, Jr., MD

Miriam G. Cisternas, MS

Adolfo Correa, MD. MPH, PhD

Felicia Cosman, MD

Janet D. Cragan, MD, MPH

Kristen D'Andrea, BA

Nancy Doernberg

John P. Dormans, MD, FACS

Ann L. Elderkin, PA

Zarina Fershteyn, MPH

Aimee J. Foreman, MA

Steven Gitelis, MD

Steve M. Gnatz, MD, MHA

Robert H. Haralson, III, MD, MBA

Charles G. (Chad) Helmick, MD

Serena Hu, MD

Jeffrey N. Katz, MD

Toby King, CAE

Ron Kirk, MA, DC

Steven M. Kurtz, PhD

Nancy Lane, MD

Assia Miller, MD, MPH

Reba L. Novich, MSW

Richard Olney, MD, MPH

Peter Panopalis, MD

David J. Pasta, MS

Andrew N. Pollak, MD

J. Edward Puzas, PhD

B. Steven Richards, III, MD

John P. Sestito, JD, MS

Csaba Siffel, MD, PhD

Paul D. Sponseller, MD

E. William St. Clair, MD

Andrew Stuart, MA

Kimberly J. Templeton, MD

George Thompson, MD

Laura Tosi, MD

William G. Ward, Sr., MD

Sylvia I. Watkins-Castillo, PhD

Stuart L. Weinstein, MD

James G. Wright, MD, MPH, FRCSC

Edward H. Yelin, PhD

Bone and Joint Decade

The Bone and Joint Decade is an international collaborative movement sanctioned by the United Nations/World Health Organization and **working to improve the quality of life for people with musculoskeletal conditions and to advance the understanding, prevention and treatment of these conditions.**

Officially proclaimed by the U.S. President, the United States Bone and Joint Decade (USBJD) 2002-2011 has been endorsed by all 50 States and more than one hundred national health care professional, patient and public organizations, all 125 U.S. medical schools and many colleges of medicine.

The goal of the United States Bone and Joint Decade is to improve bone and joint health by enhancing collaborative efforts among individuals and organizations in order to raise awareness of the growing burden of musculoskeletal disorders on society, to promote wellness and prevent musculoskeletal disease, and to advance research that will lead to improvements in prevention, diagnosis and treatment.

www.usbjd.org
usbjd@usbjd.org
Phone: 847-384-4010

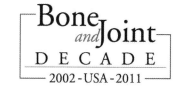

Table of Contents

Preface

It is with pleasure that I introduce you to this publication of the *Burden of Musculoskeletal Diseases in the United States*, the timely result of a partnership between the American Academy of Orthopaedic Surgeons and a number of other organizations supporting the U.S. Bone and Joint Decade (2002-2011). The level of disease recognition that the Decade has provided has done much to push the state of the science forward, and this new publication presents a snapshot of how far we have come since its predecessor, the 1999 *Musculoskeletal Conditions in the United States*, was released.

Although many advances have been made, musculoskeletal conditions remain common, chronic, and costly—and potentially disabling—to an increasingly graying population with high expectations of the health system. With the National Center for Health Statistics' 2005 National Health Interview Survey as a solid base, this publication examines such issues as spinal problems, arthritis and joint pain, osteoporosis, injuries, congenital conditions, neoplasms, and health care utilization and costs. The biomedically inclined reader will find within these pages both food for thought and a call to action.

The plight of millions of Americans whose lives are affected by the physical, financial, and emotional demands of musculoskeletal conditions make the findings of *Burden* difficult to ignore. I encourage you to read and digest its contents, and to appropriate for yourself those parts within your specific areas of interest or expertise.

Stephen I. Katz, MD, PhD
Director
National Institute of Arthritis and
Musculoskeletal and Skin Diseases
National Institutes of Health
Bethesda, Maryland
January 10, 2008

Foreword

Musculoskeletal disorders and diseases are the leading cause of disability in the United States and account for more that one-half of all chronic conditions in people over 50 years of age in developed countries. The economic impact of these conditions is also staggering. In 2004, the sum of the direct expenditures in health care costs and the indirect expenditures in lost wages for persons with a musculoskeletal disease diagnosis has been estimated to be $849 billion dollars, or 7.7% of the national gross domestic product.

Beyond these statistics, the human toll in terms of the diminished quality of life is immeasurable. This situation is unlikely to improve in the foreseeable future and will likely be intensified by current demographic trends, including the graying of the baby boomer population, the epidemic of morbid obesity, and the higher recreational activity levels of our elderly population.

Despite these compelling facts, the investment in musculoskeletal research in the United States lags behind other chronic conditions. While musculoskeletal diseases are common, disabling and costly, they remain under-appreciated, under recognized, and under-resourced by our national policy makers.

In March 2002, President George W. Bush declared the years 2002–2011 the National Bone and Joint Decade. The mission of the U.S. Bone and Joint Decade is to "promote and facilitate collaboration among organizations committed to improving bone and joint health through education and research."

This volume serves the mission of the decade in that several professional organizations concerned with musculoskeletal health have collaborated to tabulate up-to-date data on the burden of musculoskeletal diseases to educate health care professionals, policy makers, and the public. The information presented here is an update of two previous editions entitled *Musculoskeletal Conditions in the United States*, published in 1992 and 1999 by the American Academy of Orthopaedic Surgeons. The present volume, renamed *The Burden of Musculoskeletal Diseases in the United States,* represents a true collaboration of a coalition of professional organizations committed to the mission of the U.S. Bone and Joint Decade.

These data should stimulate increased investment in basic, translational, clinical, and health policy research to delineate the underlying mechanisms of these diseases and their response to treatment. Through such research, novel preventive and therapeutic approaches with protential to mitigate the societal and personal impact of musculoskeletal disease will emerge.

Joshua J. Jacobs, MD
Chair, Management Oversight Team, *Burden of Musculoskeletal Diseases in the United States,* American Academy of Orthopaedic Surgeons

John P. Dormans, MD
Scoliosis Research Society

Steve M. Gnatz, MD, MHA
American Academy of Physical Medicine and Rehabilitation

Nancy Lane, MD
United States Bone and Joint Decade

Edward J. Puzas, PhD
Orthopaedic Research Society

E. William St. Clair, MD
American College of Rheumatology

Chapter 1

Burden of Musculoskeletal Disease Overview

Musculoskeletal conditions are among the most disabling and costly conditions suffered by Americans. In March 2002, President George W. Bush proclaimed the years 2002–2011 as the United States Bone and Joint Decade, providing national recognition to the fact that musculoskeletal disorders and diseases are the leading cause of physical disability in this country.[1,2]

As the U.S. population rapidly ages in the next 25 years, musculoskeletal impairments will increase because they are most prevalent in the older segments of the population. By the year 2030, the number of individuals in the United States older than the age of 65 is projected to double, with persons aged 85 and over the most rapidly expanding segment of society. In Europe, by 2010, for the first time there will be more people older than 60 years of age than people younger than 20 years of age.[3] Health care services worldwide will be facing severe financial pressures in the next 10 to 20 years due to the escalation in the numbers of people affected by musculoskeletal diseases. Bone and joint disorders account for more than one-half of all chronic conditions in people older than 50 years of age in developed countries, and are the most common cause of severe, long-term pain and disability.[4]

The goal of the United States Bone and Joint Decade is to improve the quality of life for people with musculoskeletal conditions and to advance understanding and treatment of these conditions through research, prevention, and education. The cornerstone of the Bone and Joint Decade movement is the burden of musculoskeletal disease, defined as the incidence and prevalence

of musculoskeletal conditions; the resources used to prevent, care, and cure for them; and the impact on individuals, families, and society. The impact of musculoskeletal diseases includes loss of productivity for persons who live with a musculoskeletal condition that reduces their ability to work and perform activities of daily living, and those persons who die prematurely from a musculoskeletal condition. It also takes into consideration the quality of life, pain, discomfort, and disability for disabled persons and their relatives and friends. Direct costs of the burden of musculoskeletal disease include hospital inpatient, hospital emergency and outpatient services, physician outpatient services, other practitioner services, home health care, prescription drugs, nursing home cost, prepayment and administration and non-health sector costs. Indirect cost relates to morbidity and mortality, including the value of productivity losses due to premature death due to a disease and the value of lifetime earnings.

Musculoskeletal conditions are not among the top ten health conditions funded by research.[5] In spite of the widespread prevalence of musculoskeletal conditions, this is primarily due to the low mortality from musculoskeletal conditions in comparison with other health conditions. However, the morbidity cost of musculoskeletal conditions is tremendous, as musculoskeletal conditions often restrict activities of daily living, cause lost work days, and are the source of lifelong pain.

In 1998, the Institute of Medicine wrote that "in setting national priorities NIH should strengthen its analysis in the use of health data, such as burdens of disease, and of data on the impact of research and the health of the public."[6] National health data in several countries show that musculoskeletal conditions rank among the top health concerns for citizens in the United States and worldwide. By current estimates, over 40% of the disabling conditions of persons aged 18 years and over are musculoskeletal related, yet research funding to alleviate this major health condition remains substantially below that of other major health conditions, such as cancer, respiratory, and circulatory (e.g., heart) diseases. Funding for the National Institute of Arthritis and Musculoskeletal and Skin Diseases (NIAMS) began in 1987. In subsequent years, research funding for these conditions has declined and since 2000 routinely less than 2% of the National Institutes of Health (NIH) budget has been appropriated to musculoskeletal disease research annually. (Table 1.1)

Clearly, musculoskeletal conditions are common, disabling, and costly. Yet they remain under-recognized, under-appreciated, and under-resourced. This book provides a strong case for the immediate and ongoing need to understand and support musculoskeletal conditions and reduce the burden it brings to our people.

Section 1.1: Prevalence of Select Medical Conditions in the U.S. Population

Musculoskeletal medical conditions were reported by 107.67 million adults in the U.S. in 2005 in the National Health Interview Survey (NHIS), representing nearly one in two persons aged 18 and over of the estimated 2005 population. The rate of chronic musculoskeletal conditions found in the adult population is nearly twice that of chronic circulatory conditions, which include coronary and heart conditions, and more than twice that of all chronic respiratory

conditions. On an age adjusted basis, which accounts for differences in the age distribution of the health care database sample and the actual population, musculoskeletal conditions are reported by more than 48% of the population, or 48.3 persons per 100 population. This compares to a rate of 27.8 and 23.6 per 100 population for circulatory and respiratory conditions, respectively. (Table 1.2 and Graph 1.1.1) The NHIS annual survey of self-reported health conditions is used throughout this chapter to highlight chronic health conditions of the U.S. population.

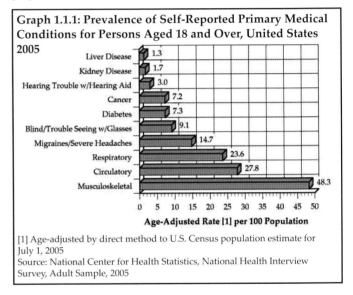

Graph 1.1.1: Prevalence of Self-Reported Primary Medical Conditions for Persons Aged 18 and Over, United States 2005

Condition	Age-Adjusted Rate [1] per 100 Population
Liver Disease	1.3
Kidney Disease	1.7
Hearing Trouble w/Hearing Aid	3.0
Cancer	7.2
Diabetes	7.3
Blind/Trouble Seeing w/Glasses	9.1
Migraines/Severe Headaches	14.7
Respiratory	23.6
Circulatory	27.8
Musculoskeletal	48.3

[1] Age-adjusted by direct method to U.S. Census population estimate for July 1, 2005
Source: National Center for Health Statistics, National Health Interview Survey, Adult Sample, 2005

Musculoskeletal conditions are found among all age groups, with the proportion of persons reporting these conditions increasing with age. Musculoskeletal conditions are reported by nearly three of four (72%) persons aged 75 years and over, compared to approximately 69% reporting circulatory conditions. (Table 1.2)

Females, in general, on an age-adjusted basis, report a higher rate of occurrence than males for most major medical conditions. Among females, musculoskeletal conditions are reported at a rate of 52.5 cases per 100 population, while among males the rate is 46.1 per 100. (Table 1.3)

Musculoskeletal conditions are reported proportionally between all race groups, with the exception of persons of the Asian race, where one in three, compared to the one in two of other race groups, is likely to report a musculoskeletal condition. (Table 1.4)

Section 1.1.1: Musculoskeletal, Circulatory, and Respiratory Conditions

On an age-adjusted basis, musculoskeletal conditions are reported equal to or more frequently than other common chronic or serious medical conditions related to the circulatory or respiratory systems by persons aged 18 and older. Three of the four most common medical conditions reported in 2005 were musculoskeletal conditions: low back pain, chronic joint pain, and arthritis. The other most commonly reported medical condition is chronic hypertension. (Table 1.5 and Graph 1.1.2)

Low back pain, the most frequently cited musculoskeletal condition, is reported by nearly 62.0 million adults, with an age-adjusted rate of 27.8 in 100 persons aged 18 or older reporting this condition. Among persons reporting low back pain, more than 20.3 million, or one-third, also reported pain radiating down the leg below the knee. Cervical/neck pain is also a commonly reported musculoskeletal disease, and was reported by 32.3 million adults.

Chronic joint pain, defined as joint pain lasting three months or longer, was reported by 58.9 million adults aged 18 and older (26.4 of 100), while 46.9 million (21.1 in 100) reported having been diagnosed with arthritis. Chronic joint pain and arthritis are not mutually exclusive and may be reported by the same individual. Age is the general predictor of the occurrence of chronic health conditions, with the exception of respiratory conditions, which are found as frequently among younger adults as among the elderly.

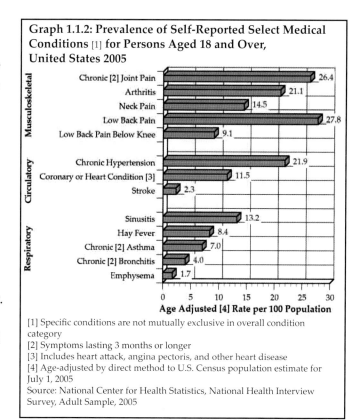

Graph 1.1.2: Prevalence of Self-Reported Select Medical Conditions [1] for Persons Aged 18 and Over, United States 2005

[1] Specific conditions are not mutually exclusive in overall condition category
[2] Symptoms lasting 3 months or longer
[3] Includes heart attack, angina pectoris, and other heart disease
[4] Age-adjusted by direct method to U.S. Census population estimate for July 1, 2005
Source: National Center for Health Statistics, National Health Interview Survey, Adult Sample, 2005

Chronic hypertension, defined as hypertension diagnosed at two or more physician visits, is the only other medical condition that approaches the rate of chronic musculoskeletal conditions. Among adults aged 18 and older, 46.9 million persons reported chronic hypertension in 2005, an age-adjusted rate of 21.9 in 100 persons. Chronic respiratory ailments, while common, are reported in significantly lower numbers, with sinusitis, reported by 29.5 million (13.2 in 100) persons, the most common condition.

Gender is a greater predictor of chronic musculoskeletal conditions than of chronic circulatory or respiratory conditions, with females more likely to report a specific musculoskeletal condition than males. Among chronic circulatory and respiratory conditions, with the exception of sinusitis, males and females report specific conditions in about equal proportions. (Table 1.6)

As is seen with chronic musculoskeletal conditions, chronic circulatory and respiratory conditions are reported at lower rates by persons of the Asian race than other races. (Table 1.7)

Section 1.1.2: Chronic Joint Pain

Among the nearly 59 million persons reporting chronic joint pain, knee pain is the most frequently cited, with more than 36.2 million persons reporting knee pain in 2005. Knee pain is reported by all age groups in the age 18 and over population. Shoulder pain, reported by 18.3 million persons aged 18 and older, is the second most common joint for chronic pain, and is reported more frequently by persons aged 45 to 64 than by other age groups. Pain in the toes and/or fingers is reported by more than 17.7 million persons, again more frequently reported in the 45 to 64 age group. Chronic hip pain is reported by 14.2 million persons. Overall, persons aged 65 and older report chronic joint pain more

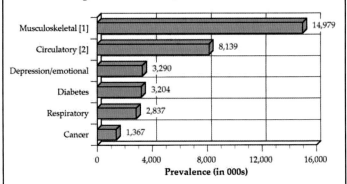

Graph 1.2.1: Self-Reported Prevalance of Impairment in Activities of Daily Living Due to Select Medical Conditions for Persons Aged 18 and Older, United States 2005

[1] Includes arthritis/rheumatism condition, back or neck problem, fracture/bone/joint injury, musculoskeletal/connective tissue condition, missing or amputated limb/finger/digit.
[2] Includes heart or hypertension, stroke, circulation problem.
Source: National Center for Health Statistics, National Health Interview Survey, Person Sample, 2005

daily living due to medical conditions. More than 29 million adults aged 18 years and over, or 13% of the population, report they have difficulty performing routine daily activities of life without assistance due to medical conditions. An additional 5.27 million children between the ages of 1 and 17 years are reported by their parents as needing assistance in daily activities expected for their age due to a medical condition. (Table 1.9)

The most frequently cited medical condition for which persons report limitations in the activities of daily life is musculoskeletal. Nearly 15 million adults aged 18 and over are limited by one or more musculoskeletal conditions, including arthritis or rheumatism, back or neck problems, fracture or bone/joint injury, a missing or amputated limb, or a musculoskeletal connective tissue condition. (Graph 1.2.1) Overall, 13% of adults aged 18 and over have reduced quality of life due to medical conditions, and more than one-half of these are due to musculoskeletal conditions. (Graph 1.2.2)

Graph 1.1.3: Proportion of Population [1] Reporting Joint Pain [2], United States 2005

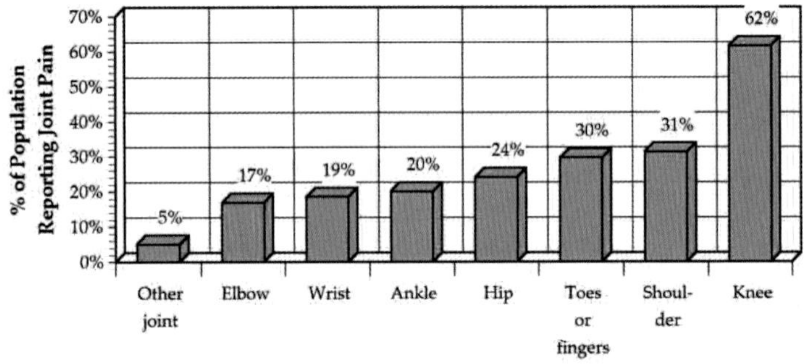

[1] Age-adjusted to July 1, 2005 U.S. Census population estimates
[2] Symptoms lasting 3 months or longer
Source: National Center for Health Statistics, National Health Interview Survey, Adult Sample, 2005

frequently than younger persons. (Table 1.8 and Graph 1.1.3)

Section 1.2: Activity Limitation Due to Select Medical Conditions

Participants in the 2005 NHIS survey were asked about limitations they experience in activities of

Reflecting the overall prevalence of medical conditions in females, females are also more

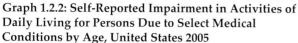

Graph 1.2.2: Self-Reported Impairment in Activities of Daily Living for Persons Due to Select Medical Conditions by Age, United States 2005

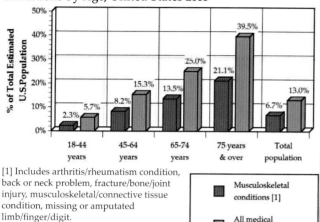

[1] Includes arthritis/rheumatism condition, back or neck problem, fracture/bone/joint injury, musculoskeletal/connective tissue condition, missing or amputated limb/finger/digit.
Source: National Center for Health Statistics, National Health Interview Survey, Person Sample, 2005

likely to report impairment in activities of daily living than are males. This is particularly true for musculoskeletal conditions, with 62% of female adults aged 18 and over reporting they are limited in activities of daily living. (Table 1.10)

Members of the white, black/African American, and "other race" populations report limitations due to medical conditions in approximately the same proportions. Members of the Asian race are somewhat less likely to report limitations in activities of daily living due to a medical condition. (Table 1.11)

Section 1.3: Lost Work Days and Bed Days

Musculoskeletal conditions are also the greatest cause of total lost work days and medical bed days in the U.S.. One in six persons (16%) employed in the previous 12 months in the U.S. at the time of the survey reported lost work days totaling nearly 437.6 million days as a result of musculoskeletal conditions. Chronic circulatory conditions accounted for 236 million lost work days, while chronic respiratory conditions accounted for 216 million. On average, workers lost 12 days in a 12 month period due to musculoskeletal conditions. (Table 1.12)

More than one in five persons (21%) reported at least one bed day in the previous 12 months due to a musculoskeletal condition, with total bed days due to musculoskeletal conditions reported at more than 810.3 million. An average 40 bed days per person was reported. (Table 1.13)

Musculoskeletal conditions accounted for one-half of both lost work days and bed days due to

Graph 1.3.1: Proportion of Total Lost Work Days for Persons Aged 18 and Over by Major Medical Condition, United States 2005

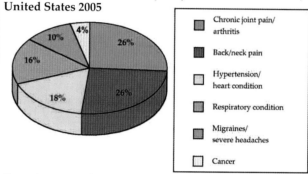

Respondents reported "Yes" when asked "Are you limited in any way in any activities because of physical, mental or emotional problems."

Respondents reporting a limitation reported "Yes" when asked if limitation was caused by "arthritis/rheumatis; back/neck problem; fracture/bone/joint injury; other injury; heart problem; stroke; hypertension."

Lost work days due to multiple conditions possible.

Source: National Center for Health Statistics, National Health Interview Survey, Adult Sample, 2005

Graph 1.3.2: Proportion of Total Bed Days for Persons Aged 18 and Over by Major Medical Condition, United States 2005

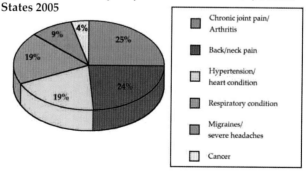

Respondents reported "Yes" when asked "Are you limited in any way in any activities because of physical, mental or emotional problems."

Respondents reporting a limitation reported 'Yes' when asked if limitation was caused by "arthritis/rheumatis; back/neck problem; fracture/bone/joint injury; other injury; heart problem; stroke; hypertension."

Bed days due to multiple conditions possible.

Source: National Center for Health Statistics, National Health Interview Survey, 2005

major medical conditions in 2005. (Graphs 1.3.1 and 1.3.2) Compared to circulatory and respiratory conditions, musculoskeletal conditions accounted for more than twice the number of lost work days of either of these two conditions, and 36% and 45% more bed days than circulatory and respiratory conditions, respectively. (Graph 1.3.3)

Graph 1.3.3: Total Productivity Loss Due to Select Medical Conditions [1,2] **for Persons Aged 18 and Over, United States, 2005**

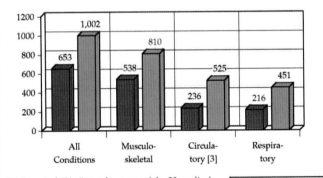

[1] Reported "Yes" to at least one of the 23 medical conditions (70% of the weighted population). Multiple conditions resulting in bed days possible.
[2] Symptoms lasting 3 months or longer OR 2 or more physician visits
[3] Includes heart attack, angina pectoris, and other heart disease
Source: National Center for Health Statistics, National Health Interview Survey, Adult Sample, 2005

Graph 1.3.4: Total Productivity Loss Due to Select Musculoskeletal Conditions [1,2] **for Persons Aged 18 and Over, United States 2005**

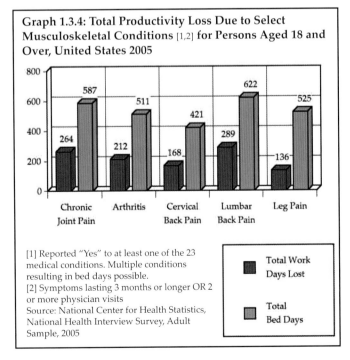

[1] Reported "Yes" to at least one of the 23 medical conditions. Multiple conditions resulting in bed days possible.
[2] Symptoms lasting 3 months or longer OR 2 or more physician visits
Source: National Center for Health Statistics, National Health Interview Survey, Adult Sample, 2005

Major musculoskeletal causes of lost work days and medical bed days are chronic joint pain, arthritis, and cervical/neck and low back pain. (Graph 1.3.4) Persons reporting low back pain that radiates below the knee reported one of the highest average number of lost work days (30.1) and the highest average number of medical bed days (47.4). Circulatory conditions reported as the cause of lost work days, on average, resulted in a slightly higher average number of work days lost per worker than did musculoskeletal conditions (15.3 versus 12.3, respectively), but accounted for substantially lower average bed days (21.4 versus 39.5, respectively). (Tables 1.12 and 1.13)

Overall, the high proportion of workers reporting lost work days or bed days as a result of a musculoskeletal condition results in an economic burden on the economy that is twice that reported for chronic circulatory or chronic respiratory conditions.

Section 1.4: Summary Health Care Utilization and Economic Cost of Musculoskeletal Diseases

The annual average proportion of the U.S. population with a musculoskeletal condition requiring medical care has increased by more than two percentage points over the past decade and now constitutes more than 30% of the population. The increasing prevalence of musculoskeletal conditions, along with a growing and aging population, has resulted in a more than 41% increase in total aggregate direct cost to treat persons with a musculoskeletal condition. In 2002-2004, the annual average cost, in 2004 dollars, for musculoskeletal health care was estimated to be $510 billion, the equivalent of 4.6% of the national gross domestic product (GDP). Indirect cost, expressed primarily as wage losses for persons aged 18 to 64 with a work history, added another $339 billion, or 3.1% of the GDP, to the cost associated with these conditions. Estimated incremental cost, that proportion of total direct cost associated with treatment incurred beyond that of persons of similar demographic and health characteristics but who do not have one or more musculoskeletal diseases (i.e., likely attributable to a musculoskeletal disease), is estimated to be $156.7 billion, with an annual indirect incremental cost estimate of $110.5 billion.

Treatments that mitigate the long-term impacts of musculoskeletal conditions and return persons to full and active lives are needed.

1. Weinstein S: 2000-2010: The Bone and Joint Decade. *J Bone Joint Surg Am* 2000;82:1-3.

2. A Proclamation by the President of the United States of America: National Bone and Joint Decade Proclamation: National Bone and Joint Decade, 2002-2011. Office of the Press Secretary, 2002.

3. Murray CJL, Lopez AD: *The Global Burden of Disease: A Comprehensive Assessment of Mortality and Disability from Diseases, Injuries, and Risk Factors in 1990 and Projected to 2020.* Cambridge, MA: Harvard University Press, 1996.

4. Conference proceedings: The bone and joint decade 2000-2010 for prevention and treatment of musculoskeletal disorders. Lund, Sweden. *Acta Orthop. Scand. Suppl.*; 1998:218.

5. Michaud CM, Murray CJL, Bloom BR: Burden of disease: implications for future research. *JAMA* 2001;285:535-539.

6. Committee on the NIH Research Priority-Setting Process, Institute of Medicine: Scientific opportunities and public needs: Improving setting and public input. Institute of Medicine of the National Academies, 1998.

Section 1.5: Burden of Musculoskeletal Diseases Overview Data Tables

Table 1.1: National Institutes of Health (NIH) Funding, 2000-2006

National Institutes of Health (NIH) Organizations		Mean % of Total NIH Funding 2000-2006
NCI	National Cancer Institute	17.5%
NIAID	National Institute of Allergy and Infectious Diseases	12.6%
NHLBI	National Heart, Lung, and Blood Institute	10.7%
NIGMS	National Institute of General Medical Sciences	7.1%
NIDDK	National Institute of Diabetes and Digestive and Kidney Diseases	6.6%
NINDS	National Institute of Neurological Disorders and Stroke	5.5%
NIMH	National Institute of Mental Health	5.1%
NICHD	National Institute of Child Health and Human Development	4.6%
NCRR	National Center for Research Resources	4.0%
NIA	National Institute on Aging	3.7%
NIDA	National Institute on Drug Abuse	3.7%
NIEHS	National Institute of Environmental Health Sciences	2.6%
NEI	National Eye Institute	2.4%
NIAMS	**National Institute of Arthritis and Musculoskeletal and Skin Diseases**	**1.9%**
NHGRI	National Human Genome Research Institute	1.8%
NIAAA	National Institute on Alcohol Abuse and Alcoholism	1.6%
NIDCR	National Institute of Dental and Craniofacial Research	1.4%
NIDCD	National Institute on Deafness and Other Communication Disorders	1.4%
NLM	National Library of Medicine	1.1%
NIBIB	National Institute of Biomedical Imaging and Bioengineering	0.7%
NCMHD	National Center on Minority Health and Health Disparities	0.6%
NINR	National Institute of Nursing Research	0.5%
NCCAM	National Center for Complementary and Alternative Medicine	0.4%
FIC	John E. Fogarty International Center for Advanced Study in the Health Sciences	0.2%
OD	Office of the Director (includes Office of AIDS Research and Office of Research on Women's Health)	1.2%
Total Funding (in 000s)		$ 24,783,710

Source: NIH Almanac-Appropriations. Available at: http://www.nih.gov/about/almanac/appropriations/index.htm Accessed: October 15, 2007.

Table 1.2: Prevalence and Age-Adjusted Rate of Self-Reported Select Medical Conditions by Age, United States 2005

Medical Condition	Prevalence Aged 18 & Over (in millions)					Age-Adjusted Rate [5] Per 100 Total Population
	18-44	45-64	65-74	75+	Total	
Musculoskeletal [1]	41.949	41.486	12.265	11.969	107.668	48.30
Circulatory [2]	11.990	27.316	11.032	11.553	61.891	27.76
Respiratory [3]	23.452	19.882	52.920	3.964	52.590	23.59
Migraines or Severe Headaches	20.281	10.319	1.366	0.860	32.827	14.72
Blind or Trouble Seeing w/Glasses	6.073	8.105	2.434	3.644	20.255	9.09
Diabetes	2.640	7.596	3.421	2.529	16.186	7.26
Cancer [4]	2.430	5.961	3.518	4.086	15.995	7.18
Hearing Trouble w/Hearing Aid	0.627	1.326	1.323	3.352	6.628	2.97
Kidney Disease	0.931	1.305	0.675	0.880	3.791	1.70
Liver Disease	0.738	1.721	0.321	0.185	2.965	1.33

Medical Condition	Proportion of Population in Age Group Reporting Condition				
	18-44	45-64	65-74	75+	Total
Musculoskeletal [1]	38.0%	57.4%	66.5%	72.1%	49.4%
Circulatory [2]	10.9%	37.8%	59.8%	69.6%	28.4%
Respiratory [3]	21.2%	27.5%	28.7%	23.9%	24.1%
Migraines or Severe Headaches	18.4%	14.3%	7.4%	5.2%	15.1%
Blind or Trouble Seeing w/Glasses	5.5%	11.2%	13.2%	22.0%	9.3%
Diabetes	2.4%	10.5%	18.5%	15.2%	7.4%
Cancer [4]	2.2%	8.2%	19.1%	24.6%	7.3%
Hearing Trouble w/Hearing Aid	0.6%	1.8%	7.2%	20.2%	3.0%
Kidney Disease	0.8%	1.8%	3.7%	5.3%	1.7%
Liver Disease	0.7%	2.4%	1.7%	1.1%	1.4%

[1] Includes arthritis, chronic joint symptoms (more than 3 months in duration), pain in lower back or neck (more than 3 months duration)

[2] Includes coronary heart disease, angina pectoris, heart attack, stroke, chronic hypertension, heart disease

[3] Includes emphysema, chronic asthma, hay fever, sinusitis, chronic bronchitis

[4] Includes all types of cancer

[5] Age-adjusted by direct method to US Census population estimate for July 1, 2005

Source: National Center for Health Statistics, National Health Interview Survey, Adult Sample, 2005

Table 1.3: Prevalence of Self-Reported Select Medical Conditions by Gender, United States 2005

	Prevalence Age 18 & Over (in millions)		
Medical Condition	**Male**	**Female**	**Total**
Musculoskeletal [1]	48.402	59.266	107.668
Circulatory [2]	28.563	33.328	61.891
Respiratory [3]	20.351	32.239	52.590
Migraines or Severe Headaches	9.857	22.970	32.827
Blind or Trouble Seeing w/Glasses	8.074	12.181	20.255
Diabetes	7.896	8.290	16.186
Cancer [4]	6.778	9.217	15.995
Hearing Trouble w/Hearing Aid	3.885	2.743	6.628
Kidney Disease	1.736	2.055	3.791
Liver Disease	1.571	1.395	2.965

	Proportion of Population by Sex Reporting Condition		
Medical Condition	**Male**	**Female**	**Total**
Musculoskeletal [1]	46.1%	52.5%	49.4%
Circulatory [2]	27.2%	29.5%	28.4%
Respiratory [3]	19.4%	28.6%	24.1%
Migraines or Severe Headaches	9.4%	20.4%	15.1%
Blind or Trouble Seeing w/Glasses	7.7%	10.8%	9.3%
Diabetes	7.5%	7.3%	7.4%
Cancer [4]	6.5%	8.2%	7.3%
Hearing Trouble w/Hearing Aid	3.7%	2.4%	3.0%
Kidney Disease	1.7%	1.8%	1.7%
Liver Disease	1.5%	1.2%	1.4%

[1] Includes arthritis, chronic joint symptoms (more than 3 months in duration), pain in lower back or neck (more than 3 months duration)

[2] Includes coronary heart disease, angina pectoris, heart attack, stroke, chronic hypertension, heart disease

[3] Includes emphysema, chronic asthma, hay fever, sinusitis, chronic bronchitis

[4] Includes all types of cancer

Source: National Center for Health Statistics, National Health Interview Survey, Adult Sample, 2005

Table 1.4: Prevalence of Self-Report Selected Medical Conditions by Race, United States, 2005

Prevalence Age 18 & Over (in millions)

Medical Condition	White	Black/ African American	Asian	Other or Mixed Race	Total
Musculoskeletal [1]	92.130	10.431	2.764	2.343	107.668
Circulatory [2]	51.271	7.961	1.547	1.112	61.891
Respiratory [3]	44.564	5.719	1.097	1.210	52.590
Migraines or Severe Headaches	27.461	3.621	0.864	0.880	32.827
Blind or Trouble Seeing w/Glasses	16.760	2.538	0.404	0.553	20.255
Diabetes	12.886	2.513	0.437	0.351	16.186
Cancer [4]	14.776	0.816	0.241	0.163	15.995
Hearing Trouble w/Hearing Aid	6.210	0.232	0.129	0.056	6.628
Kidney Disease	2.967	0.570	0.104	0.149	3.791
Liver Disease	2.484	0.314	0.081	0.086	2.965

Proportion of Population by Race Reporting Condition

Medical Condition	White	Black/ African American	Asian	Other or Mixed Race	Total
Musculoskeletal [1]	51.0%	42.0%	33.9%	54.2%	49.4%
Circulatory [2]	28.4%	32.1%	19.0%	25.7%	28.4%
Respiratory [3]	24.7%	23.0%	13.5%	28.0%	24.1%
Migraines or Severe Headaches	15.2%	14.6%	10.6%	20.3%	15.1%
Blind or Trouble Seeing w/Glasses	9.3%	10.2%	5.0%	12.8%	9.3%
Diabetes	7.1%	10.1%	5.4%	8.1%	7.4%
Cancer [4]	8.2%	3.3%	3.0%	3.8%	7.3%
Hearing Trouble w/Hearing Aid	3.4%	0.9%	1.6%	1.3%	3.0%
Kidney Disease	1.6%	2.3%	1.3%	3.4%	1.7%
Liver Disease	1.4%	1.3%	1.0%	2.0%	1.4%

[1] Includes arthritis, chronic joint symptoms (more than 3 months in duration), pain in lower back or neck (more than 3 months duration)

[2] Includes coronary heart disease, angina pectoris, heart attack, stroke, chronic hypertension, heart disease

[3] Includes emphysema, chronic asthma, hay fever, sinusitis, chronic bronchitis

[4] Includes all types of cancer

Source: National Center for Health Statistics, National Health Interview Survey, Adult Sample, 2005

Table 1.5: Prevalence of Most Frequently Reported Medical Conditions by Age, United States 2005

Medical Condition	Prevalence Age 18 & Over (in millions)					Age-Adjusted Rate [4] per 100 Total Population
	18-44	45-64	65-74	75+	Total	
Musculoskeletal [1 2]	41.949	41.486	12.265		107.668	48.30
Chronic [2] Joint Pain	17.161	25.426	8.313	7.963	58.863	26.40
Arthritis	8.624	20.780	8.609	8.927	46.941	21.06
Neck Pain (Cervical Back Pain)	14.076	13.018	2.906	2.293	32.293	14.49
Lower Back Pain (Lumbar Back Pain)	27.632	22.784	5.906	5.64	61.965	27.79
Lower Back Pain Spreading Below Knee	7.007	9.030	2.267	2.042	20.346	9.13
Circulatory	11.990	27.316	11.032		61.891	27.76
Chronic Hypertension	8.067	22.521	9.127	9.044	48.759	21.87
Coronary or Heart Condition [3]	4.763	9.822	4.927	6.071	25.587	11.48
Stroke	0.401	1.558	1.144	2.063	5.165	2.32
Respiratory	23.452	19.882	52.920		52.590	23.59
Sinusitis	12.875	11.831	2.683	2.126	29.517	13.24
Hay Fever	8.566	7.750	1.438	0.897	18.651	8.37
Chronic [2] Asthma	7.746	5.281	1.600	1.07	15.697	7.04
Chronic [2] Bronchitis	3.504	3.544	1.026	0.838	8.912	4.00
Emphysema	0.341	1.430	1.070	0.951	3.791	1.70

Medical Condition	Proportion of Population in Age Group Reporting Condition				
	18-44	45-64	65-74	75+	Total
Musculoskeletal [1,2]	38.0%	57.4%	66.5%	72.1%	49.4%
Chronic [2] Joint Pain	15.5%	35.2%	45.1%	48.0%	27.0%
Arthritis	7.8%	28.7%	46.7%	53.8%	21.6%
Neck Pain (Cervical Back Pain)	12.7%	18.0%	15.8%	13.8%	14.8%
Lower Back Pain (Lumbar Back Pain)	25.0%	31.5%	32.0%	34.0%	28.5%
Lower Back Pain Spreading Below Knee	6.3%	12.5%	12.3%	12.3%	9.3%
Circulatory	10.9%	37.8%	59.8%	69.6%	28.4%
Chronic Hypertension	7.3%	31.2%	49.5%	54.5%	22.4%
Coronary or Heart Condition [3]	4.3%	13.6%	26.7%	36.6%	11.7%
Stroke	0.4%	2.2%	6.2%	12.4%	2.4%
Respiratory	21.2%	27.5%	28.7%	23.9%	24.1%
Sinusitis	11.7%	16.4%	14.5%	12.8%	13.6%
Hay Fever	7.8%	10.7%	7.8%	5.4%	8.6%
Chronic [2] Asthma	7.0%	7.3%	8.7%	6.4%	7.2%
Chronic [2] Bronchitis	3.2%	4.9%	5.6%	5.0%	4.1%
Emphysema	0.3%	2.0%	5.8%	5.7%	1.7%

[1] Specific conditions are not mutually exclusive in overall condition category

[2] Symptoms lasting 3 months or longer

[3] Includes heart attack, angina pectoris, and other heart disease

[4] Age-adjusted by direct method to US Census population estimate for July 1, 2005

Source: National Center for Health Statistics, National Health Interview Survey, Adult Sample, 2005

Table 1.6: Prevalence of Most Frequently Reported Medical Conditions by Gender, United States 2005

	Prevalence Age 18 & Over (in millions)		
Medical Condition	Males	Females	Total
Musculoskeletal [1,2]	48.402	59.266	107.668
Chronic [2] Joint Pain	25.967	32.896	58.863
Arthritis	18.261	28.681	46.941
Neck Pain (Cervical Back Pain)	13.022	19.271	32.293
Lower Back Pain (Lumbar Back Pain)	27.502	34.463	61.965
Lower Back Pain Spreading Below Knee	8.481	11.865	20.346
Circulatory	28.563	33.328	61.891
Chronic Hypertension	22.171	26.588	48.758
Coronary or Heart Condition [3]	12.538	13.049	25.587
Stroke	2.239	2.926	5.165
Respiratory	20.351	32.239	52.590
Sinusitis	10.170	19.346	29.517
Hay Fever	7.983	10.668	18.651
Chronic [2] Asthma	5.348	10.349	15.697
Chronic [2] Bronchitis	2.886	6.026	8.912
Emphysema	2.061	1.730	3.791

	Proportion of Population by Sex Reporting Condition		
Medical Condition	Males	Females	Total
Musculoskeletal [1,2]	46.1%	52.5%	49.4%
Chronic [2] Joint Pain	24.7%	29.1%	27.0%
Arthritis	17.4%	25.4%	21.6%
Neck Pain (Cervical Back Pain)	12.4%	17.1%	14.8%
Lower Back Pain (Lumbar Back Pain)	26.2%	30.5%	28.5%
Lower Back Pain Spreading Below Knee	8.1%	10.5%	9.3%
Circulatory	27.2%	29.5%	28.4%
Chronic Hypertension	21.1%	23.6%	22.4%
Coronary or Heart Condition [3]	12.0%	11.6%	11.7%
Stroke	2.1%	2.6%	2.4%
Respiratory	19.4%	28.6%	24.1%
Sinusitis	9.7%	17.1%	13.6%
Hay Fever	7.6%	9.5%	8.6%
Chronic [2] Asthma	5.1%	9.2%	7.2%
Chronic [2] Bronchitis	2.8%	5.3%	4.1%
Emphysema	2.0%	1.5%	1.7%

[1] Specific conditions are not mutually exclusive in overall condition category

[2] Symptoms lasting 3 months or longer

[3] Includes heart attack, angina pectoris, and other heart disease

Source: National Center for Health Statistics, National Health Interview Survey, Adult Sample, 2005

Table 1.7: Prevalence of Most Frequently Reported Medical Conditions by Race, United States 2005

| Medical Condition | Prevalence Age 18 & Over (in millions) | | | | |
	White	Black/ African American	Asian	Other or Mixed Race	Total
Musculoskeletal [1,2]	92.130	10.431	2.764	2.343	107.668
Chronic [2] Joint Pain	50.803	5.593	1.136	1.330	58.863
Arthritis	40.351	4.718	0.868	1.004	46.941
Neck Pain (Cervical Back Pain)	27.745	2.954	0.757	0.839	32.293
Lower Back Pain (Lumbar Back Pain)	52.561	6.303	1.599	1.503	61.965
Lower Back Pain Spreading Below Knee	17.031	2.308	0.467	0.540	20.346
Circulatory	51.271	7.961	1.547	1.112	61.891
Chronic Hypertension	39.414	7.097	1.372	0.876	48.759
Coronary or Heart Condition [3]	22.366	2.258	0.445	0.514	25.587
Stroke	4.213	0.706	0.118	0.127	5.165
Respiratory	44.564	5.719	1.097	1.210	52.590
Sinusitis	24.996	3.292	0.509	0.720	29.517
Hay Fever	16.225	1.502	0.569	0.355	18.651
Chronic [2] Asthma	12.895	2.048	0.337	0.416	15.697
Chronic [2] Bronchitis	7.511	1.063	0.096	0.243	8.912
Emphysema	3.503	0.180	0.024	0.084	3.791

| Medical Condition | Proportion of Population by Race Reporting Condition | | | | |
	White	Black/ African American	Asian	Other or Mixed Race	Total
Musculoskeletal [1,2]	51.0%	42.0%	33.9%	54.2%	49.4%
Chronic [2] Joint Pain	28.1%	22.5%	14.0%	30.8%	27.0%
Arthritis	22.4%	19.0%	10.6%	23.2%	21.6%
Neck Pain (Cervical Back Pain)	15.4%	11.9%	9.3%	19.4%	14.8%
Lower Back Pain (Lumbar Back Pain)	29.1%	25.4%	19.6%	34.8%	28.5%
Lower Back Pain Spreading Below Knee	9.4%	9.3%	5.7%	12.5%	9.3%
Circulatory	28.4%	32.1%	19.0%	25.7%	28.4%
Chronic Hypertension	21.8%	28.6%	16.8%	20.3%	22.4%
Coronary or Heart Condition [3]	12.4%	9.1%	5.5%	11.9%	11.7%
Stroke	2.3%	2.8%	1.4%	2.9%	2.4%
Respiratory	24.7%	23.0%	13.5%	28.0%	24.1%
Sinusitis	13.8%	13.3%	6.2%	16.6%	13.6%
Hay Fever	9.0%	6.1%	7.0%	8.2%	8.6%
Chronic [2] Asthma	7.1%	8.3%	4.1%	9.6%	7.2%
Chronic [2] Bronchitis	4.2%	4.3%	1.2%	5.6%	4.1%
Emphysema	1.9%	0.7%	0.3%	1.9%	1.7%

[1] Specific conditions are not mutually exclusive in overall condition category

[2] Symptoms lasting 3 months or longer

[3] Includes heart attack, angina pectoris, and other heart disease

Source: National Center for Health Statistics, National Health Interview Survey, Adult Sample, 2005

Table 1.8: Prevalence of Chronic Joint Pain [1] by Joint by Age, United States 2005

	Persons with Self-Reported Chronic Joint Condition (in 000s)					% of Total w/Joint Pain
	18-44	45-64	65-74	75+	All Ages	
Knee	11,064	15,411	5,111	4,666	36,252	61.6%
Shoulder	4,641	8,596	2,682	2,440	18,360	31.2%
Toes or Fingers	3,330	8,535	2,902	2,673	17,440	29.6%
Hip	2,980	6,462	2,395	2,369	14,207	24.1%
Ankle	3,742	5,184	1,526	1,335	11,787	20.0%
Wrist	3,330	4,879	1,462	1,208	10,878	18.5%
Elbow	2,951	4,904	1,211	857	9,924	16.9%
Other Joint	735	1,270	501	409	2,916	5.0%
All Chronic Joint	17,161	25,426	8,313	7,963	58,863	
% of Age Group [2] w/Joint Pain	15.1%	34.9%	44.6%	43.9%	26.4%	

[1] Symptoms lasting 3 months or longer

[2] Age-adjusted to July 1, 2005 U.S. Census population estimates

Source: National Center for Health Statistics, National Health Interview Survey, Adult Sample, 2005

Table 1.9: Self-Reported Impairment in Activities of Daily Living for Persons Due to Select Medical Conditions by Age, United States 2005

Prevalence of Reported Impairment (in 000s)

Condition	1-17	18-44	45-64	65-74	75+	Total Aged 18 & Over
Musculoskeletal [1]	227	2,618	6,003	2,523	3,836	14,979
Circulatory [2]	*	6,610	3,042	1,710	2,778	8,139
Depression/Anxiety/Emotional Problem [3]	743	1,238	1,604	180	268	3,290
Diabetes	*	303	1,448	733	720	3,204
Respiratory (Lung Breathing Problem)	488	493	1,108	549	676	2,827
Nervous System [4]/Sensory Organ	95	865	1,096	354	373	2,689
Vision Problem	153	249	706	392	797	2,144
Hearing Problem	187	165	366	228	637	1,396
Cancer	*	135	537	323	373	1,367
Birth Ddefect/Mental Retardation/Developmental	904	NA	NA	NA	NA	NA
Total All Conditions	5,270	6,512	11,160	4,662	7,175	29,059

% of Total 2005 U.S. Population

	1-17	18-44	45-64	65-74	75+	Total Aged 18 & Over
All Medical Conditions	7.2%	5.7%	15.3%	25.0%	39.5%	13.0%
Musculoskeletal Conditions	0.2%	2.3%	8.2%	13.5%	21.1%	6.7%

[1] Includes arthritis/rheumatism condition, back or neck problem, fracture/bone/joint injury, musculoskeletal/connective tissue condition, missing or amputated limb/finger/digit in 0-17 population defined as injury or bone/joint/muscle problem

[2] Includes heart or hypertension, stroke, circulation problem

[3] In 0-17 population, defined as emotional/behavioral problem

[4] In 0-17 population, defined as epilepsy/seizures

* Reported number does not meet sample size reliability

Source: National Center for Health Statistics, National Health Interview Survey, Person Sample, 2005

Table 1.10: Self-Reported Impairment in Activities of Daily Living for Persons Aged 18 and Over Due to Select Medical Conditions by Gender, United States 2005

Prevalence of Reported Impairment for Persons Age 18 and Over (in 000s)

Condition	Males Prevalence	Males % of Total	Females Prevalence	Females % of Total	Total Prevalence
Musculoskeletal [1]	5,692	38.0%	9,287	62.0%	14,979
Circulatory	3,768	46.3%	4,371	53.7%	8,139
Depression/Anxiety/Emotional Problem	1,324	40.2%	1,966	59.8%	3,290
Diabetes	1,318	41.1%	1,886	58.9%	3,204
Respiratory	1,213	42.9%	1,614	57.1%	2,827
Nervous System/Sensory Organ	1,065	39.6%	1,624	60.4%	2,689
Vision Problem	887	41.4%	1,257	58.6%	2,144
Hearing Problem	721	51.6%	674	48.3%	1,396
Cancer	657	48.1%	710	51.9%	1,367

[1] Includes arthritis/rheumatism condition, back or neck problem, fracture/bone/joint injury, musculoskeletal/connective tissue condition, missing or amputated limb/finger/digit

Source: National Center for Health Statistics, National Health Interview Survey, Person Sample, 2005

Table 1.11: Self-Reported Impairment in Activities of Daily Living for Persons Aged 18 and Over Due to Select Medical Conditions by Race, United States 2005

Prevalence of Reported Impairment for Persons Age 18 and Over (in 000s)

Condition	White Prevalence	White % of Total	Black/African American Prevalence	Black/African American % of Total	Asian Prevalence	Asian % of Total	Other or Mixed Race Prevalence	Other or Mixed Race % of Total	Total Prevalence
Musculoskeletal [1]	12,606	7.0%	1,757	7.0%	277	3.0%	338	8.1%	14,979
Circulatory	6,632	3.7%	1,162	4.8%	190	2.2%	155	4.0%	8,139
Depression/Anxiety/Emotional Problem	2,726	1.5%	384	1.5%	56	0.6%	124	3.0%	3,290
Diabetes	2,472	1.4%	562	2.3%	93	1.0%	77	1.8%	3,204
Respiratory	2,373	1.3%	352	1.4%	22	0.2%	80	1.9%	2,827
Nervous System/Sensory Organ	2,239	1.2%	337	1.4%	44	0.5%	70	1.7%	2,689
Vision Problem	1,774	1.0%	266	1.1%	55	0.6%	49	1.2%	2,144
Hearing Problem	1,198	0.7%	112	0.4%	44	0.5%	43	1.0%	1,396
Cancer	1,182	0.7%	149	0.6%	19	0.2%	17	0.4%	1,367

[1] Includes arthritis/rheumatism condition, back or neck problem, fracture/bone/joint injury, musculoskeletal/connective tissue condition, missing or amputated limb/finger/digit

Source: National Center for Health Statistics, National Health Interview Survey, Person Sample, 2005

Table 1.12: Lost Work Days from Self-Reported Select Medical Conditions for Persons Aged 18 and Over, United States 2005

Condition	Total # w/ Condition (in 000s)	% U. S. Population Reporting Lost Work Days as a Result of Medical Condition	Total # Reporting Lost Work Days (in 000s)	Total Work Days Lost (in 000s)	Average Work Days Lost per Condition
All Conditions [1]	152,543	31.3%	68,222	652,984	9.6
Musculoskeletal	107,668	16.4%	35,655	437,593	12.3
Circulatory	31,190	7.1%	15,461	236,158	15.3
Respiratory	52,589	9.0%	19,617	216,040	11.0
Musculoskeletal Conditions					
Chronic [2] Joint Pain	58,863	8.2%	17,948	263,647	14.7
Arthritis	46,941	5.6%	12,191	211,516	17.4
Neck Pain (Cervical Back Pain)	32,294	5.4%	11,805	167,757	14.2
Lower Back Pain (Lumbar Back Pain)	61,965	9.9%	21,657	288,789	13.3
Lower Back Pain Spreading Below Knee	20,346	2.9%	6,230	135,922	21.8
Circulatory					
Chronic [2] Hypertension	24,207	5.4%	11,723	175,845	15.0
Coronary or Heart Condition [3]	25,583	2.7%	5,854	104,992	17.9
Stroke	5,166	0.2%	533	16,057	30.1
Respiratory					
Sinusitis	59,517	5.5%	12,011	143,017	11.9
Hay Fever	18,651	3.4%	7,403	82,704	11.2
Chronic [2] Asthma	15,697	2.6%	5,595	69,752	12.5
Chronic [2] Bronchitis	8,912	1.5%	3,177	55,984	17.6
Emphysema	3,791	0.2%	435	9,864	22.7
Migraines/Severe Headaches	32,826	6.6%	14,302	181,283	12.7
Cancer	15,995	1.6%	3,420	77,287	22.6

[1] Reported "Yes" to at least one of the 23 medical conditions (70% of the weighted population). Multiple conditions resulting in lost work days possible.

[2] Symptoms lasting 3 months or longer OR 2 or more physician visits

[3] Includes heart attack, angina pectoris, and other heart disease

Source: National Center for Health Statistics, National Health Interview Survey, Adult Sample Level File, 2005

Table 1.13: Bed Days from Self-Reported Select Medical Conditions for Persons Aged 18 and Over, United States 2005

Condition	% U.S. Population Reporting Bed Days as a Result of Medical Condition	Total # Reporting Bed Days	Total Bed Days (in 000s)	Average Bed Days per Condition
All Conditions [1]	35.0%	76,170	1,001,761	13.2
Musculoskeletal	20.9%	20,492	810,366	39.5
Circulatory	11.3%	24,596	525,267	21.4
Respiratory	11.5%	25,039	450,594	18.0
Musculoskeletal Conditions				
Chronic [2] Joint Pain	12.0%	26,120	587,049	22.5
Arthritis	9.4%	20,492	510,573	24.9
Neck Pain (Cervical Back Pain)	7.4%	16,105	420,628	26.1
Lower Back Pain (Lumbar Back Pain)	13.3%	28,966	622,283	21.5
Lower Back Pain Spreading Below Knee	5.1%	11,074	525,267	47.4
Circulatory				
Chronic [2] Hypertension	8.6%	18,767	414,510	22.1
Coronary or Heart Condition [3]	5.4%	11,824	306,294	25.9
Stroke	1.1%	2,472	109,606	44.3
Respiratory				
Sinusitis	6.8%	14,779	286,716	19.4
Hay Fever	3.9%	8,531	153,153	18.0
Chronic [2] Asthma	3.7%	8,099	181,761	22.4
Chronic [2] Bronchitis	2.4%	5,181	142,190	27.4
Emphysema	0.9%	1,909	85,571	44.8
Migraines/Severe Headaches	8.5%	18,415	386,144	21.0
Cancer	2.9%	6,408	187,650	29.3

[1] Reported "Yes" to at least one of the 23 medical conditions (70% of the weighted population). Multiple conditions resulting in bed days possible.

[2] Symptoms lasting 3 months or longer OR 2 or more physician visits

[3] Includes heart attack, angina pectoris, and other heart disease

Source: National Center for Health Statistics, National Health Interview Survey, Adult Sample Level File, 2005

Chapter 2

Spine: Low Back and Neck Pain

Lumbar/low back pain and cervical/neck pain are among the most common physical conditions requiring medical care and affecting an individual's ability to work and manage the daily activities of life. Back pain is also the most common physical condition for which patients visit their doctor. In a given year, between 12% and 15% of the United States population will visit their physician with a complaint of back pain. Over the past 7 years, this rate has shown a slow, but steady, increase. In 2004, more than 44.6 million patients visited a physician with a complaint of back pain.

Joint pain, also called musculoskeletal pain, from mild strains to severe disabling conditions, affects many. In the United States, two major annual health care surveys are conducted by the National Center for Health Statistics to identify the incidence and prevalence of select health conditions. One of the conditions included is referred to as "joint pain." In reality it is not pain arising from a joint, but rather a musculoskeletal pain in a defined body area. Joint pain is among the most frequently reported conditions in both surveys.

Back pain, including cervical/neck pain and lumbar/low back pain, is more common than severe headaches or allergies resulting from hay fever or sinus conditions. In recent years, between 43%[1] and 60%[2] of adult persons in the United States reported experiencing neck or low back pain in the previous 3 months, while severe headache or migraine was reported by 15%. Hay fever or sinusitis was reported by 9% and 14%, respectively, in a previous 12-month period. Back pain is also reported more frequently than other musculoskeletal pain, including pain in the arm, shoulder, hip, or knee. Low back pain prevalence increases with age, while neck pain tends to peak in the 45 to 64 age range.

Eleven percent (11%) of the population aged 18 or older report they have a physical, mental, or emotional problem or illness that precludes work; 20% of persons with either low back or neck pain report they cannot work, while 33% of persons with multiple back pain sites are unable to work. Back pain also greatly limits the type and duration of work a person can do. Three of four persons with multiple back pain sites report work limitations.

Estimated annual direct medical costs for all spine related conditions for the years 2002-2004 were $193.9 billion, with $30.3 billion estimated as the incremental cost directly related to spine pain. (Chapter 9: Health Care Utilization and Economic Cost of Musculoskeletal Diseases.) In addition, annual indirect costs of $14.0 billion in lost wages were incurred as a result of spine disorders.

Back pain often results from complex conditions that are not easily understood. Many are probably related to degeneration, but the actual underlying cause of a back pain episode is often uncertain. Thus, in reviewing administrative data sets for prevalence of conditions, it is important to realize that diagnostic categories may be inaccurate, reflecting the probable diagnosis rather than the definitive diagnosis.

Section 2.1: Low Back and Joint Pain

In 2004, between 30% and 40% of people in the United States report they experienced low back pain in a previous 3 month period in the two self-reported health conditon national health surveys. (Tables 2.1 and 2.2 and Graph 2.1.1) Among those persons reporting low back pain, approximately 25% also experienced pain radiating into the leg. An additional 15% to 20% of persons reported experiencing neck pain. Overall, about one in two

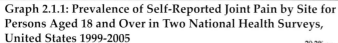

Graph 2.1.1: Prevalence of Self-Reported Joint Pain by Site for Persons Aged 18 and Over in Two National Health Surveys, United States 1999-2005

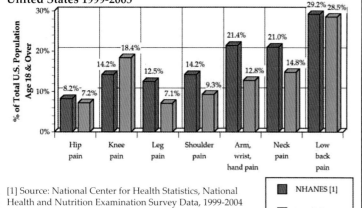

[1] Source: National Center for Health Statistics, National Health and Nutrition Examination Survey Data, 1999-2004
[2] Source: National Center for Health Statistics, National Health Interview Survey, Adult Sample, 2005

NHANES [1]
NHIS [2]

persons report experiencing back pain at least once a year. This is a greater rate of pain than is reported for hips, knees, legs, shoulders, and the upper limb (arm, elbow, wrist, and hands). Approximately one-half of all persons reporting joint pain experience it in more than one site. This is true for persons reporting back pain and for persons reporting joint pain other than back pain. The most frequently reported single site of joint pain is in the lower back.

Graph 2.1.2: Distribution of Back Pain by Site for Persons Aged 18 and Over, United States 1999-2004

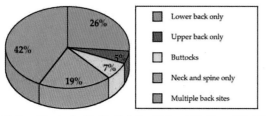

Lower back only
Upper back only
Buttocks
Neck and spine only
Multiple back sites

Source: National Center for Health Statistics, National Health and Nutrition Examination Survey, 1999-2004

Graph 2.1.3: Distribution of Joint Pain Other than Back Pain by Site for Persons Aged 18 and Over, United States 1999-2004

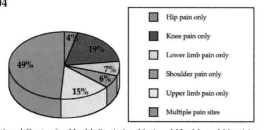

Hip pain only
Knee pain only
Lower limb pain only
Shoulder pain only
Upper limb pain only
Multiple pain sites

Source: National Center for Health Statistics, National Health and Nutrition Examination Survey, 1999-2004

Back pain is reported in similar rates by females and males. The rates are also similar in all age groups over the age of 18 (Graphs 2.1.2 and 2.1.3) and in all racial groups. (Tables 2.3 and 2.4) Back pain is not selective, but is a major health concern for persons of all ages and ethnic backgrounds in the United States. On average, nearly 5% of all annual health care visits to physicians, emergency departments, outpatient clinics, as well as hospitalizations are for treatment of back pain.

The epidemiology of low back pain is not well understood and the overall prevalence, as supported by health care assessment databases, remains unclear. In 2005, 40.5 million patient visits to hospitals and physician offices had low back pain as the first diagnosis. More than 3 out of 4 visits were to a physician's office, but 4% entailed hospitalization. (Tables 2.5 and 2.5a and Graph 2.1.4) The two major diagnostic categories in patients with low back pain are disc degeneration and "back injury."

Graph 2.1.4: Distribution of Health Care Visits for Low Back Pain, United States 2004

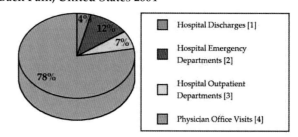

Hospital Discharges [1]
Hospital Emergency Departments [2]
Hospital Outpatient Departments [3]
Physician Office Visits [4]

[1] Source: Agency for Healthcare Research and Quality, Healthcare Cost and Utilization Project, Nationwide Inpatient Sample, 2004
[2] Source: National Center for Health Statistics, National Hospital Ambulatory Medical Care Survey, Hospital Emergency, 2004
[3] Source: National Center for Health Statistics, National Hospital Ambulatory Medical Care Survey, Outpatient, 2004
[4] Source: National Center for Health Statistics, National Ambulatory Medical Care Survey, 2004

The most common diagnosis in patients with low back pain is disc degeneration. Until recently, degenerative back pain was thought to be primarily the result of use or wear and tear. Recent studies, however, have shown a strong genetic link.[3] Intervertebral disc degeneration is a common and natural process of the human spine. Degeneration occurs gradually with aging and can alter the biomechanics and function of the spine. Although these changes go unnoticed in many persons, in others they manifest in back pain and sometimes even neurological compromise.

In this discussion we are dividing the diagnostic codes into three groups: back disorders, disc disorders, and back injuries. This approach was chosen to allow comparison to earlier editions of this text. Back disorders include inflammatory spine conditions, spondylosis, spinal stenosis, lumbago, sciatica, backache, and disorders of the sacrum (ICD-9-CM codes 720, 721, and 724). Disc

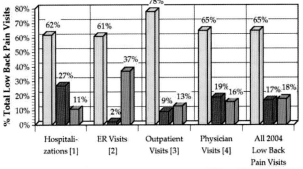

Graph 2.1.5: Distribution of Health Care Resource Use for Low Back Pain by Type of Diagnosis, United States, 2004

[1] Source: Agency for Healthcare Research and Quality, Healthcare Cost and Utilization Project, Nationwide Inpatient Sample, 2004
[2] Source: National Center for Health Statistics, National Hospital Ambulatory Medical Care Survey, Hospital Emergency, 2004
[3] Source: National Center for Health Statistics, National Hospital Ambulatory Medical Care Survey, Outpatient, 2004
[4] Source: National Center for Health Statistics, National Ambulatory Medical Care Survey, 2004

disorders include herniations, disc degeneration, and post laminectomy syndromes (ICD-9-CM code 722). Back injuries include fractures, dislocation, and sprains (ICD-9-CM codes 805, 806, 839, 846, and 847). This division, while useful in analyzing the databases, may not always accurately reflect the primary diagnosis. Further there is some overlap. For example, a patient with back pain of unknown origin could be given a diagnosis of lumbago, placing him or her in the back disorder category; a diagnosis of disc degeneration, falling into the disc disorder category; or a diagnosis of back strain, falling into

the back injury category. Unfortunately, databases do not permit diagnostic verification, and sometimes a diagnosis is provided primarily for reimbursement purposes.

Back disorders accounted for 65% of 2004 low back pain health care resource visits. Both physician office visits and outpatient hospital visits in 2004 were predominantly for back disorders, and 62% of hospitalizations were for back disorders. (Table 2.5a and Graph 2.1.5)

Disc disorders, which include disc displacement (herniation) and degeneration, accounted for about one-half (17%) of the remaining low back pain resource visits. Disc disorders comprised 27% of the hospitalizations in 2004, but only 2% of emergency room visits.

Back injury, which includes fractures, sprains, and strains, often reported as caused by over-exertion or overuse, accounted for the remaining 18% of 2004 low back pain resource visits. Back injuries accounted for 27% of emergency room visits in 2004, but only 11% of hospitalizations.

The incidence of low back pain is greatest in persons of young adult and middle age. In 2004, 74% of all health care visits for low back pain were made by persons between the ages of 18 and 64. (Table 2.5 and Graph 2.1.6) Low back pain in this group is often accompanied by reduced ability to work or inability to work at all. The socioeconomic impact of low back pain, including both direct and indirect costs of health care and

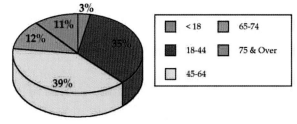

Graph 2.1.6: Distribution of Low Back Pain Health Care Resource Visits by Age, United States 2004

Sources: Agency for Healthcare Research and Quality, Healthcare Cost and Utilization Project, Nationwide Inpatient Sample, 2004; National Center for Health Statistics, National Hospital Ambulatory Medical Care Survey, Hospital Emergency, 2004; National Center for Health Statistics, National Hospital Ambulatory Medical Care Survey, Outpatient, 2004; National Center for Health Statistics, National Ambulatory Medical Care Survey, 2004

disability attendant to the disorder, has been estimated to exceed $100 billion each year.[4]

Back disorders are found more frequently among persons aged 75 and over than in any other age group, accounting for 81% of health care visits in this age group in 2004. (Table 2.5a and Graph 2.1.7) This is probably a reflection of the prevalence of spinal stenosis in elderly patients. Among the small percentage of persons with low back pain who are younger than 18, back disorders represented 76% of their visits; the

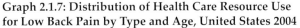
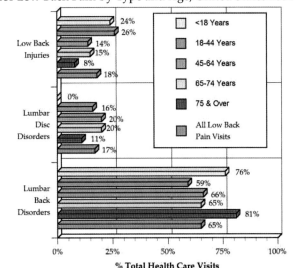

Graph 2.1.7: Distribution of Health Care Resource Use for Low Back Pain by Type and Age, United States 2004

Sources: Agency for Healthcare Research and Quality, Healthcare Cost and Utilization Project, Nationwide Inpatient Sample, 2004; National Center for Health Statistics, National Hospital Ambulatory Medical Care Survey, Hospital Emergency, 2004; National Center for Health Statistics, National Hospital Ambulatory Medical Care Survey, Outpatient, 2004; National Center for Health Statistics, National Ambulatory Medical Care Survey, 2004

balance of visits for low back pain among the young were due to back injuries. Disc herniations and disc degeneration are rare in this age group. Lumbar back injuries accounted for 28% of the health care visits among persons aged 18 to 44, the highest proportion of all age groups. Disc disorders were seen most frequently among persons aged 45 to 74, accounting for 20% of 2004 health care visits for low back pain in that age group.

The average age of persons hospitalized in 2004 for low back pain was 59.8 years. This compares to an average age of 42.0 years for persons

visiting an emergency department, 48.1 years for visits to an outpatient department, and 51.7 years for visits to a physician. (Table 2.5)

Persons hospitalized for low back pain in 2004 spent an average of 4½ days in the hospital. (Table 2.8 and Graph 2.1.8) Persons hospitalized

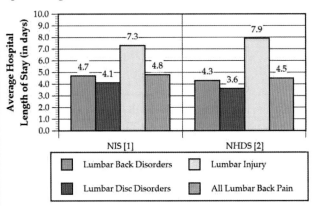

Graph 2.1.8: Average Length of Hospital Stay for Lumbar Spine Diagnosis, United States 2004

[1] Source: Agency for Healthcare Research and Quality, Healthcare Cost and Utilization Project, Nationwide Inpatient Sample, 2004
[2] Source: National Center for Health Statistics, National Hospital Discharge Survey, 2004

for lumbar back injuries were hospitalized for the longest period of time, an average of more than seven days.

Low back pain is found more frequently among females than males, with females representing 56% of the 2004 health care visits. Males were seen more often for low back injuries (19% of visits) and disc disorders (22%) than were females; 70% of the female visits for low back pain were diagnosed as back disorders. Again, this is probably a reflection of the prevalence of spinal stenosis. (Table 2.5 and Graph 2.1.9)

Overall, lumbar/low back pain accounted for 1 in 25 health care resource visits in 2004. The staggering impact of low back pain on both the health care resources in the United States and the disability inflicted on the individual is difficult to fully quantify.

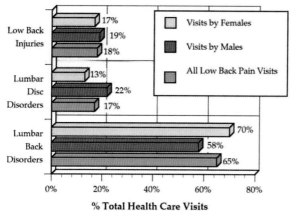

Graph 2.1.9: Distribution of Health Care Resource Use for Low Back Pain by Type and Gender, United States 2004

Sources: Agency for Healthcare Research and Quality, Healthcare Cost and Utilization Project, Nationwide Inpatient Sample, 2004; National Center for Health Statistics, National Hospital Ambulatory Medical Care Survey, Hospital Emergency, 2004; National Center for Health Statistics, National Hospital Ambulatory Medical Care Survey, Outpatient, 2004; National Center for Health Statistics, National Ambulatory Medical Care Survey, 2004

Section 2.2: Cervical/Neck Pain

Cervical/neck pain is a very common reason for visiting a doctor. In 2004, 16.4 million patient visits, or 1.5% of all health care visits to hospitals and physician offices, were for neck pain. Four out of five (80%) of the visits were to physician offices, while only 3% of patients with cervical/neck pain were hospitalized. (Table 2.6a and Graph 2.2.1)

In presenting health care resource utilization for cervical pain, three categories of cervical pain are addressed. One is labeled cervical disc disorders, and includes disc displacements, herniations, and disc degeneration (ICD-9-CM code 722). A second group is cervical injuries, and includes sprains, strains, and fractures (ICD-9-CM codes 805, 806, 839, and 847). A third group, referred to as cervical disorders, includes pain caused by other disease entities, including cervical spondylosis and stenosis (ICD-9-CM codes 721 and 723).

Cervical disorders accounted for 59% of health care visits for upper back pain in 2004. (Table 2.6a) Patients with cervical disorders are treated primarily in outpatient settings, accounting for 67% of cervical pain patient visits in hospital

outpatient settings and 63% of physicians office visits.

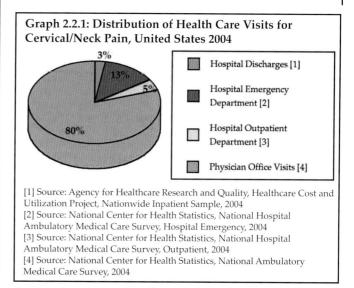

Graph 2.2.1: Distribution of Health Care Visits for Cervical/Neck Pain, United States 2004

Hospital Discharges [1]
Hospital Emergency Department [2]
Hospital Outpatient Department [3]
Physician Office Visits [4]

[1] Source: Agency for Healthcare Research and Quality, Healthcare Cost and Utilization Project, Nationwide Inpatient Sample, 2004
[2] Source: National Center for Health Statistics, National Hospital Ambulatory Medical Care Survey, Hospital Emergency, 2004
[3] Source: National Center for Health Statistics, National Hospital Ambulatory Medical Care Survey, Outpatient, 2004
[4] Source: National Center for Health Statistics, National Ambulatory Medical Care Survey, 2004

Cervical disc disorders accounted for only 11% of all neck pain health care visits in 2004, but were responsible for 31% of hospitalizations. (Table 2.6a and Graph 2.2.2) Neck injuries accounted for 30% of all neck pain. This is a much higher percentage than found in low back pain injuries. The majority of patients with cervical injuries were treated in an outpatient setting, and accounted for 69% of all emergency department visits for cervical/ neck pain.

Graph 2.2.2: Distribution of Health Care Resource Use for Cervical/Neck Pain by Diagnosis Type, United States, 2004

Cervical Back Disorders
Cervical/ Neck Injury
Cervical Disc Disorders

[1] Source: Agency for Healthcare Research and Quality, Healthcare Cost and Utilization Project, Nationwide Inpatient Sample, 2004
[2] Source: National Center for Health Statistics, National Hospital Ambulatory Medical Care Survey, Hospital Emergency, 2004
[3] Source: National Center for Health Statistics, National Hospital Ambulatory Medical Care Survey, Outpatient, 2004
[4] Source: National Center for Health Statistics, National Ambulatory Medical Care Survey, 2004

Inpatient care for cervical/neck pain is, on average, utilized primarily by older persons. The average age for persons hospitalized for cervical/neck pain in 2004 was 58.2 years, with persons having a neck injury being somewhat younger at 47.9 years. (Table 2.6) The average age of persons treated in an emergency department for neck injury was 33.0 years. The overall average age of emergency room patients with a neck pain diagnosis was 39.0 years. Hospital outpatient and physician office patients were, on average, 46.0 and 48.4 years old, respectively.

Four out of five neck pain diagnoses (81%) in 2004 were for persons between the ages of 18 and 64. (Table 2.6a and Graph 2.2.3) Only 4% of

Graph 2.2.3: Distribution of Cervical/Neck Pain Health Care Resource Visits by Age, United States 2004

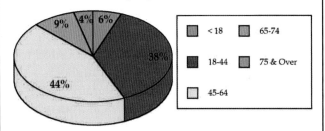

Sources: Agency for Healthcare Research and Quality, Healthcare Cost and Utilization Project, Nationwide Inpatient Sample, 2004; National Center for Health Statistics, National Hospital Ambulatory Medical Care Survey, Hospital Emergency, 2004; National Center for Health Statistics, National Hospital Ambulatory Medical Care Survey, Outpatient, 2004; National Center for Health Statistics, National Ambulatory Medical Care Survey, 2004

patients were over the age of 75, with 6% younger than 18 years of age. Among persons aged 18 to 44 years, cervical injuries (40%) and cervical disorders (49%) accounted for nearly all health care visits for upper back pain. (Table 2.6a and Graph 2.2.4) Health care visits for neck injuries by persons under the age of 18 accounted for a larger share of total visits than was found in any other age group (45%). Cervical disc disorders, as the first diagnosis for neck pain, was found most frequently in persons aged 45 to 64 years.

Persons hospitalized for neck pain in 2004 spent an average of just under 5 days in the hospital. (Table 2.8 and Graph 2.2.5) Persons hospitalized for neck injuries were hospitalized for the longest period of time, an average of 8 to 10 days.

Graph 2.2.4: Distribution of Health Care Resource Use for Cervical/Neck Pain by Type and Age, United States 2004

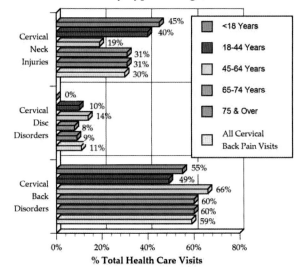

Sources: Agency for Healthcare Research and Quality, Healthcare Cost and Utilization Project, Nationwide Inpatient Sample, 2004; National Center for Health Statistics, National Hospital Ambulatory Medical Care Survey, Hospital Emergency, 2004; National Center for Health Statistics, National Hospital Ambulatory Medical Care Survey, Outpatient, 2004; National Center for Health Statistics, National Ambulatory Medical Care Survey, 2004

Females accounted for 59% of the health care visits for neck pain in 2004, a slightly higher proportion than was found with low back pain. (Table 2.6a and Graph 2.2.6) Cervical disorders accounted for 62% of visits by females, with injuries accounting for 27%. Among males, 34% of health care visits for cervical/neck pain were the result of neck injuries, with cervical neck disorders accounting for 54% of the visits.

Graph 2.2.5: Average Length of Hospital Stay for Cervical Spine Diagnosis, United States 2004

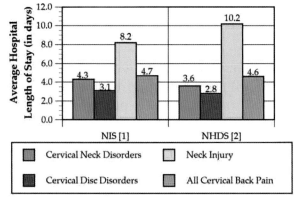

[1] Source: Agency for Healthcare Research and Quality, Healthcare Cost and Utilization Project, Nationwide Inpatient Sample, 2004
[2] Source: National Center for Health Statistics, National Hospital Discharge Survey, 2004

Graph 2.2.6: Distribution of Health Care Resource Use for Cervical/Neck Pain by Type and Gender, United States 2004

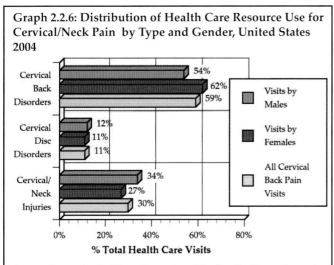

Sources: Agency for Healthcare Research and Quality, Healthcare Cost and Utilization Project, Nationwide Inpatient Sample, 2004; National Center for Health Statistics, National Hospital Ambulatory Medical Care Survey, Hospital Emergency, 2004; National Center for Health Statistics, National Hospital Ambulatory Medical Care Survey, Outpatient, 2004; National Center for Health Statistics, National Ambulatory Medical Care Survey, 2004

Graph 2.3.1: Spine Diagnosis Visits as a Proportion of All Health Care Visits, United States 2004

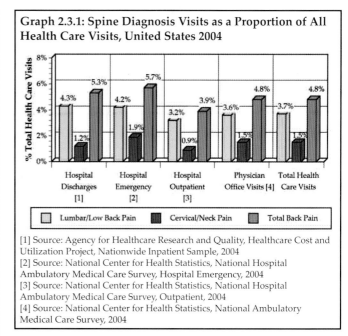

[1] Source: Agency for Healthcare Research and Quality, Healthcare Cost and Utilization Project, Nationwide Inpatient Sample, 2004
[2] Source: National Center for Health Statistics, National Hospital Ambulatory Medical Care Survey, Hospital Emergency, 2004
[3] Source: National Center for Health Statistics, National Hospital Ambulatory Medical Care Survey, Outpatient, 2004
[4] Source: National Center for Health Statistics, National Ambulatory Medical Care Survey, 2004

Section 2.3: Burden of Back Pain

While lumbar/low back pain is more common than cervical/neck pain, together they accounted for 5%, or 1 in 20, health care visits in 2004. (Tablas 2.7 and 2.7a and Graph 2.3.1) The majority of visits (78%) were physician office visits. Over the past 7 years, physician office visits for back pain have increased steadily. In 1998, 12% of the population aged 18 and over visited a physician for back pain, accounting for 32 million visits. In 2004, the proportion of the population visiting their physician for back pain had increased to more than 15%, and the total number of visits increased to nearly 45 million. (Table 2.9 and Graph 2.3.2)

The financial cost associated with back pain is obviously enormous and unfortunately rising. Greater understanding of the causes of back pain and its resultant disability is needed to thwart and reduce this rising trend. Understanding why disc degeneration causes pain in some yet not in others is needed to address the burden of pain and disability and the significant economic impact low back pain treatment creates on health care resources each year.

Graph 2.3.2: Trend in Number and Proportion of the Population with Physician Visits for Back Pain, United States 1998-2004

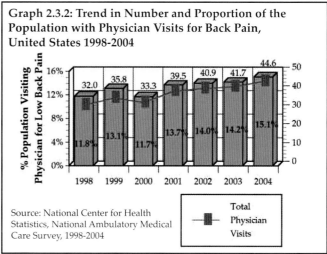

Source: National Center for Health Statistics, National Ambulatory Medical Care Survey, 1998-2004

Section 2.3.1: Limitations Resulting from Back Pain

More than one in ten persons (11%) over the age of 18 in the United States report health care problems limit their ability to work, and one in three (32%) report their health limits the amount or type of work they can perform. An additional 8% of the population report that their ability to walk is impacted by their health. Pain is a major cause of these limitations. Back pain is cited more frequently than any other pain entity (e.g., head, shoulder, leg, foot) by persons reporting work or walking limitations. (Table 2.10 and Graph 2.3.3)

Graph 2.3.3: Proportion of Persons Aged 18 and Over Reporting Pain Limits Ability to Walk or Work by Pain Site, United States 1999-2004

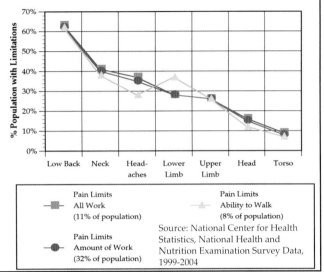

Source: National Center for Health Statistics, National Health and Nutrition Examination Survey Data, 1999-2004

report they cannot work at all due to health limitations; among this group, 24% to 43% report back pain as the cause. This compares to only 10% of persons in this age group with total work restrictions who report they have no back pain. Among the 32% of the population reporting limitations in the amount or type of work they can perform, the differences are even greater. Between 55% and 84% report back pain, while only 29% of those with no back pain report work restrictions. (Table 2.11 and Graphs 2.3.4a-b)

In another national study, bed days and lost work days were reported for persons self-reporting back pain in the previous 3 months. Of the total 144.1 million persons reporting back pain, approximately one in four (33.7 million) reported they spent one or more days in bed due to back

Between 1999 and 2004, an average of 62% of the population who reported work or walking limitations also reported they had low back pain. During this same time period, 38% to 41% reported they had neck pain. Low back pain was reported nearly twice as often as headaches or lower limb joint pain (hip, leg, foot) as the cause of work or walking limitations.

Work limitations due to back pain are reported in similar proportion by males and females. The presence of back pain in more than one site (e.g., low back, upper back, buttocks, neck, and spine) is more likely to be the cause of work limitations than back pain that is localized.

Back pain severe enough to keep people from working at any occupation is most likely to be reported by individuals aged 65 to 74, and may be the cause of involuntary early retirement. However, individuals in the prime working ages of 45 to 64 frequently report back pain as the cause of their inability to work at all; they also report that the pain places limitations on the amount or type of work they can do in nearly the same proportion as those aged 65 and older. Overall, 14% of the population aged 45 to 64

Graph 2.3.4a: Proportion of Persons Aged 18 or Older with Work History for Whom Pain Limits Their Ability to Work by Age, United States 1999-2004

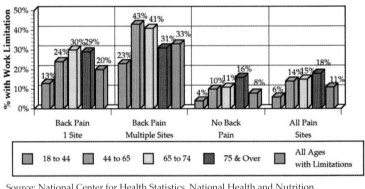

Source: National Center for Health Statistics, National Health and Nutrition Examination Survey Data, 1999-2004

Graph 2.3.4b: Proportion of Persons Aged 18 or Older with Work History for Whom Pain Limits the Amount of Work They Can Perform by Age, United States 1999-2004

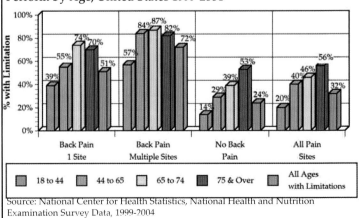

Source: National Center for Health Statistics, National Health and Nutrition Examination Survey Data, 1999-2004

pain. With an average of 9.3 days bed days reported, persons in the United States spent a total of 313.5 million days in bed due to back pain in 2004. In addition, 25.9 million persons reporting back pain also reported losing an average of 7.2 work days. (Table 2.12 and Graphs 2.3.5a-b) Hence, in 2004, an estimated 186.7 million work days were lost due to back pain.

The most severe pain, resulting in the highest average number of bed and lost work days, was reported by persons with low back pain and radiating leg pain. This group of 20.3 million persons spent an average of 19.9 days in bed and lost an average of 12.9 work days. They probably

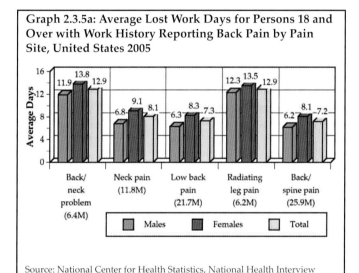

Graph 2.3.5a: Average Lost Work Days for Persons 18 and Over with Work History Reporting Back Pain by Pain Site, United States 2005

Source: National Center for Health Statistics, National Health Interview Survey, 2005

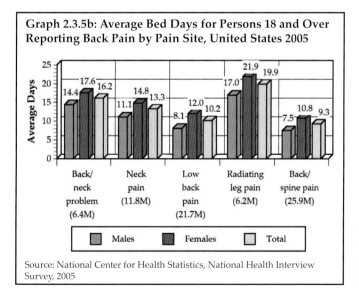

Graph 2.3.5b: Average Bed Days for Persons 18 and Over Reporting Back Pain by Pain Site, United States 2005

Source: National Center for Health Statistics, National Health Interview Survey, 2005

include most patients with disc herniation and symptomatic spinal stenosis. In all instances, females reported higher levels of back pain and more bed and lost work days than did males.

Section 2.4: Spine Procedures

While nonsurgical treatment for back pain is the treatment of choice, when back pain becomes so disabling that patients can no longer function in the activities of daily living, spine surgery may be performed. Three procedures account for 83% of spine procedures. The most frequently performed spine procedure in 2004 was a diskectomy, accounting for 34% of spine procedures performed in an inpatient setting. Spinal fusion procedures accounted for 32% of all spine procedures performed in 2004, and were performed on more than one-half of spine pain patients hospitalized. (Table 2.13 and Graph 2.4.1) Spinal decompression, which may or may not be performed in conjunction with a spinal fusion, accounted for 17% of all spine procedures.

Section 2.4.1: Spinal Fusion

The rate of spinal fusion procedures has risen rapidly over the past several decades. Spinal fusion is performed either alone or in conjunction with decompression and/or reduction of a spine deformity. Fusion is performed on the cervical, thoracic and lumbar regions of the spine. The increase in spinal fusion rates has been documented by several authors, with increased rates of 55% between 1979 and 1990[5]; 220% between 1990 and 2001[6]; and 250% between 1990 and 2003[7] cited. Revision fusion rates have been reported at increased rates of 180% between 1990 and 2003.[7]

Increased rates of spinal fusion have been noted since the 1980s. Likely explanations for these increases are advances in technology, including the development of new diagnostic techniques and new implant devices that allow for better surgical management; increased training in spinal surgery; and the aging of the population with inherent medical problems.

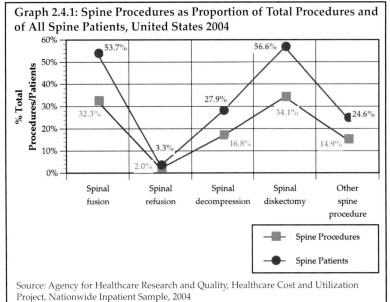

Graph 2.4.1: Spine Procedures as Proportion of Total Procedures and of All Spine Patients, United States 2004

Source: Agency for Healthcare Research and Quality, Healthcare Cost and Utilization Project, Nationwide Inpatient Sample, 2004

100,000 persons of 81.2 in 1998 and 114.8 in 2004. However, data from 2004 showed a slight decline from 2003 in this growth curve. Whether this is an indication of a slowing of the spinal fusion procedures rate or an anomaly in the 2004 data remains to be seen in future years.

Between 1998 and 2004, the rate of revision fusion procedures increased by 70%. The revision rate over this 7 year period had a fluctuating rate, but overall continued growth. In 1998, revision spinal fusions were performed at a rate of 4.4 per 100,000 persons. By 2004, the rate had increased to 6.9 per 100,000 persons.

During this 1998 to 2004 period, the cost of performing spinal fusion procedures increased by 111% for a primary spinal fusion and 145% for a

Lumbar spinal fusion rates have increased more rapidly than the rates for cervical or thoracic fusion and are increasingly being performed on an older population. Rates of lumbar fusion vary dramatically among geographic regions, hospitals, and even between surgeons in the same hospital, indicating that the outcomes and indications for lumbar fusion vary.[8] The primary diagnosis for several conditions have shown increased rates of fusion, with disc degeneration outpacing those of spondylolysis/spondylolisthesis and spinal stenosis.[6]

Since the mid-1980s, cervical spinal fusion rates have been reported at 25% of the rates of lumbar fusion. Wide geographic variation is found in the rates of both cervical and lumbar fusion.[9] However, cervical rates may have been affected by reporting procedures, as it was not until 1995 that multilevel spinal procedures were reported with more than one procedural code. Between 1985 and 1996, cervical spinal fusion procedures were reported at an increate rate of 310%, while the same author reports increased rates of 286% in lumbar and 358% in thoracic fusion rates.[9]

In more recent years, 1998 to 2004, spinal fusion rates based on the Nationwide Inpatient Sample (NIS) have shown a continued rise, increasing by 54%. (Table 2.14 and Graph 2.4.2) This growth reflects a primary fusion procedure rate per

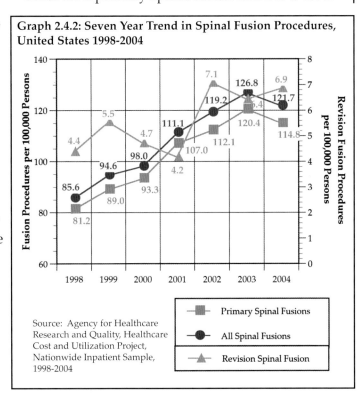

Graph 2.4.2: Seven Year Trend in Spinal Fusion Procedures, United States 1998-2004

Source: Agency for Healthcare Research and Quality, Healthcare Cost and Utilization Project, Nationwide Inpatient Sample, 1998-2004

revision spinal fusion procedure. In 2004, the mean hospital cost, as reported in the National Inpatient Sample for a primary spinal fusion was $56,000 and a revision spinal fusion was $63,000.

Combining the increased rate of procedures with the increasing cost of performing them, the

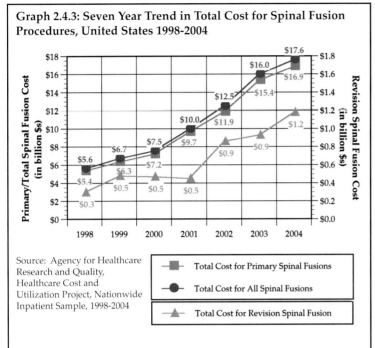

Graph 2.4.3: Seven Year Trend in Total Cost for Spinal Fusion Procedures, United States 1998-2004

Source: Agency for Healthcare Research and Quality, Healthcare Cost and Utilization Project, Nationwide Inpatient Sample, 1998-2004

- ■ Total Cost for Primary Spinal Fusions
- ● Total Cost for All Spinal Fusions
- ▲ Total Cost for Revision Spinal Fusion

on males and females; however, patients between the ages of 18 and 64 were significantly more likely to have the procedure than those under age 18 and those 65 years and older. (Table 2.16)

Spinal fusion is most frequently performed following a diagnosis of cervical disc pain, accounting for 19% of first diagnosis of spinal fusion patients in 2004. (Table 2.17) Lumbar disc degeneration and lumbar disc displacement were the second and third most frequent first diagnosis, accounting for 13% and 11% of first diagnoses, respectively.

The introduction of motion preservation options in the past few years will most certainly have an impact on spinal fusion as the preferred treatment option.

Section 2.4.2: Ruptured Spine Diagnosis and Diskectomy Procedures

estimated cost of primary spinal fusion procedures increased by 215% between 1998 and 2004, totaling $16.9 billion in 2004. An additional $1.2 billion was spent on revision spinal procedures, an increase of 292% between 1998 and 2004. (Table 2.14 and Graph 2.4.3)

Mean charges for lumbar spinal fusion procedures in 2004 were $63,520, based on an average hospital stay of 4.7 days. The average cost of a cervical spinal fusion procedure was nearly 40% less, $39,300, based on an average hospital stay of 3.5 days. (Table 2.14)

In 2004, 327,000 spinal fusion procedures were performed on patients with lumbar/low back pain or cervical/neck pain. The number of primary lumbar fusion procedures was slightly higher than cervical procedures (150,000 versus 135,000, respectively), accounting for 46% versus 41% of all fusion procedures. (Table 2.15 and Graph 2.4.4) Because many more are patients operated on for low back pain problems requiring decompression only (e.g., disc herniations, some spinal stenosis), the percentage of patients who were fused in the low back group was lower (9.5%) than in the neck group (31.3%). Spinal fusion procedures were performed about equally

A diskectomy was the most frequent inpatient spine procedure performed in 2004, accounting for more than 325,300 procedures. Two-thirds (66%) of diskectomy procedures were performed on patients with a ruptured disc diagnosis, primarily for a lumbar disc. (Tables 2.18 and 2.19) The average age at which a diskectomy was performed in 2004 was 50.8 years. Patients

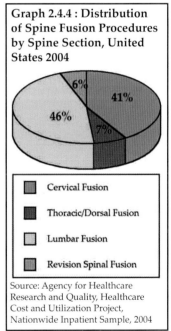

Graph 2.4.4 : Distribution of Spine Fusion Procedures by Spine Section, United States 2004

- Cervical Fusion
- Thoracic/Dorsal Fusion
- Lumbar Fusion
- Revision Spinal Fusion

Source: Agency for Healthcare Research and Quality, Healthcare Cost and Utilization Project, Nationwide Inpatient Sample, 2004

spent a mean of 2.9 days in the hospital, at a mean cost of $34,580 per patient. Total health care cost for inpatient diskectomy procedures in 2004 was $11.25 billion.

Although the majority of persons with a ruptured disc diagnosis undergoing surgery were hospitalized in 2004, the health care impact and cost of a ruptured, or herniated, disc is much more severe due to only 7% of patients with this diagnosis being hospitalized. The majority of the total 5 million persons diagnosed with a ruptured disc in 2004 were seen in a physician's office. (Table 2.18 and Graph 2.4.5) A ruptured disk

Graph 2.4.5: Health Care Visits for Ruptured Spine by Location, United States 2004

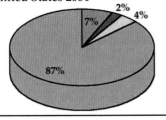

- Hospital Discharges [1]
- Hospital Emergency Departments [2]
- Hospital Outpatient Departments [3]
- Physician Office Visits [4]

[1] Source: Agency for Healthcare Research and Quality, Healthcare Cost and Utilization Project, Nationwide Inpatient Sample, 2004
[2] Source: National Center for Health Statistics, National Hospital Ambulatory Medical Care Survey, Hospital Emergency, 2004
[3] Source: National Center for Health Statistics, National Hospital Ambulatory Medical Care Survey, Outpatient, 2004
[4] Source: National Center for Health Statistics, National Ambulatory Medical Care Survey, 2004

Graph 2.4.6: Health Care Visits for Ruptured Spine by Age, United States 2004

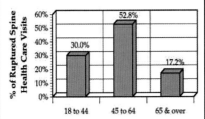

Sources: Agency for Healthcare Research and Quality, Healthcare Cost and Utilization Project, Nationwide Inpatient Sample, 2004; National Center for Health Statistics, National Hospital Ambulatory Medical Care Survey, Hospital Emergency, 2004: National Center for Health Statistics, National Hospital Ambulatory Medica Care Survey, Outpatient, 2004; National Center for Health Statistics, National Ambulatory Medical Care Survey, 2004

occurs primarily between the ages of 18 and 64 (83% of diagnoses); rarely does it occur in persons under the age of 18 or over the age of 75. (Graph 2.4.6)

The mean number of diskectomy procedures reported by the National Hospital Discharge Survey over the past 10 years is 299,000 per year, with a range of 279,000 to 324,000 fluctuating around this mean. (Table 2.20 and Graph 2.4.7)

Graph 2.4.7: Ten-Year Trend in Spinal Diskectomy Procedures, United States 1996-2005

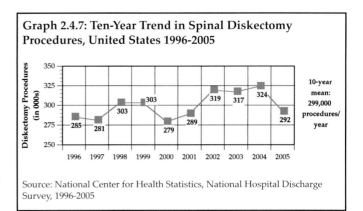

Source: National Center for Health Statistics, National Hospital Discharge Survey, 1996-2005

Section 2.5: Neuromusculoskeletal Conditions

The spinal column is an extremely complex biomechanical structure with intimate neurological, muscular, and ligamentous interfaces. Functional and structural disorders of the spine often produce symptomatology affecting contiguous structures and regions. The resultant types of disorders affecting multiple domains have been referred to as neuromusculoskeletal or spine-related disorders. Included in this group are spinal subluxations, spinal sprains and strains, cervical, thoracic, lumbar and pelvic symptoms and ill-defined conditions; and spine-related (cervico-genic) headaches. These types of conditions are prevalent, disturbing, and compromising to patients' functional abilities. In 2004, over 111 million patient visits were attributed to disorders in the neuromusculoskeletal category. In part, the reason for the ill-defined nature of some of these conditions may lie in the intrinsic complexity of the spinal column and the multiple structures and systems with which it interfaces. For example, individuals with chronic lumbar and pelvic pain may also complain of depression, digestive problems, and sexual dysfunction. Many patients with chronic cervical symptoms suffer from headaches as well.

Since 1999, neuromusculoskeletal complaints have shown a steady increase in incidence. This increase may be associated with the increasingly sedentary lifestyle of Americans and the marked increase in occupational and recreational use of computers with attendant ergonomic risks. The proportionate rise in cervical and thoracic and lumbar spine symptoms and ill-defined conditions has been similar in distribution since 1999. In 2004, the number of patient visits related to cervical spine symptoms and ill-defined conditions (34.1 million) were approximately equal in number to visits for similar lumbar spine disorders (34.9 million). In 2004, thoracic symptoms and ill-defined disorders numbered 18.3 million, while pelvic disorders numbered 13.2 million. Females are more prone than males to these spine-related disorders across a range of categories.

Section 2.6: Economic Cost of Spine Conditions

Chapter 9 summarizes the cost of musculoskeletal conditions based on analysis of the Medical Expenditures Panel Survey (MEPS) from 1996 to 2004. The MEPS, which began in 1996, is a set of large-scale surveys of families and individuals, their medical providers (doctors, hospitals, pharmacies, etc.), and their employers. MEPS collects data on the specific health services that Americans use, how frequently they use them, the cost of these services, and how they are paid for, as well as data on the cost, scope, and breadth of health insurance held by and available to U.S. workers. Currently MEPS collects data from two major components: households and insurance companies. The Household Component (MEPS-HC) provides data from individual households and their members, which is supplemented by data from their medical providers. The Insurance Component (MEPS-IC) is a separate survey of employers that provides data on employer-based health insurance. MEPS also includes a Medical Provider Component (MEPS-MPC), that covers hospitals, physicians, home health care providers, and pharmacies identified by MEPS-HC respondents. Its purpose is to supplement and/or replace information received from the MEPS-HC respondents.[10]

As with the National Health Interview Survey (NHIS), data in the household component is self-reported. Self-reported data from available databases indicates a range in the prevalence of all specific conditions. As noted earlier in this chapter, more than 44.6 million persons visited their physician with a complaint of back pain in 2004, while 94.3 persons self-reported low back or neck pain in 2005 in the NHIS. Economic projections are based on the MEPS self-reported spine conditions, or 32.7 million incidences.

The estimated annual cost for medical care of spine conditions, discussed in Chapter 9, both as a primary condition and secondary to another condition, in 2004 was $193.9 billion or an average of $5,923 for each of the 32.7 million persons who reported having a spine condition. Of this total, $30.3 billion is estimated as the incremental cost directly related to spine conditions. A breakdown of the $193.9 billion cost due to spine conditions shows 34% for ambulatory care, 32% for emergency room or inpatient care, 20% for prescription drugs, and 14% for other expenses. The cost of spine conditions, in 2004 dollars, rose from $130.2 billion in 1996 to $193.9 billion in 2004, an increase of 49%. The increasing cost of prescription drugs accounts for the largest percentage of this total cost increase, rising from 13% of total cost to 20% over the 9-year period. Earnings loss, or indirect costs, due to spine conditions for persons between the ages of 18 to 64 years with a work history was estimated at $22.4 billion per year between 2000 and 2004.

1. National Center for Health Statistics: National Health Interview Survey, Adult Sample Level File, 2005.

2. National Center for Health Statistics: National Health and Nutrition Examination Survey Data, 1998-2004.

3. Battie MC, Videman T: Lumbar disc degeneration: Epidemiology and genetics. *J Bone Joint Surg Am* 2006;88:3-9.

4. Katz J: Lumbar disc disorders and low-back pain: socioeconomic factors and consequences. *J Bone Joint Surg Am* 2006;88:21-24.

5. Katz J: Lumbar spinal fusion: Surgical rates, costs, and complications. *Spine* 1995;20:78S-83S.

6. Deyo R: Epidemiology of spinal surgery: Rates and trends. Center for Cost and Outcomes Research, University of Washington; available at: http://depts.washington.edu/ccor/studies/SpineSurgEpi.shtml. Accessed May 2, 2007.

7. Ong KL, Lau E, Kurtz SM, et al: Cervical, thoracic, and lumbar fusion rates in the U.S.: Perspective from two health databases. Paper presented at: 53rd Annual Meeting, Orthopaedic Research Society; 2007;San Diego, CA.

8. Abraham DJ, Herkowitz HN, Katz JN: Indications for thoracic and lumbar spine fusion and trends in use. *Orthop Clin North Am* 1998;29:803-811.

9. Abraham DJ, Herkowitz HN, Katz JN: Indications and trends in use in cervical spinal fusions. *Orthop Clin North Am* 1998;29:731-744.

10. Agency for Health Care Research and Quality: Medical Expenditure Panel Survey Background. 2007. Available at: http://www.meps.ahrq.gov/mepsweb/about_meps/survey_back.jsp. Accessed May 7, 2007.

Section 2.7: Spine: Low Back and Neck Pain Data Tables

Table 2.1: Self-Reported Prevalence of Joint Pain by Site of Joint and Selected Demographic Characteristics for Persons Aged 18 and Over, United States 2005

Prevalence of Pain by Site (rate per 100 persons)

		Lower Back [1]	Neck [2]	Back w/ Radiating Leg Pain [3]	Upper Limb [4]	Shoulder [5]	Lower Limb [6]	Knee [7]	Hip [8]
Gender	Male	26.2	12.4	8.1	11.3	9.3	6.1	16.7	5.3
	Female	30.5	17.1	9.4	14.2	9.4	8.1	20.0	8.9
Age	18-44 years	25.0	12.7	7.7	6.7	4.9	4.5	11.6	3.2
	45-64 years	31.5	18.0	9.7	18.3	12.9	9.6	23.2	9.7
	65-74 years	32.0	15.8	9.9	21.4	15.7	10.3	29.6	13.7
	75 & over	34.0	13.8	10.5	20.4	16.0	10.1	30.5	15.5
Race	White	29.1	15.4	9.0	13.5	9.8	7.4	18.9	7.6
	Black	25.4	11.9	7.8	9.0	7.1	5.6	17.1	5.4
	Asian	19.6	9.3	6.0	7.5	4.6	3.4	9.4	1.8
	Other	34.7	19.4	10.7	14.8	11.9	10.0	22.6	8.2
Total		28.5	14.8	8.8	12.8	9.3	7.1	18.4	7.2

[1] "During the PAST THREE MONTHS, did you have …Low back pain?"

[2] "During the PAST THREE MONTHS, did you have …Neck pain?"

[3] If low back pain, "Did this pain spread down either leg to areas below the knees?"

"DURING THE PAST 30 DAYS, have you had any symptoms of pain, aching, or stiffness in or around a joint?"

[4] Hand, wrist, fingers

[5] Shoulder

[6] Ankle, foot

[7] Knee, right/left

[8] Hip, right/left

Source: National Center for Health Statistics, National Health Interview Survey, Adult Sample Level File, 2005

Table 2.2: Self-Reported Prevalence of Joint or Back Pain by Site and Selected Demographic Characteristics for Persons Aged 18 and Over, United States 2005

Prevalence of Pain by Site (rate per 100 persons)

		Lower Back [1]	Neck [2]	Back w/ Radiating Leg Pain [3]	Upper Limb [4]	Shoulder [5]	Lower Limb [6]	Knee [7]	Hip [8]
Gender	Male	36.7	18.8	9.0	19.4	14.4	10.4	14.4	6.1
	Female	41.4	23.0	11.7	23.3	14.0	14.5	14.0	10.2
Age	18-44 years	38.0	19.8	8.0	15.6	10.2	9.1	10.2	4.8
	45-64 years	41.5	24.0	13.8	28.5	19.4	16.3	19.4	11.5
	65-74 years	37.0	19.9	12.1	26.6	16.7	16.5	16.7	12.2
	75 & over	39.7	17.0	10.3	26.8	17.9	16.4	17.9	14.6
Race	White	40.2	21.9	10.3	23.2	15.1	13.3	15.1	9.4
	Black/African American	36.6	16.5	11.3	14.3	11.8	11.9	11.8	6.4
	Mexican American	33.3	18.2	9.1	17.6	9.6	8.6	9.6	4.2
	Other Hispanic	31.6	16.4	9.2	18.6	11.8	8.5	11.8	4.2
	Other	43.8	25.2	12.5	20.3	15.0	11.8	15.0	5.9
Total		39.2	21.0	10.4	21.4	14.2	12.5	14.2	8.2

[1] "During the PAST THREE MONTHS, did you have …Low back pain?"

[2] "During the PAST THREE MONTHS, did you have ...Neck pain?"

[3] If low back pain, "Did this pain spread down either leg to areas below the knees?"

"DURING THE PAST 30 DAYS, have you had any symptoms of pain, aching, or stiffness in or around a joint?"

[4] Hand, wrist, fingers

[5] Shoulder

[6] Ankle, foot

[7] Knee, right/left

[8] Hip, right/left

Source: National Center for Health Statistics, National Health and Nutrition Examination Survey, 1999-2004

Table 2.3: Distribution of Back Pain by Site and Selected Demographic Characteristics for Persons Aged 18 and Over, United States 1999-2004

| | | Proportion of Persons Reporting Back Pain | | | | |
		Lower Back Pain Only [1]	Upper Back Pain Only [2]	Buttocks [3]	Neck and Spine Only [4]	Multiple Back Pain Sites [5]
Gender	Male	28%	5%	6%	22%	40%
	Female	25%	5%	9%	17%	44%
Age	18-44 years	28%	6%	4%	20%	42%
	45-64 years	23%	5%	10%	18%	44%
	65-74 years	26%	4%	12%	21%	38%
	75 & over	33%	6%	11%	14%	36%
Race	White	25%	5%	7%	20%	43%
	Black/African American	39%	3%	7%	15%	36%
	Mexican American	27%	3%	8%	23%	40%
	Other Hispanic	25%	8%	8%	17%	43%
	Other	28%	3%	4%	23%	42%
Total		26%	5%	7%	19%	42%

[1] "With respect to pain problem, located in …low back pain?"

[2] "With respect to pain problem, located in …upper back pain?"

[3] "With respect to pain problem, located in …buttocks?"

[4] "With respect to pain problem, located in …neck and spine?"

[5] "With respect to pain problem, located in …multiple sites of back"

Source: National Center for Health Statistics. National Health and Nutrition Examination Survey Data, 1999-2004.

Table 2.4: Distribution Joint Pain by Site and Selected Demographic Characteristics for Persons Aged 18 and Over, United States 1999-2004

		Proportion of Persons Reporting Joint Pain (excluding back pain)					
		Hip Pain Only [1]	Knee Pain Only [2]	Lower Limb Pain Only [3]	Shoulder Pain Only [4]	Upper Limb Pain Only [5]	Multiple Pain Sites [6]
Gender	Male	3%	21%	7%	8%	16%	45%
	Female	5%	18%	7%	5%	14%	52%
Age	18-44 years	3%	22%	8%	8%	17%	42%
	45-64 years	4%	18%	6%	5%	13%	53%
	65-74 years	5%	16%	8%	5%	13%	54%
	75 & over	6%	15%	6%	5%	13%	54%
Race	White	4%	18%	7%	6%	15%	49%
	Black/African American	5%	26%	10%	7%	10%	43%
	Mexican American	3%	17%	5%	5%	19%	50%
	Other Hispanic	5%	21%	4%	9%	20%	41%
	Other	4%	15%	5%	10%	13%	52%
Total		4%	19%	7%	6%	15%	49%

[1] "With respect to pain problem, located in ...hip pain?"

[2] "With respect to pain problem, located in ...knee pain?"

[3] "With respect to pain problem, located in ...leg, foot pain?"

[4] "With respect to pain problem, located in ...shoulder pain?"

[5] "With respect to pain problem, located in ...elbow, wrist or finger pain"

[6] "With respect to pain problem, located in ...multiple joint pain sites"

Source: National Center for Health Statistics. National Health and Nutrition Examination Survey Data, 1999-2004.

Table 2.5: Prevalence of Lumbar and Low Back Disorders by Gender and Age, United States 2004

	Total	Gender		Age (in years)					Ave Age
		Male	Female	<18	18-44	45-64	65-74	75 & over	for Dx
Hospital Discharges [1]	Total Number of Hospital Discharges for Low Back Disorders (in 000s)								
Back Disorders	1,051	418	631	*	195	340	194	314	61.8
Disc Disorders	456	204	250	*	126	172	73	84	56.5
Back Injury	181	85	96	*	54	37	21	63	57.8
All Lumbar and Low Back Pain	1,585	665	915	14	356	516	269	428	59.8
Hospital Emergency Room Visits [2]	Total Number of Emergency Room Visits for Low Back Disorders (in 000s)								
Back Disorders	2,985	1,427	1,558	85	1,589	933	170	208	43.3
Disc Disorders	114	58	56	*	54	56	*	*	45.5
Back Injury	1,792	803	989	89	1,125	429	66	84	39.0
All Lumbar and Low Back Pain	4,646	2,156	2,490	168	2,617	1,342	232	287	42.0
Hospital Outpatient Visits [3]	Total Number of Outpatient Department Visits for Low Back Disorders (in 000s)								
Back Disorders	2,269	909	1,360	69	902	835	281	182	48.8
Disc Disorders	270	111	159	*	115	102	38	*	49.8
Back Injury	368	168	200	*	236	84	24	*	42.4
All Lumbar and Low Back Pain	2,760	1,140	1,620	74	1,179	975	329	204	48.1
Physician Office Visits [4]	Total Number of Physician Visits for Low Back Disorders (in 000s)								
Back Disorders	21,813	8,306	13,507	679	6,171	9,067	2,765	3,130	52.7
Disc Disorders	6,497	3,893	2,604	*	2,074	3,056	951	416	52.2
Back Injury	5,454	2,601	2,853	167	2,461	1,913	664	249	47.2
All Lumbar and Low Back Pain	31,540	13,752	17,788	846	9,907	12,926	4,219	3,641	51.7

Total Health Care Visits for Lumbar and Low Back Pain, 2004

	Total	Male	Female	<18	18-44	45-64	65-74	75 & over	
	Total Number of Health Care Visits for Low Back Disorders (in 000s)								
Back Disorders	28,118	11,060	17,056	833	8,857	11,175	3,410	3,834	
Disc Disorders	7,337	4,266	3,069	*	2,369	3,386	1,062	500	
Back Injury	7,795	3,657	4,138	256	3,876	2,463	775	396	
All Lumbar and Low Back Pain	40,531	17,713	22,813	1,102	14,059	15,759	5,049	4,560	
Percent of Total		44%	56%	3%	35%	39%	12%	11%	
Hospital Discharges [1]	1,585	665	915	14	356	516	269	428	59.8
Hospital Emergency Room Visits [2]	4,646	2,156	2,490	168	2,617	1,342	232	287	42.0
Hospital Outpatient Visits [3]	2,760	1,140	1,620	74	1,179	975	329	204	48.1
Physician Office Visits [4]	31,540	13,752	17,788	846	9,907	12,926	4,219	3,641	51.7
All Lumbar and Low Back Pain Diagnoses	40,531	17,713	22,813	1,102	14,059	15,759	5,049	4,560	
Percent of Total		44%	56%	3%	35%	39%	12%	11%	

* Estimate does not meet standards for reliability

[1] Source: Agency for Healthcare Research and Quality, Healthcare Cost and Utilization Project, Nationwide Inpatient Sample, 2004

[2] Source: National Center for Health Statistics, National Hospital Ambulatory Medical Care Survey, Hospital Emergency, 2004

[3] Source: National Center for Health Statistics, National Hospital Ambulatory Medical Care Survey, Outpatient, 2004

[4] Source: National Center for Health Statistics, National Ambulatory Medical Care Survey, 2004

Table 2.5a: Prevalence Rate of Lumbar and Low Back Disorders by Gender and Age, United States 2004

	Total	Male	Female	≤18	18-44	45-64	65-74	75 & over
Hospital Discharges [1]		Proportion of Hospital Discharges for Low Back Disorders						
Back Disorders	62%	59%	65%	*	52%	62%	67%	68%
Disc Disorders	27%	29%	26%	*	34%	31%	25%	18%
Back Injury	11%	12%	10%	*	14%	7%	7%	14%
All Lumbar/Low Back Pain (in 000s)	1,585	665	915	14	356	516	269	428
Hospital Emergency Room Visits [2]		Proportion of Emergency Room Visits for Low Back Disorders						
Back Disorders	61%	62%	60%	49%	57%	66%	72%	71%
Disc Disorders	2%	3%	2%	*	2%	4%	*	*
Back Injury	37%	35%	38%	51%	41%	30%	28%	29%
All Lumbar/Low Back Pain (in 000s)	4,646	2,156	2,490	168	2,617	1,342	232	287
Hospital Outpatient Visits [3]		Proportion of Hospital Outpatient Department Visits for Low Back Disorders						
Back Disorders	78%	77%	79%	100%	72%	82%	82%	100%
Disc Disorders	9%	9%	9%	*	9%	10%	11%	*
Back Injury	13%	14%	12%	*	19%	8%	7%	*
All Lumbar/Low Back Pain (in 000s)	2,760	1,140	1,620	74	1,179	975	329	204
Physician Office Visits [4]		Proportion of Physician Office Visits for Low Back Disorders						
Back Disorders	65%	56%	71%	80%	58%	65%	63%	82%
Disc Disorders	19%	26%	14%	*	19%	22%	22%	11%
Back Injury	16%	18%	15%	20%	23%	14%	15%	7%
All Lumbar/Low Back Pain (in 000s)	31,540	13,752	17,788	846	9,907	12,926	4,219	3,641
Total Health Care Visits for Lumbar and Low Back Pain, 2004		Proportion of Health Care Visits for Low Back Disorders						
Back Disorders	65%	58%	70%	76%	59%	66%	65%	81%
Disc Disorders	17%	22%	13%	*	16%	20%	20%	11%
Back Injury	18%	19%	17%	24%	26%	14%	15%	8%
All Lumbar/Low Back Pain (in 000s)	40,531	17,713	22,813	1,102	14,059	15,759	5,049	4,560

	Total Diagnoses	Low Back Disorders as % of Total	Low Back Disorders	All Medical Conditions
		% by Resource		
Hospital Discharges [1]	36,626	4.3%	3.9%	3.3%
Hospital Emergency Room Visits [2]	110,216	4.2%	11.5%	10.0%
Hospital Outpatient Visits [3]	84,994	3.2%	6.8%	7.7%
Physician Office Visits [4]	868,560	3.6%	77.8%	78.9%
All Lumbar and Low Back Pain Diagnoses (in 000s)	1,100,396	3.7%	40,531	1,100,396

* Estimate does not meet standards for reliability

[1] Source: Agency for Healthcare Research and Quality, Healthcare Cost and Utilization Project, Nationwide Inpatient Sample, 2004

[2] Source: National Center for Health Statistics, National Hospital Ambulatory Medical Care Survey, Hospital Emergency, 2004

[3] Source: National Center for Health Statistics, National Hospital Ambulatory Medical Care Survey, Outpatient, 2004

[4] Source: National Center for Health Statistics, National Ambulatory Medical Care Survey, 2004

Table 2.6: Prevalence of Neck and Cervical Spine Disorders by Gender and Age, United States 2004

		Gender			Age (in years)				Ave Age
	Total	Male	Female	≤18	18-44	45-64	65-74	75 & over	for Dx
Hospital Dischargess [1]	Total Number of Hospital Discharges for Cervical Pain Disorders (in 000s)								
Cervical Disorders	252	114	138	*	49	104	44	51	58.2
Cervical Disc Disorders	145	66	78	*	42	72	16	15	53.4
Neck Injury	73	42	30	*	30	18	*	13	47.9
All Cervical Back Pain	431	203	227	9	112	173	62	75	55.2
Hospital Emergency Room Visits [2]	Total Number of Emergency Room Visits for Cervical Pain Disorders (in 000s)								
Cervical Disorders	654	277	377	76	350	168	*	*	39.0
Cervical Disc Disorders	*	*	*	*	*	*	*	*	*
Neck Injury	1,490	657	833	212	919	267	63	29	33.0
All Cervical Back Pain	2,127	927	1,200	276	1,265	430	104	52	35.0
Hospital Outpatient Visits [3]	Total Number of Outpatient Department Visits for Cervical Pain Disorders (in 000s)								
Cervical Disorders	523	234	289	21	225	207	54	*	45.1
Cervical Disc Disorders	120	47	72	*	38	72	*	*	51.3
Neck Injury	137	60	77	20	62	24	*	*	46.5
All Cervical Back Pain	763	330	433	42	321	297	66	36	46.0
Physician Office Visits [4]	Total Number of Physician Visits for Cervical Pain Disorders (in 000s)								
Cervical Disorders	8,638	3,235	5,403	437	2,481	4,571	842	307	49.5
Cervical Disc Disorders	1,690	727	962	*	581	957	115	38	50.2
Neck Injury	3,445	1,653	1,792	204	1,543	1,136	422	140	45.5
All Cervical Back Pain	13,104	5,293	7,811	641	4,475	6,249	1,274	466	48.4

Total Health Care Visits for Lumbar and Low Back Pain, 2004

	Total	Male	Female	≤18	18-44	45-64	65-74	75 & over	for Dx
	Total Number of Health Care Visits for Cervical Pain Disorders (in 000s)								
Cervical Disorders	10,067	3,860	6,207	534	3,105	5,050	940	358	
Cervical Disc Disorders	1,955	840	1,112	*	661	1,101	131	53	
Neck Injury	5,145	2,412	2,732	436	2,554	1,445	485	182	
All Cervical (Neck) Back Pain	16,425	6,753	9,671	968	6,173	7,149	1,506	629	
Percent of Total		41%	59%	6%	38%	44%	9%	4%	
Hospital Discharges [1]	431	203	227	9	112	173	62	75	55.2
Hospital Emergency Room Visits [2]	2,127	927	1,200	276	1,265	430	104	52	35.0
Hospital Outpatient Visits [3]	763	330	433	42	321	297	66	36	46.0
Physician Office Visits [4]	13,104	5,293	7,811	641	4,475	6,249	1,274	466	48.4
All Cervical (Neck) Back Pain Diagnoses	16,425	6,753	9,671	968	6,173	7,149	1,506	629	
Percent of Total		41%	59%	6%	38%	44%	9%	4%	

* Estimate does not meet standards for reliability

[1] Source: Agency for Healthcare Research and Quality, Healthcare Cost and Utilization Project, Nationwide Inpatient Sample, 2004

[2] Source: National Center for Health Statistics, National Hospital Ambulatory Medical Care Survey, Hospital Emergency, 2004

[3] Source: National Center for Health Statistics, National Hospital Ambulatory Medical Care Survey, Outpatient, 2004

[4] Source: National Center for Health Statistics, National Ambulatory Medical Care Survey, 2004

Table 2.6a: Prevalence Rate of Neck and Cervical Spine Disorders by Gender and Age, United States 2004

	Total	Male	Female	≤18	18-44	45-64	65-74	75 & over
Hospital Discharges [1]	Proportion of Hospital Discharges for Cervical Pain Disorders							
Cervical Disorders	54%	51%	56%	*	40%	54%	73%	65%
Cervical Disc Disorders	31%	30%	32%	*	35%	37%	27%	19%
Neck Injury	16%	19%	12%	*	25%	9%	*	16%
All Cervical Back Pain	431	203	227	9	112	173	62	75
Hospital Emergency Room Visits [2]	Proportion of Emergency Room Visits for Cervical Pain Disorders							
Cervical Disorders	31%	30%	31%	26%	28%	39%	*	*
Cervical Disc Disorders	*	*	*	*	*	*	*	*
Neck Injury	69%	70%	69%	74%	72%	61%	100%	100%
All Cervical Back Pain	2,127	927	1,200	276	1,265	430	104	52
Hospital Outpatient Visits [3]	Proportion of Outpatient Department Visits for Cervical Pain Disorders							
Cervical Disorders	67%	69%	66%	51%	69%	68%	100%	*
Cervical Disc Disorders	15%	14%	16%	*	12%	24%	*	*
Neck Injury	18%	18%	18%	*	19%	8%	*	*
All Cervical Back Pain	763	330	433	42	321	297	66	36
Physician Office Visits [4]	Proportion of Physician Visits for Cervical Pain Disorders							
Cervical Disorders	63%	58%	66%	68%	54%	69%	61%	63%
Cervical Disc Disorders	12%	13%	12%	*	13%	14%	8%	8%
Neck Injury	25%	29%	22%	32%	34%	17%	31%	29%
All Cervical Back Pain	13,104	5,293	7,811	641	4,475	6,249	1,274	466

Total Health Care Visits for Lumbar and Low Back Pain, 2004

	Total	Male	Female	≤18	18-44	45-64	65-74	75 & over
	Proportion of Health Care Visits for Cervical Pain Disorders							
Cervical Disorders	59%	54%	62%	55%	49%	66%	60%	60%
Cervical Disc Disorders	11%	12%	11%	*	10%	14%	8%	9%
Neck Injury	30%	34%	27%	45%	40%	19%	31%	31%
All Cervical (Neck) Back Pain	16,425	6,753	9,671	968	6,173	7,149	1,506	629

	Total Diagnoses	Cervical Disorders as % of Total	Cervical Disorders	All Medical Conditions
			% by Resource	
Hospital Discharges [1]	36,626	1.2%	2.6%	3.3%
Hospital Emergency Room Visits [2]	110,216	1.9%	12.9%	10.0%
Hospital Outpatient Visits [3]	84,994	0.9%	4.6%	7.7%
Physician Office Visits [4]	868,560	1.5%	79.8%	78.9%
All Cervical (Neck) Back Pain Diagnoses	1,100,396	1.5%	16,425	1,100,396

* Estimate does not meet standards for reliability

[1] Source: Agency for Healthcare Research and Quality, Healthcare Cost and Utilization Project, Nationwide Inpatient Sample, 2004

[2] Source: National Center for Health Statistics, National Hospital Ambulatory Medical Care Survey, Hospital Emergency, 2004

[3] Source: National Center for Health Statistics, National Hospital Ambulatory Medical Care Survey, Outpatient, 2004

[4] Source: National Center for Health Statistics, National Ambulatory Medical Care Survey, 2004

Table 2.7: Summary of Resource Allocation of Total Health Care Occurrences for Back Pain and Related Conditions by Gender and Age, United States 2004

	Total	Male	Female	<18	18-44	45-64	65-74	75 & over	Ave Age at DX	All Conditions (in 000s)	Spine as % of All Diagnoses
Lumbar (Low) Back Pain	**Total Number of Lumbar/Low Back Diagnoses** (in 000s)										
Hospital Discharges [1]	1,585	665	915	*	356	516	269	428	59.8	36,626	4.3%
Hospital Emergency Room Visits [2]	4,646	2,156	2,490	168	2,617	1,342	232	287	42.0	110,216	4.2%
Hospital Outpatient Visits [3]	2,760	1,140	1,620	74	1,179	975	329	204	48.1	84,994	3.2%
Physician Office Visits [4]	31,540	13,752	17,788	846	9,907	12,926	4,219	3,641	51.7	868,560	3.6%
All Lumbar and Low Back Pain Diagnoses	40,531	17,713	22,813	1,088	14,059	15,759	5,049	4,560		1,100,396	3.7%
Percent of Total		44%	56%	3%	35%	39%	12%	11%			
Cervical Back Pain (Neck)	**Total Number of Cervical/Neck Diagnoses** (in 000s)										
Hospital Discharges [1]	431	203	227	*	112	173	62	75	55.2	36,626	1.2%
Hospital Emergency Room Visits [2]	2,127	927	1,200	276	1,265	430	104	52	35.0	110,216	1.9%
Hospital Outpatient Visits [3]	763	330	433	42	321	297	66	36	46.0	84,994	0.9%
Physician Office Visits [4]	13,104	5,293	7,811	641	4,475	6,249	1,274	466	48.4	868,560	1.5%
All Cervical (Neck) Back Pain Diagnoses	16,425	6,753	9,671	959	6,173	7,149	1,506	629		1,100,396	1.5%
Percent of Total		41%	59%	6%	38%	44%	9%	4%			
Total Back Pain (Lumbar and Cervical) Diagnoses [5]	**Total Number of Spinal Diagnoses** (in 000s)										
Hospital Discharges [1]	1,937	833	1,099	22	447	659	319	488	58.9	36,626	5.3%
Hospital Emergency Room Visits [2]	6,314	2,873	3,441	393	3,595	1,667	323	336	40.2	110,216	5.7%
Hospital Outpatient Visits [3]	3,332	1,380	1,953	114	1,396	1,209	374	239	47.9	84,994	3.9%
Physician Office Visits [4]	41,444	17,883	23,562	1,339	13,345	17,576	5,161	4,023	50.9	868,560	4.8%
All Back Pain Diagnoses	53,027	22,969	30,055	1,868	18,783	21,111	6,177	5,086		1,100,396	4.8%
Percent of Total		43%	57%	4%	35%	40%	12%	10%			

* Estimate does not meet standards for reliability

[1] Source: Agency for Healthcare Research and Quality, Healthcare Cost and Utilization Project, Nationwide Inpatient Sample, 2004

[2] Source: National Center for Health Statistics, National Hospital Ambulatory Medical Care Survey, Hospital Emergency, 2004

[3] Source: National Center for Health Statistics, National Hospital Ambulatory Medical Care Survey, Outpatient, 2004

[4] Source: National Center for Health Statistics, National Ambulatory Medical Care Survey, 2004

[5] Diagnosis with both lumbar and cervical pain possible.

Table 2.7a: Summary of Resource Allocation as a Proportion of Total Health Care Occurrences for Back Pain and Related Conditions by Gender and Age, United States 2004

		Gender		Age (in years)					Ave Age at DX	Spine as % of All Diagnoses
	Total	Male	Female	<18	18-44	45-64	65-74	75 & over		
Lumbar (Low) Back Pain		**Proportion of Total Lumbar/Low Back Diagnoses**								
Hospital Discharges [1]	3.9%	3.8%	4.0%	*	2.5%	3.3%	5.3%	9.4%	59.8	4.3%
Hospital Emergency Room Visits [2]	11.5%	12.2%	10.9%	15.4%	18.6%	8.5%	4.6%	6.3%	42.0	4.2%
Hospital Outpatient Visits [3]	6.8%	6.4%	7.1%	6.8%	8.4%	6.2%	6.5%	4.5%	48.1	3.2%
Physician Office Visits [4]	77.8%	77.6%	78.0%	77.8%	70.4%	82.0%	83.6%	79.8%	51.7	3.6%
All Lumbar and Low Back Pain Diagnoses	40,531	17,713	22,813	1,088	14,059	15,759	5,049	4,560		3.7%
Percent of Total		44%	56%	3%	35%	39%	12%	11%		
Cervical Back Pain (Neck)		**Proportion of Total Cervical/Neck Diagnoses**								
Hospital Discharges [1]	2.6%	3.0%	2.3%	*	1.8%	2.4%	4.1%	11.9%	55.2	1.2%
Hospital Emergency Room Visits [2]	12.9%	13.7%	12.4%	28.8%	20.5%	6.0%	6.9%	8.3%	35.0	1.9%
Hospital Outpatient Visits [3]	4.6%	4.9%	4.5%	4.4%	5.2%	4.2%	4.4%	5.7%	46.0	0.9%
Physician Office Visits [4]	79.8%	78.4%	80.8%	66.8%	72.5%	87.4%	84.6%	74.1%	48.4	1.5%
All Cervical (Neck) Back Pain Diagnoses	16,425	6,753	9,671	959	6,173	7,149	1,506	629		1.5%
Percent of Total		41%	59%	6%	38%	44%	9%	4%		
Total Back Pain (Lumbar and Cervical) Diagnoses [5]		**Proportion of Total Spinal Diagnoses**								
Hospital Discharges [1]	3.7%	3.6%	3.7%	1.2%	2.4%	3.1%	5.2%	9.6%	58.9	5.3%
Hospital Emergency Room Visits [2]	11.9%	12.5%	11.4%	21.0%	19.1%	7.9%	5.2%	6.6%	40.2	5.7%
Hospital Outpatient Visits [3]	6.3%	6.0%	6.5%	6.1%	7.4%	5.7%	6.1%	4.7%	47.9	3.9%
Physician Office Visits [4]	78.2%	77.9%	78.4%	71.7%	71.0%	83.3%	83.6%	79.1%	50.9	4.8%
All Back Pain Diagnoses	53,027	22,969	30,055	1,868	18,783	21,111	6,177	5,086		4.8%
Percent of Total		43%	57%	4%	35%	40%	12%	10%		

* Estimate does not meet standards for reliability

[1] Source: Agency for Healthcare Research and Quality, Healthcare Cost and Utilization Project, Nationwide Inpatient Sample, 2004

[2] Source: National Center for Health Statistics, National Hospital Ambulatory Medical Care Survey, Hospital Emergency, 2004

[3] Source: National Center for Health Statistics, National Hospital Ambulatory Medical Care Survey, Outpatient, 2004

[4] Source: National Center for Health Statistics, National Ambulatory Medical Care Survey, 2004

[5] Diagnosis with both lumbar and cervical pain possible.

Table 2.8: Average Length of Hospital Stay (LOS) for Lumbar Spine Diagnosis, United States 2004

	Average LOS (in days)	
	NIS [1]	NHDS [2]
Spinal Deformity & Related Conditions	5.5	5.1
Back Pain (Lumbar and Low Back)		
Back Disorders	4.7	4.3
Disc Disorders	4.1	3.6
Back Injury	7.3	7.9
All Lumbar and Low Back Pain	4.8	4.5
Cervical Back Pain (Neck)		
Neck Disorders	4.3	3.6
Cervical Disc Disorders	3.1	2.8
Neck Injury	8.2	10.2
All Cervical Back Pain	4.7	4.6
Total	4.8	4.6

[1] Source: Agency for Healthcare Research and Quality, Healthcare Cost and Utilization Project, Nationwide Inpatient Sample, 2004

[2] Source: National Center for Health Statistics, National Hospital Discharge Survey, 2004

Table 2.9: Trends in Physician Visits for Back Pain, United States 1998-2004

Physician Visits for Back Pain

Total Number of Patients (in 000s)

	1998	1999	2000	2001	2002	2003	2004
Physician Visits for Back Pain (Lumbar and Low Back)							
Back Disorders	15,885	14,787	16,151	21,195	20,040	22,446	21,813
Disc Disorders	3,004	4,563	3,728	5,318	4,997	4,095	6,497
Back Injury	5,252	8,027	6,835	5,152	7,351	5,728	5,454
Total, Back Pain	23,037	25,499	25,019	29,917	29,146	31,028	31,540
Physician Visits for Cervical Back Pain (Neck)							
Neck Disorders	4,337	5,430	4,8074	5,161	6,692	5,868	8,638
Disk Disorders	568	1,917	868	1,646	1,266	1,933	1,690
Neck Injury	4,324	3,804	2,936	3,223	4,777	3,306	3,445
Total, Cervical Back Pain	8,922	10,342	8,266	9,554	11,727	10,720	13,104
Physician Visits for Back Pain (Lumbar and Cervical)							
Total Visits	31,959	35,842	33,285	39,4714	40,872	41,748	44,644

Physician Visits for Back Pain as Proportion of Total Population

Proportion of Total U.S. Population [1]

	1998	1999	2000	2001	2002	2003	2004
Physician Visits for Back Pain (Lumbar and Low Back)							
Back Disorders	5.9%	5.4%	5.7%	7.4%	6.9%	7.6%	7.4%
Disc Disorders	1.1%	1.7%	1.3%	1.8%	1.7%	1.4%	2.2%
Back Injury	1.9%	2.9%	2.4%	1.8%	2.5%	2.0%	1.8%
Total, Back Pain	8.5%	9.4%	8.8%	10.4%	10.0%	10.6%	10.6%
Physician Visits for Cervical Back Pain (Neck)							
Cervical Disorders	1.6%	2.0%	1.7%	1.8%	2.3%	2.0%	2.9%
Disk Disorders	0.2%	0.7%	0.3%	0.6%	0.4%	0.7%	0.6%
Neck Injury	1.6%	1.4%	1.0%	1.1%	1.6%	1.1%	1.2%
Total, Cervical Back Pain	3.3%	3.8%	2.9%	3.3%	4.0%	3.7%	4.4%
Physician Visits for Back Pain (Lumbar and Cervical)							
Total Visits	11.8%	13.1%	11.7%	13.7%	14.0%	14.2%	15.1%

[1] Proportion of total population based on U.S. Census Population Estimates as of July 1 for each year.

Source: National Center for Health Statistics, National Ambulatory Medical Care Survey,1998- 2004

Table 2.10: Work Limitations with Reported Joint or Back Pain for Persons Aged 18 and Over, United States 1999-2004

| | % Reporting Site Pain | | |
| | Pain Limits All Work (11% of population) | Pain Limits Amount of Work (32% of population) | Pain Limits Ability to Walk (8% of population) |
Pain Site Reported			
Low back Pain	63%	62%	62%
Neck Pain	41%	40%	38%
Headaches	37%	35%	28%
Lower Limb (Leg, Foot)	28%	28%	37%
Upper limb (Shoulder, Girdle, Arm, Hand)	26%	26%	26%
Head	16%	15%	12%
Torso (Sternum, Chest, Abdomen)	9%	8%	7%

Source: National Center for Health Statistics. National Health and Nutrition Examination Survey Data, 1999-2004.

Table 2.11: Limitation in Work Due to Back Pain by Gender and Age for Persons Age 18 and Over, United States 1999-2004

| | | Proportion of Persons Reporting Work Limitations | | | | | | | |
| | | Pain Keeps from Working [1] | | | | Back Pain Limits Amount of Work Can Do [2] | | | |
Status of Back Pain		With Back Pain in One Site [3]	With Back Pain in Multiple Sites [4]	No Back Pain Reported	All Pain Sites	With Back Pain in One Site [3]	With Back Pain in Multiple Sites [4]	No Back Pain Reported	All Pain Sites
Gender	Male	18%	33%	8%	10%	51%	69%	25%	31%
	Female	21%	33%	8%	11%	51%	75%	31%	34%
Age	18-44 years	13%	23%	4%	6%	39%	57%	14%	20%
	45-64 years	24%	43%	10%	14%	55%	84%	29%	40%
	65-74 years	30%	41%	11%	15%	74%	87%	39%	46%
	75 & over	29%	31%	16%	18%	70%	82%	53%	56%
Total		20%	33%	8%	11%	51%	72%	25%	32%

[1] 11% of the population reports a long-term physical, mental or emotional problem keeps them from working.

[2] 32% of the population reports a long-term physical, mental or emotional problem limits the kind or amount of work they can do.

[3] "With respect to pain problem, located in …Low back pain, upper back pain, buttocks, neck and spine?"

[4] "With respect to pain problem, located in …multiple sites of back"

Source: National Center for Health Statistics. National Health and Nutrition Examination Survey Data, 1999-2004.

Table 2.12: Bed and Lost Work Days Associated with Back Pain, United States 2005

	Incidence of Reported Condition (in 000s)	Incidence of Bed Days (in 000s)	Average Number of Bed Days	Total Bed Days (in 000s)	Incidence of Lost Work Days (in 000s)	Average Number of Work Days Lost	Total Lost Work Days (in 000s)
Back/Neck Problem Causes Difficulty with Activity							
Male	8,542	4,118	14.4	59,299	2,823	11.9	33,594
Female	11,268	6,514	17.6	114,646	3,537	13.8	48,811
Total	19,810	10,632	16.2	172,238	6,360	12.9	82,044
Neck Pain in Past 3 Months							
Male	13,022	5,998	11.1	66,578	4,774	6.8	32,463
Female	19,271	10,107	14.8	149,584	7,031	9.1	63,982
Total	32,294	16,105	13.3	214,197	11,805	8.1	95,621
Low Back Pain in Past 3 Months							
Male	27,502	11,357	8.1	91,992	9,844	6.3	62,017
Female	34,463	17,609	12.0	211,308	11,813	8.3	98,048
Total	61,965	28,966	10.2	295,453	21,657	7.3	158,096
Radiating Leg Pain (with Low Back Pain)							
Male	8,480	4,172	17.0	70,924	2,623	12.3	32,263
Female	11,865	6,902	21.9	151,154	3,608	13.5	48,708
Total	20,346	11,074	19.9	220,373	6,230	12.9	80,367
All Spine Pain or Problems							
Male	72,361	13,070	7.5	98,025	11,532	6.2	71,498
Female	71,810	20,644	10.8	222,955	14,394	8.1	116,591
Total	144,171	33,714	9.3	313,540	25,927	7.2	186,674

Source: National Center for Health Statistics, National Health Interview Survey, 2005

Table 2.13: Select Spine Procedures as a Proportion of All Spine Procedures and Spine Patients, United States 2004

Procedure	All Spine Procedures [1]		
	Number	% of Total Spine Procedures	% of Total Spine Patients
Spinal diskectomy	325,332	34.1%	56.8%
Spinal fusion	307,878	32.3%	53.7%
Spinal decompression	160,169	16.8%	27.9%
Spinal refusion	18,935	2.0%	3.3%
Kyphoplasty	6,221	0.7%	1.1%
Vertebroplasty	3,344	0.4%	0.6%
Other procedure	131,411	13.8%	22.9%
All spine procedures	953,290	100.0%	166.3%
Total spine procedure patients	573,170		

[1] Multiple procedures performed on some patients

Source: Agency for Healthcare Research and Quality, Healthcare Cost and Utilization Project, Nationwide Inpatient Sample, 2004

Table 2.14: Seven-Year Trend in Spinal Fusion Procedures, United States 1998-2004

ICD-9-CM	Description	Year	Number of Patients	Rate of Year-to-Year Increase in Patients	Number of Procedures [1]	Rate of Year-to-Year Increase in Procedures	Mean Age of Patient	Mean Length of Stay	Mean Hospitalization Charge [2]	Rate of Year-to-Year Increase in Mean Charge	Total Hospitalization Charges (in billions)	Rate of Year-to-Year Increase in Total Hospital Charges
		1998	204,000		220,000		49.0	4.7	$26,000		$5.35	
		1999	224,000	10%	243,000	11%	48.7	4.6	$29,000	10%	$6.34	19%
		2000	242,000	8%	263,000	8%	49.4	4.3	$32,000	10%	$7.18	13%
81.00-81.08	Spinal Fusion	2001	277,000	14%	305,000	16%	49.4	4.3	$35,000	10%	$9.66	35%
		2002	289,000	5%	323,000	6%	50.2	4.4	$42,000	17%	$11.87	23%
		2003	310,000	7%	350,000	8%	51.3	4.3	$50,000	21%	$15.35	29%
		2004	307,000	-1%	307,000	-12%	51.8	4.5	$56,000	11%	$16.87	10%
	7-Year Change			50%		40%				111%		215%
		1998	12,000		12,000		47.1	4.6	$26,000		$0.30	
		1999	14,000	23%	15,000	28%	48.6	4.9	$34,000	31%	$0.48	60%
		2000	13,000	-9%	13,000	-12%	49.0	5.4	$39,000	13%	$0.47	-2%
81.30-81.393	Spinal Refusion [3]	2001	11,000	-14%	12,000	-11%	50.2	4.3	$40,000	4%	$0.45	-4%
		2002	19,000	66%	20,000	71%	50.0	4.4	$46,000	14%	$0.86	91%
		2003	17,000	-8%	19,000	-8%	51.0	4.4	$55,000	19%	$0.93	8%
		2004	19,000	10%	19,000	2%	52.7	4.8	$63,000	16%	$1.18	26%
	7-Year Change			62%		61%				145%		292%
		1998	214,000		231,000		48.9	4.7	$26,000		$5.59	
		1999	236,000	10%	258,000	11%	48.6	4.6	$29,000	11%	$6.71	20%
		2000	253,000	7%	277,000	7%	49.4	4.3	$32,000	10%	$7.53	12%
81.00-81.08 + 81.30-81.393	Total	2001	285,000	13%	317,000	15%	49.5	4.3	$35,000	10%	$9.97	32%
		2002	304,000	7%	343,000	8%	50.2	4.3	$42,000	17%	$12.50	25%
		2003	324,000	6%	369,000	7%	51.3	4.2	$50,000	21%	$16.01	28%
		2004	321,000	-1%	327,000	-11%	51.8	4.5	$56,000	11%	$17.87	12%
	7-Year Change			50%		41%				112%		220%

[1] Up to 15 diagnosis per patient were included multiple spine procedures per patient can be coded

[2] "Charge" refers to hospitalization charges and does not include professional (i.e., physician fees), drugs or non-covered charges

[3] Prior to 2002, spinal refusion procedures were coded to the single code, 81.09. In 2002, this code was dropped and multiple codes implemented.

Source: Agency for Healthcare Research and Quality, Healthcare Cost and Utilization Project, Nationwide Inpatient Sample, 1998-2004

Table 2.15: Distribution of Spine Fusion Procedures by Spine Section, United States 2004

		Spine Fusion Procedures [1]		
	Number	% of Total Spine Fusion Procedures	% of Total Spine Fusion Patients	% of Total Spine Patients
Cervical Fusion	134,761	41.2%	44.3%	6.6%
Thoracic or Dorsal Fusion	23,601	7.2%	7.8%	1.2%
Lumbar Fusion	149,516	45.7%	49.2%	7.3%
Spine Refusion Procedures	18,935	5.8%	6.2%	0.9%
Total Spinal Fusion or Refusion Procedures	326,813	100.0%	107.5%	16.1%
Total Spine Fusion Patients	303,904			
All Spine Diagnosed Patients	2,036,165			

[1] Multiple procedures performed on some patients

Source: Agency for Healthcare Research and Quality, Healthcare Cost and Utilization Project, Nationwide Inpatient Sample, 2004

Table 2.16: Proportion of Back Pain Diagnoses with Spinal Fusion Procedure by Gender and Age, United States 2004

	Total Number of Spinal Diagnoses (in 000s)								Average Age for Fusion	Mean Length of Stay (in days)	Mean Charges
		Gender			Age (in Years)						
	Total	Male	Female	≤18	18-44	45-64	65-74	75 & over			
Lumbar/Low Back Pain											
All Lumbar/Low Back Pain Diagnoses	1,585	665	915	14	356	516	269	428	59.8		
Total Lumbar Spinal Fusion Procedures	150	66	84	*	39	65	27	16	54.3	4.7	$ 63,520
% Diagnoses with Spinal Fusion Procedure	9.5%	9.9%	9.2%	*	11.0%	12.6%	10.0%	3.7%			
Cervical/Neck Pain											
All Cervical (Neck) Back Pain Diagnoses	431	203	227	9	112	173	62	75	55.2		
Total Cervical Spinal Fusion Procedures	135	66	68	*	41	71	15	7	51.2	3.5	$ 39,300
% Diagnoses with Spinal Fusion Procedure	31.3%	32.5%	30.0%	*	36.6%	41.0%	24.2%	9.3%			
All Back Pain											
All Back Pain Diagnoses	1,937	833	1,099	22	447	659	319	488	58.9		
Total Spinal Fusion Procedures	321	141	163	*	86	140	44	24	51.8	4.4	$ 54,020
% Diagnoses with Spinal Fusion Procedure	16.6%	16.9%	14.8%	*	19.2%	21.2%	13.8%	4.9%			

* Estimate does not meet standards for reliability

Source: Agency for Healthcare Research and Quality, Healthcare Cost and Utilization Project, Nationwide Inpatient Sample, 2004

Table 2.17: Primary (1st) Diagnosis for Spinal Fusion Procedures, United States 2004

Diagnosis	Number of Diagnoses	% of Total Spinal Fusion Procedures
Cervical Disc Displacement	49,667	19.4%
Lumbar Disc Degeneration	33,396	13.1%
Lumbar Disc Displacement	28,398	11.1%
Lumbar Spinal Stenosis	23,499	9.2%
Cervical Spondylosis	20,375	8.0%
Cervical Spondylosis with Myelopathy	16,841	6.6%
Lumbosacral Spondylosis	14,623	5.7%
Cervical Disc Displacement with Myelopathy	12,914	5.0%
Cervical Spinal Stenosis	8,496	3.3%
Cervical Disc Degeneration	7,756	3.0%
Idiopathic Scoliosis	6,724	2.6%
FX Lumbar Vertebra-Closed	3,204	1.3%
Lumbar Postlaminectomy Syndrome	2,325	0.9%
Scoliosis NEC	2,104	0.8%
All Other Diagnoses	25,595	10.0%
All Spine 1st Diagnoses	255,907	100.0%

Source: Agency for Healthcare Research and Quality, Healthcare Cost and Utilization Project, Nationwide Inpatient Sample, 2004

Table 2.18: Health Care Visits for Ruptured Spine and Spinal Diskectomy Procedures, United States 2004

Total Number of Spinal Diagnosis (in 000s)

Health Care Visits for Ruptured (Herniated) Spine Diagnosis [1]	Total	Gender		Age (in years)				75 & over	Average Age	% of Total Visits
		Male	Female	<18	18-44	45-64	65-74			
Hospital Discharges [2]	347.5	170.4	175.1	0.8	126.8	145.5	42.4	31.2	51.4	7.0%
Hospital Emergency Department Visits [3]	113.6	53.9	59.7	0.0	66.5	38.9	8.3	0.0	42.0	2.3%
Hospital Outpatient Visits [4]	198.9	69.1	129.8	0.0	78.7	96.7	19.9	3.6	48.7	4.0%
Physician Office Visits [5]	4,338.6	2,484.3	1,854.3	0.0	1,226.2	2,356.2	674.6	81.5	50.0	86.8%
All Ruptured Spine Diagnoses	4,998.6	2,777.7	2,218.9	0.8	1,498.2	2,637.3	745.2	116.3		100.0%
Percent of Total		55.6%	44.4%	0.0%	30.0%	52.8%	14.9%	2.3%		

Spinal Diskectomy Procedure [6]	Total	Male	Female	<18	18-44	45-64	65-74	75 & over	Average Age	Mean Length of Stay (in days)	Mean Charges
Hospital Discharges [2]	325.3	163.2	159.8	1.90	112.9	148.6	40.3	20.7	50.8	2.9	$ 34,580
Physician Office Visits [5]*	164.1	*	*	*	*	*	*	*	*	NA	NA
Diskectomy Procedures		163.2	159.8	1.9	112.9	148.6	40.3	20.7			
Percent of Total		50.5%	49.5%	0.6%	34.8%	45.8%	12.4%	6.4%			
Proportion of Inpatient [1] Diskectomy Procedures with Ruptured Spine Diagnosis	66%	70%	62%	67%	71%	69%	58%	40%			

* Estimate does not meet standards for reliability

[1] ICD-9-CM diagnosis codes: 722.00, 722.10, 722.11, 722.20, 722.70, 722.71, 722.72, 722.73

[2] Source: Agency for Healthcare Research and Quality, Healthcare Cost and Utilization Project, Nationwide Inpatient Sample, 2004

[3] Source: National Center for Health Statistics, National Hospital Ambulatory Medical Care Survey, Hospital Emergency, 2004

[4] Source: National Center for Health Statistics, National Hospital Ambulatory Medical Care Survey, Outpatient, 2004

[5] Source: National Center for Health Statistics, National Ambulatory Medical Care Survey, 2004

[6] ICD-9-CM procedure codes: 805.00, 805.10

Table 2.19: First Diagnosis for Spine Diskectomy Procedures, United States 2004

Diagnosis		Diskectomy Procedures (in 000s)	
		Number	% of Total
722.10	Displacement of lumbar intervertebral disc without myelopathy	135.5	41.7%
722.00	Displacement of cervical intervertebral disc without myelopat	49.9	15.3%
722.52	Degeneration of lumbar intervertebral disc	22.4	6.9%
721.00	Cervical spondylosis without myelopathy	17.8	5.5%
724.02	Spinal stenosis: lumbar region	13.2	4.1%
721.10	Cervical spondylosis with myelopathy	11.9	3.7%
722.71	Intervertebral disc disorder with myelopathy: cervical	11.5	3.5%
721.30	Lumbosacral spondylosis without myelopathy	7.6	2.3%
738.40	Acquired spondylolisthesis	7.5	2.3%
722.40	Degeneration of cervical intervertebral disc	7.1	2.2%
723.00	Spinal stenosis of cervical region	6.5	2.0%
722.73	Intervertebral disc disorder with myelopathy: lumbar	4.3	1.3%
	All Other diagnoses	30.2	9.3%
All Primary 1st Diagnoses		325.2	100.0%

Source: Agency for Healthcare Research and Quality, Healthcare Cost and Utilization Project, Nationwide Inpatient Sample, 2004

Table 2.20: Diskectomy Procedure Trends, United States 1996-2005

Year	1996	1997	1998	1999	2000	2001	2002	2003	2004	2005	10-Year Mean
Procedures [1] (to nearest 000)	285,000	281,000	303,000	303,000	279,000	289,000	319,000	317,000	324,000	292,000	299,000

[1] ICD-9-CM Procedure Codes: 501.00

Source: National Center for Health Statistics Centers for Disease Control and Prevention, National Hospital Discharge Survey, 1996-2005. Data extracted and analyzed by AAOS Dept. of Research and Scientific Affairs.

Chapter 3

Spinal Deformity and Related Conditions

The term spinal deformity includes several conditions in which the spine is abnormally curved or aligned. One of the more frequent spinal deformities is scoliosis, or a side to side abnormal curvature of the spine. Spinal deformity and scoliosis can be found at birth due to genetic causes, develop during childhood, or develop late in life due to degenerative disc and joint disease.

Common signs of scoliosis are a prominent shoulder, shoulder blade, or chest wall asymmetry. Another sign is uneven hips with one hip seemingly higher than the other. (Figure 3.0.1) It is important not to confuse scoliosis with poor

degree to which the condition manifests initially in pain or disability. Estimated prevalence of spinal deformity conditions has been cited in numerous studies. (Table 3.1)

Section 3.1: Scoliosis and Spinal Deformity in Children

There are several different types of scoliosis. The most common type of scoliosis is idiopathic, meaning the cause of the curve is unknown. Approximately 80 to 85% of scoliosis cases are idiopathic.[1] Idiopathic scoliosis can initially occur

Figure 3.0.1: Scoliosis

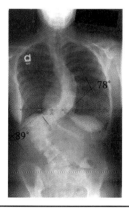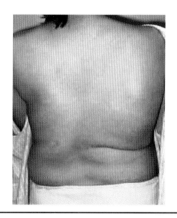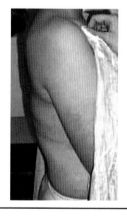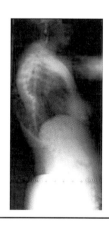

posture and to realize that scoliosis will usually not disappear with age. Other deformities include kyphosis, an exaggerated rounding of the back that may occur by itself or in conjunction with osteoporosis, and spondylolisthesis, a slippage of one vertebra onto its neighboring vertebra. A variety of other spinal deformity conditions will be discussed in this chapter including spondylolysis and Scheuermann kyphosis.

In spite of the severity of these conditions and the impact they have on the lives of children and adults, the prevalence of spinal deformities in children under the age of 18 is difficult to determine due to relatively low numbers and the

as early as the first 3 years of life (infantile idiopathic scoliosis), from 4 to 10 years of age (juvenile idiopathic scoliosis), or from 10 years of age to skeletal maturity (adolescent idiopathic scoliosis). Adolescent idiopathic scoliosis is the most common type.

Scoliosis, if severe enough (>25°), is usually treated with bracing if the child is growing or with surgery if the curvature is more severe (>45°-50°). The standard radiographic/x-ray measurement technique for all forms of scoliosis is the Cobb angle measurement technique (Figure 3.1.1), measured from the end-plates of the maximally tilted end vertebral bodies in a

The Burden of Musculoskeletal Diseases in the United States - Copyright © 2008

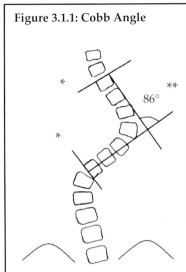

Figure 3.1.1: Cobb Angle

86°

*Both lines are drawn along the end of the vertebrae that are most tilted from the horizontal.
**The Cobb angle is the angle formed by the intersection of these two lines.

standing radiograph.[2] Whether the curve is >25° or >40°-45°, the treatment is preventative in nature, helping to avoid progression of the curve and more significant future problems if left untreated. While this preventative aspect is hugely valuable and intuitively important, its benefit is difficult to measure from a public health standpoint, especially for rare conditions of childhood, such as juvenile and adolescent pediatric scoliosis.

Section 3.1.1: Adolescent Idiopathic Scoliosis

According to the Scoliosis Research Society (SRS), idiopathic scoliosis is diagnosed when a patient has asymmetry on forward bending combined with a curve of at least 10°.[3] By this definition, the prevalence of adolescent idiopathic scoliosis in children from 10 to 16 years of age is 2%-3%. (Table 3.2 and Graph 3.1.1) Though the male-to-female ratio for smaller curves is about equal, larger curves seem to be more common in females. Similar results were found in a study

conducted in 1985, where 29,195 children were screened for idiopathic scoliosis.[4]

Several studies have investigated the natural history and natural course of curve progression in adolescent idiopathic scoliosis. All report the strongest predictive factors in the development of idiopathic scoliosis are age, magnitude of curve, and gender.[5-9] Girls are more likely to have adolescent idiopathic scoliosis than boys, and some studies report the onset is earlier in girls than boys. A factor highly correlated with curve progression is age at diagnosis; patients diagnosed at a younger age have a greater risk of curve progression. It should be noted, however, that those diagnosed at a younger age seem to have a more favorable response to milder forms

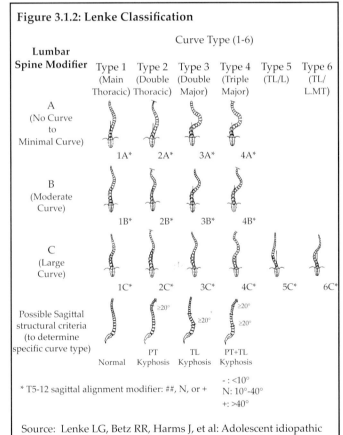

Figure 3.1.2: Lenke Classification

Source: Lenke LG, Betz RR, Harms J, et al: Adolescent idiopathic scoliosis: A new classification to determine extent of spinal arthrodesis. *J Bone Joint Surg Am* 2001;83(8):1169-81.

of treatment, supporting school screening to detect and lead to earlier diagnosis for those children with a smaller degree of curvature.

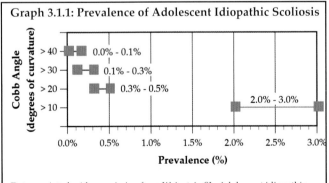

Graph 3.1.1: Prevalence of Adolescent Idiopathic Scoliosis

Data reprinted with permission from Weinstein SL. Adolescent idiopathic scoliosis: Prevalence and natural history. *Instr Course Lect* 1988;38:115–126.

Within the past several years, a two-dimensional classification system, the Lenke classification system, was developed to assess the type of a curve for adolescent idiopathic scoliosis. (Figure 3.1.2)

The three components included in this system include curve type, lumbar spine modifier, and sagittal thoracic modifier.[10] A study conducted in 2001 evaluated the prevalence of six curve types in 606 adolescent patients diagnosed with idiopathic scoliosis. Approximately one-half (51%) of the patients were found to have a Type 1, or main thoracic, curve.

Treatment decisions for individuals with adolescent idiopathic scoliosis are made based on location, shape, pattern, and cause of the curve. The treatment choice is also a function of the patient's future growth potential. Treatment choices include observation, bracing, and surgery. Observation is usually reserved for patients who have curves ≤25°. Bracing, which is used to stop curve progression (rather than for lasting correction of the curve), is usually used for patients who have curves ≥25° and who are still growing. Surgery is generally used for patients with curves ≥45°. (Figure 3.1.3)

While technical outcomes of surgery are well known and show obvious benefits for those with significant deformity, long-term health related outcomes have yet to be precisely documented. The paucity of quality, long-term studies of sufficient size hampers our understanding of the mortality and morbidity rates for patients with congenital and idiopathic scoliosis, both with and without treatment. Fifty years of follow-up studies of children and adolescents with untreated scoliosis have shown conflicting results, with some studies indicating a higher risk of mortality and respiratory compromise.[11,12] Another study shows compromise only in patients with early reduced lung function and a large curvature.[13] Yet another study has shown no differences in untreated childhood scoliosis and a control group.[14] Several articles from the 1960s and one recent article report that low back pain does not occur more frequently in untreated scoliosis patients than in the general population.[14-16] unless the curvature is greater than 40°.[17,18] It has also been shown that persons treated with surgery, rather than bracing, for adolescent idiopathic scoliosis have less pain at 10 to 20 year follow-up, although function remains similar.[19,20] The cosmetic/self-image aspect of scoliosis is obvious and important, and often a major factor affecting the lives of individuals with this condition.

Figure 3.1.3: Idiopathic Scoliosis

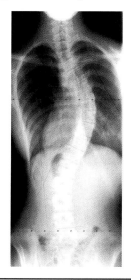 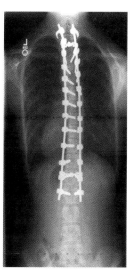 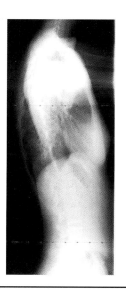 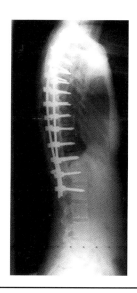

Section 3.1.2: Juvenile Idiopathic Scoliosis

In 12% to 21% of idiopathic scoliosis cases, the diagnosis is made between 4 and 10 years of age. When diagnosed at this age the condition is called juvenile idiopathic scoliosis.[21] Between the ages of 4 and 6, the female-to-male ratio of juvenile idiopathic scoliosis is 1:1; however, the ratio of female to male cases rises to between 2:1 and 4:1 in children between the ages of 4 and 10, and to 8:1 in children who are 10 years of age.[21] Both right and left curves are found with equal frequency for patients younger than 6 years, but rise to a 3:1 ratio of right versus left thoracic curves after the age of 6.[22]

Observation is the main treatment for patients with a small curve less than 20° to 25°. Follow-up visits are recommended every 4, 6, 9, or 12 months depending on the patient's age, the degree of the curve, and the characteristics of the clinical deformity.[21]

Curves between 25° and 50° are usually treated with bracing in this age group. Bracing can be done either on a part-time or full-time basis, depending on the size of the curve as well as the age of the child.[21] A study completed in 1982 evaluating the success of bracing reported an excellent prognosis when part-time bracing was utilized for patients with a curve of ≤35° and rib-vertebra angle difference (RVAD)[i] of ≤20°; however, curves ≥45° and RVAD of ≥20° had a less favorable prognosis for successful treatment with bracing.[21]

Overall, the curve patterns in patients with juvenile idiopathic scoliosis are similar to those with adolescent idiopathic scoliosis. Approximately 70% of patients with juvenile idiopathic scoliosis exhibit curve progression and

require some form of treatment. In a study conducted in 1981, 55 of 98 patients (56%) with juvenile idiopathic scoliosis required spinal surgery.[21] The most common and traditional surgery is posterior instrumentation and fusion.[21]

Section 3.1.3: Infantile Idiopathic Scoliosis

Infantile scoliosis currently accounts for less than 1% of all cases of idiopathic scoliosis in the United States. Boys are affected by infantile idiopathic scoliosis at a higher rate than girls (3:2 ratio).[23] Infantile scoliosis curves tend to be left-sided (75%-90%). Past studies have indicated this rare type of scoliosis occurs more frequently in Europe than in North America.[24]

Treatment for patients with infantile idiopathic scoliosis is determined by anticipated or actual curve progression.[23] In addition to measuring the Cobb angle, the RVAD is used as a common predictor of curve progression.[25] Patients with a Cobb angle of ≤25° and a RVAD of ≤20° are at a low risk for progression and should be re-evaluated every 4 to 6 months.[23]

Nonoperative treatment, such as bracing or casting, will be initiated if a curve progression of ≥ 10° occurs. Surgical treatment should be considered when nonoperative measures, including both bracing and casting, are not successful.[23] Surgical treatment is utilized when a curve is ≥ 45° and progressive in an immature child.[23] Overall, surgical methods are continually evolving with the goal of obtaining and maintaining curve correction while simultaneously preserving or encouraging spinal and trunk growth.

Surgical options currently utilized include various types of spinal fusion or hemiepiphysiodesis, a minimally invasive implant procedure to slow progression of curve growth. Additional techniques include growing-rod instrumentation (rods that expand and support the deformed spine) and vertical expandable (telescoping) prosthetic titanium rib (VEPTR) instrumentation.[ii] (Figure 3.1.4) The goal

---

[i] **RVAD - Rib Vertebral Angle Degree**: The angle formed on each side between the apical thoracic vertebra and its corresponding rib. The rib-vertebra angle difference is the difference between the rib-vertebral angle on the convexity of the curve subtracted from that on the concavity and may be either a positive or negative value. In a normal spine the rib-vertebra angle difference at any vertebra is zero. Resolving curves are nearly always thoracic and when first seen the rib-vertebral angle difference is less than 20° in 80% of patients. The usual pattern is for the rib-vertebral angle difference to decrease as the curve resolves. (Bradford Book, 1986) Available at: http://www.infantilescoliosis.org/terms.htm. Accessed October 3, 2007.

Figure 3.1.4: Infantile Idiopathic Scoliosis

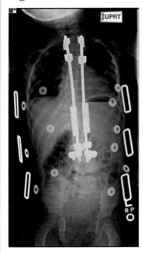

Growing Rod

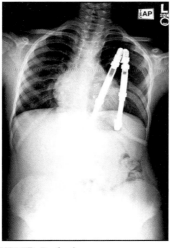

VEPTR: Back view

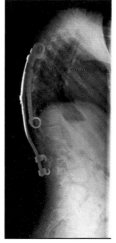

VEPTR: Side view

scoliosis are bracing and/or surgery, and are similar to those discussed for idiopathic scoliosis. Bracing is not as effective for congenital scoliosis as it is for idiopathic scoliosis.

Major abnormal spinal deformity presenting during infancy or early childhood poses a clinical problem because of the anticipated long growth period (at least 10 years); variable presentation and treatment methods; and the length of time that must pass before meaningful outcome results can be assessed in the small number of patients for definitive studies. Curves that result from

of using surgical methods is to halt the progression of the curve and gain correction of the deformity, allowing maximum growth of the spine, lungs, and thoracic cage.[23]

Section 3.1.4: Congenital Scoliosis

Congenital scoliosis is believed to affect approximately 1 child for every 1000 live births.[26] The cause is unknown in most cases but in some cases it is associated with various syndromes. (Figure 3.1.5) Diagnosis is occasionally made during prenatal ultrasound. In cases of congenital scoliosis, additional congenital conditions, such as chest wall malformation or kidney or heart abnormalities, are often present. Treatment options for congenital

Figure 3.1.5: Congenital Anomalies

Defects of Segmentation

Block Vertebra	Block Vertebra	Unilateral Bar & Hemivertebra
Bilateral failure of segmentation	Unilateral failure of segmentation	

Defects of Formation

Hemivertebra				Wedge Vertebra
Unilateral complete failure of formation				Unilateral partial failure of formation
Fully segmented	Semi-segmented	Incarcerated	Nonsegmented	

Source: McMaster MJ: Congenital scoliosis, in: Weinstein SL (ed): *The Pediatric Spine: Principles and Practice*, ed 2. Philadelphia, PA: Lippinncott Williams & Wilkins; 2001; p 163.

congenital scoliosis are often not treated as easily as idiopathic curves because the deformity is in the bones rather than the soft tissue, causing the curve to be rigid.[27]

---

ii **Titanium Rib or VEPTR** (Vertical Expandable Prosthetic Titanium Rib): An expandable titanium metal rod placed in a vertical position alongside the spine and attached to the ribs and pelvis or the spine. The VEPTR expands and supports a deformed chest wall cavity giving the lungs room to operate and grow. Used to treat many chest wall deforming and/or spine defect diagnoses which result in Thoracic Insufficiency Syndrome. Available at: http://www.infantilescoliosis.org/terms.htm. Accessed October 3, 2007.

Section 3.1.5: Neuromuscular Scoliosis

Scoliosis also occurs in conjunction with several congenital conditions that occur in infancy or childhood. These include muscular dystrophy, cerebral palsy, spina bifida, and spinal muscular atrophy. Scoliosis associated with these conditions is referred to as neuromuscular scoliosis. Both the likelihood and the severity of the scoliosis generally increases with the severity of the underlying condition. For example, a child with severe cerebral palsy who is unable to walk is more likely to have severe scoliosis than a child with mild cerebral palsy who can walk. These conditions are also discussed in Chapter 6 (Congenital and Infantile Developmental Conditions of the Musculoskeletal System.)

Cerebral palsy (CP) is defined as a non-progressive disturbance in the developing brain of the fetus or infant. Musculoskeletal problems are frequently seen as a result of the motor disorder. The more common musculoskeletal problem is scoliosis. Besides bracing, which is usually an ineffective form of treatment for more severe muscular scoliosis, surgical procedures are frequently indicated in pediatric patients with CP. In 2005, more than 100,000 children under the age of 18 were disabled with CP, and its prevalence has increased by 18% in the past two decades.[28] In 1997, 37,000 pediatric patients were discharged from hospitals with a diagnosis of CP. Among these patients, spinal fusion with instrumentation was among the top five most commonly performed surgical procedures, and was performed on 765 patients that year in the United States. Treatment for CP with spinal fusion accounted for more than 4,000 hospital days and charges of nearly $40 million.[28]

The prevalence of spina bifida (a failure of the spine—usually, the lower spine—to close and form normally during fetal development) has decreased dramatically since the 1970s with the introduction of folic acid into the diet of pregnant women. Since 1990, the annual incidence of spina bifida has been reported at 3.2 cases per 10,000 live births, with no variation in ethnic groups observed.[29]

There are several different types of muscular dystrophy (i.e., abnormal function of muscle), but all are genetic in cause and due to a lack of protein that helps muscle cells function. The most common type is Duchenne muscular dystrophy, and it primarily affects males who inherit a defective gene through their mother.[30] Duchenne muscular dystrophy occurs in approximately 1 in 3500 live male births.[30] Many patients with Duchenne muscular dystrophy develop scoliosis by the age of 12.[31] Because muscular dystrophy is usually progressive, patients are typically treated surgically, usually with spinal fusion.[32] Potential advantages of surgery include comfort and sitting tolerance, cosmetic improvement, elimination of the need for orthopaedic braces, ease of nursing care for parents, and pain relief.

Spinal muscular atrophy (SMA) affects eight children out of every 100,000 live births. The prevalence of scoliosis for patients with SMA is directly related to the severity of the disease and the specific type of SMA that the patient has.[33] SMA equally affects both females and males.[34] There is no specific treatment for SMA, but bracing can slow the inevitable progression of a scoliotic curve and postpone surgical treatment in some cases. Surgical treatment is generally spinal fusion or a segmental spinal instrumentation, and is performed when the curve progresses to greater than 50° to 60°. The goal of surgical treatment is to improve balance and sitting capability of the patient.[33]

Section 3.2: Other Childhood Spinal Conditions

Additional spinal conditions seen in children include spondylolysis, a stress fracture of the lower end of the spine; spondylolisthesis, a condition where one of the spinal vertebrae (usually in the lower/lumbar spine) slips forward on the one below it; Scheuermann kyphosis, an often painful condition manifested in exaggerated roundness of the upper part of the spine; and others. Occasionally, children have herniated discs that require surgical intervention. Children also can have different types of spinal infections and tumors. While most of these conditions are quite rare, they can cause significant disability if not recognized early and treated appropriately. Again, the preventative nature of treatment is intuitively obvious, but difficult to measure for these rare conditions.

Section 3.2.1: Spondylolysis and Spondylolisthesis

Spondylolysis is disintegration or dissolution of a vertebra. It is usually accompanied by spondylolisthesis, a forward displacement of a lumbar vertebra on the one below it, especially the fifth lumbar vertebra on the sacrum,

Many children with spondylolysis do not experience back pain and, therefore, may not require treatment. If the child remains asymptomatic, he or she is examined every 3 to 6 months; if the child begins to experience pain, a bone scan and proper radiographs are often used to reassess the situation and confirm the diagnosis. Conservative management, such as bracing, may help. Spondylolysis that progresses or remains painful in spite of conservative measures, and which interferes with daily activities, is treated with a localized spinal fusion. A similar observation/treatment pattern is used for children with spondylolisthesis. Surgery is recommended if the slip of one vertebra over another is greater than 50%. Overall, the goal of surgery for either condition is to stabilize the spondylolytic segment, prevent further slippage, relieve pain and/or nerve root irritation, and prevent neurological deficit. When indicated, surgery can help correct

Figure 3.2.1: Spondylolysis and Spondylolisthesis

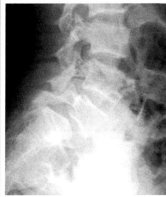 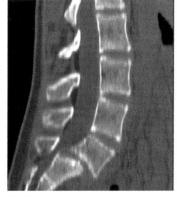 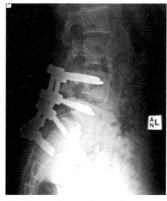

| Preoperative radiograph | CT Scan | Postoperative radiograph |

producing pain by compression of nerve roots. (Figure 3.2.1) Although spondylolysis is virtually nonexistent in newborns, by the age of 6 the incidence has reached approximately 6% for the general pediatric population. Both spondylolysis and spondylolisthesis are found at higher levels in certain populations. Examination of Eskimo skeletons indicates the incidence of spondylolysis is 13% in pediatric patients. A study conducted in 1953 found an overall incidence of 4.2% in the general pediatric population, with incidence of 6.4% in white males, 2.8% in black males, 2.3% in white females, and 1.1% in black females. Most reports have found a higher incidence of spondylolysis in males than in females (2:1 ratio, respectively), although females have a higher risk of progression.[35]

hamstring tautness, poor posture, and abnormality of gait.[34]

Section 3.2.2: Scheuermann Kyphosis

Scheuermann kyphosis affects 0.4% to 8% of healthy children. Kyphosis is an exaggerated outward curvature of the thoracic region of the spinal column resulting in a rounded upper back. (Figure 3.2.2) There is no definitive answer to whether it affects males or females at higher rates, with prevalence leaning to both sexes found in studies.[36] Patients who are skeletally mature with acceptable kyphosis (curvature) and no observable symptoms do not require treatment. If the individual is still growing and the kyphosis is severe, treatment is required, and bracing or

Figure 3.2.2: Scheuermann Kyphosis

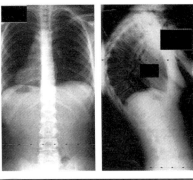

Note the increased curvature of the upper back associated with wedging and end plate irregularity of individual vertebrae at the apex.

casting is usually used, with surgery rarely indicated and only for skeletally mature patients with chronic back pain and a curve of more than 60°.[34]

Section 3.3: Adult Spinal Deformity and Degenerative Scoliosis

Deformity of the adult spine includes patients with curvature of the spine (scoliosis) of varying magnitudes caused or impacted by degenerative disc and joint disease. Adult scoliosis may be the result of persistent or progressive deformity since adolescence or a new, *de novo*, onset of deformity as a result of degeneration or "aging" of the spine. Degenerative scoliosis accounts for the majority of scoliosis cases in older populations aged 65 years and older, as reflected in the low proportion of older patients with a diagnosis of primary idiopathic scoliosis.

The prevalence of adult spinal deformity and scoliosis is not well established, with estimates ranging from 2.5% to 25% of the population.[16, 37-41] A recent study reported mild to severe adult scoliosis prevalence as high as 68% in a healthy (no known scoliosis or spine surgery) population aged 60 and over.[42] Many cases of degenerative scoliosis are undiagnosed, but elderly patients often seek care because of back and leg pain that may be caused by scoliosis and associated spinal stenosis.

Degenerative scoliosis is one of the most challenging spine conditions to treat due to the variability of the condition. It is generally thought

to originate with the degeneration of the intervertebral discs, which leads to misalignment of the vertebral column. Degenerative scoliosis, particularly in the very elderly, is often associated with other conditions, such as osteoporosis. Treatment outcomes for both nonsurgical and surgical procedures are not well documented; hence, recognition and earlier intervention are important to ward off the more complex problems of adult scoliosis. The role played by undiagnosed, mild idiopathic adolescent scoliosis on the development of degenerative scoliosis in later life is unknown.

Section 3.4: Health Care Resource Use for Spinal Deformity in 2004

While the incidence of spinal deformity among patients seeking care in any given year can be estimated, the relatively low proportion of the population seeking care for spinal deformity conditions precludes statistically reliable numbers. In addition, many persons do not seek care, or seek care for severe or disabling back or leg pain that is often caused by spinal deformity. Hence, the overall prevalence of spinal deformity in the total population is projected to be much higher than current data implies. Furthermore, degenerative scoliosis is rarely a primary, or 1st,

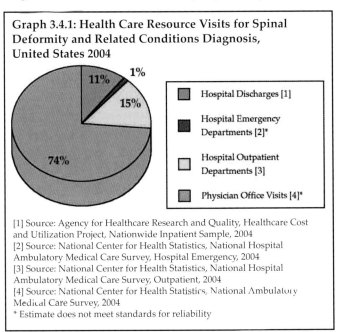

Graph 3.4.1: Health Care Resource Visits for Spinal Deformity and Related Conditions Diagnosis, United States 2004

- Hospital Discharges [1]
- Hospital Emergency Departments [2]*
- Hospital Outpatient Departments [3]
- Physician Office Visits [4]*

[1] Source: Agency for Healthcare Research and Quality, Healthcare Cost and Utilization Project, Nationwide Inpatient Sample, 2004
[2] Source: National Center for Health Statistics, National Hospital Ambulatory Medical Care Survey, Hospital Emergency, 2004
[3] Source: National Center for Health Statistics, National Hospital Ambulatory Medical Care Survey, Outpatient, 2004
[4] Source: National Center for Health Statistics, National Ambulatory Medical Care Survey, 2004
* Estimate does not meet standards for reliability

diagnosis and may not be included as a diagnosis at all.

Idiopathic and degenerative scoliosis are both found in a higher proportion of females than males.[3] As the ratio of the curve increases, indicating more severe scoliosis, the female to male ratio is reported as high as 10:1 among persons with a curve of greater than 30°.[13,43]

In 2004, an estimated 1.26 million patients utilized health care resources for care of problems associated with a spinal deformity. (Table 3.3) The majority (74%) of these care episodes were with a physician (Graph 3.4.1), and involved non-surgical and pre-surgical management of this complex patient population. In addition, nearly 200,000 persons visited hospital outpatient centers for care, while approximately 134,500 persons were hospitalized with a diagnosis of spinal deformity. Nearly all (93%) of these patients were diagnosed with scoliosis. The remainder had a diagnosis of kyphosis, a curvature of the thoracic region of the spinal column resulting in a rounded upper back, or excessive lordosis (swayback), an increased amount of curvature of the lumbar or cervical regions of the spinal column.

The overwhelming majority of spinal deformity and scoliosis patients in 2004 were female (75%),

and more than one-half (52%) were under the age of 18. However, elderly persons are more likely to be hospitalized with a spinal deformity diagnosis, with 37% of 2004 hospitalization for persons aged 75 years and older. (Graph 3.4.2)

In 2004, 62% (83,100) of patients released from a hospital with a spinal deformity or scoliosis diagnosis had a diagnosis of idiopathic scoliosis (ICD-9-CM code of 737.30). Nine percent (9%, or 7,600) of these 83,100 patients had a primary, or

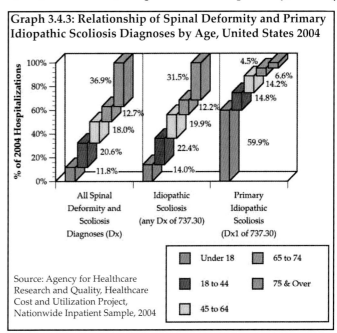

Graph 3.4.3: Relationship of Spinal Deformity and Primary Idiopathic Scoliosis Diagnoses by Age, United States 2004

Source: Agency for Healthcare Research and Quality, Healthcare Cost and Utilization Project, Nationwide Inpatient Sample, 2004

1st, diagnosis of idiopathic scoliosis; 91% had an idiopathic scoliosis diagnosis that was in addition to their primary diagnosis.

Of these 83,100 patients with idiopathic scoliosis diagnoses, 14% were under the age of 18 years, while 32% were aged 75 and over. (Table 3.4 and Graph 3.4.3) However, a primary (1st) diagnosis of idiopathic scoliosis was far more common in young persons, with 60% under the age of 18, supporting the assumption that degenerative scoliosis or spinal deformity is frequently not the primary (1st) diagnosis of elderly patients.

One-half of the young patient group (49%) were between the ages of 14 and 17 years. Another 46% were between the ages of 11 and 13, with the remainder aged 10 years or younger.

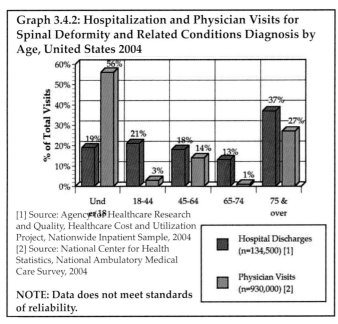

Graph 3.4.2: Hospitalization and Physician Visits for Spinal Deformity and Related Conditions Diagnosis by Age, United States 2004

[1] Source: Agency for Healthcare Research and Quality, Healthcare Cost and Utilization Project, Nationwide Inpatient Sample, 2004
[2] Source: National Center for Health Statistics, National Ambulatory Medical Care Survey, 2004

NOTE: Data does not meet standards of reliability.

Hospital Discharges (n=134,500) [1]

Physician Visits (n=930,000) [2]

Nearly all patient visits to a physician's office in 2004 with a primary (1st) diagnosis of idiopathic scoliosis (93%) were for patients under the age of 18 years. Again, the majority (74%) were between the ages of 14 and 17 years; however, children between the ages of 8 and 10 comprised 16% of the remaining patients, with the balance aged 11 to 13 years. (Table 3.5)

Although a larger proportion of persons diagnosed with a spinal deformity or scoliosis in 2004 were aged 75 and over (31%) compared to younger persons (16% under age 18), a significantly higher proportion under the age of 18 with a spinal deformity diagnosis underwent spine surgical procedures for their condition. One in three (33%) persons hospitalized with a spinal deformity or scoliosis diagnosis under the age of

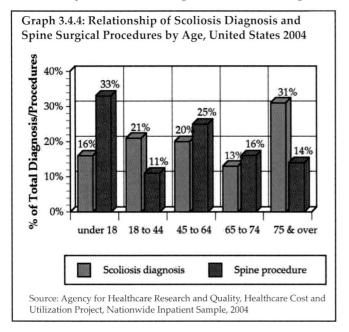

Graph 3.4.4: Relationship of Scoliosis Diagnosis and Spine Surgical Procedures by Age, United States 2004

Source: Agency for Healthcare Research and Quality, Healthcare Cost and Utilization Project, Nationwide Inpatient Sample, 2004

18 years underwent surgery, while only 1 in 7 (14%) aged 75 and over underwent surgery. (Graph 3.4.4)

Section 3.4.1: Estimated 2004 Cost for Treatment of Scoliosis and Spinal Deformity

A conservative estimate of the hospitalization cost for adult scoliosis in 2004 was $315.3 million. This estimate, which generally does not include professional fees, is based on the average cost per

hospital stay for four age groups of patients aged 18 and over with a primary (1st) diagnosis of idiopathic scoliosis. Child and adolescent primary idiopathic scoliosis hospitalization fees added an additional $373.7 million, for a total estimated hospitalization cost to treat primary idiopathic scoliosis in 2004 of $688.1 million. (Table 3.4)

Additional hospital costs of more than $2.0 billion were incurred by patients with a diagnosis of idiopathic scoliosis in addition to their primary (1st) diagnosis. It is unknown what proportion of these costs resulted directly from treatment given as a result of scoliosis; however, it can be assumed some proportion of these additional costs would not have occurred in the absence of the scoliosis condition.

In addition to health care costs associated with surgery for spinal deformity and scoliosis, significant nonsurgical resources are utilized by adults with scoliosis, increasing the burden of this condition on the health care system. A study of nonsurgical resource use, including exercise, bracing, medications, steroid injections, and formal pain management, by adults with a spinal curvature of ≥30° showed 90% of patients utilized non-surgical resources, with those patients with a high level of symptoms using more resources than those with a low level of symptoms.[44]

Overall, the cost related to spinal deformity is significant, with more than one million patient visits each year for treatment of pain due to this condition. A majority of spinal deformity cases each year are the result of degenerative scoliosis. With the aging of the U.S. population, increased awareness, identification, and treatment of spinal deformity in its earliest stages is necessary to reduce the current and future burden of this condition.

1.   National Institute of Arthritis and Musculoskeletal and Skin Diseases (NIAMS): Questions and answers about scoliosis in children and adolescents. National Institutes of Health, U.S. Department of Health and Human Services, 2007. Available at: http://www.niams.nih.gov/Health_Info/Scoliosis/default.asp. Accessed August 30, 2007.

2. Herzenberg JE, Waanders NA, Closkey RF, et al: Cobb angle versus spinous process angle in adolescent idiopathic scoliosis: The relationship of the anterior and posterior deformities. *Spine* 1990;15:874-879.

3. Lonstein J: Scoliosis: surgical versus nonsurgical treatment. *Clin Ortho Relat Res* 2006;443:248-259.

4. Morais T, Bernier M, Turcotte F: Age- and sex-specific prevalence of scoliosis and the value of school screening programs. *Am J Public Health Nations Health* 1985;75:1377-1380.

5. Bunnell W: Spinal deformity. *Pediatr Clin North Am* 1986;33:1475-1487.

6. Weinstein S: Idiopathic scoliosis: Natural history. *Spine* 1986;11:780-783.

7. Karol LA, Johnston CE 2nd, Browne RH, Madison M: Progression of the curve in boys who have idiopathic scoliosis. *J Bone Joint Surg Am* 1993;75:1804-1810.

8. Porter SB, Blount BW: Pseudotumor of infancy and congenital mascular torticollis. *Am Fam Physician* 1995;52:1731-1736.

9. Willner S: Continuous screening and treatment of teenage scoliosis is recommended. *Lakartidningen* 1994;91:22.

10. Lenke LG, Betz RR, Clements D, et al: Curve prevalence of a new classification of operative adolescent idiopathic scoliosis: Does classification correlate with treatment? *Spine* 2002;27:604-611.

11. Goldberg CJ, Gillic I, Connaughton O, et al: Respiratory function and cosmesis at maturity in infantile-onset scoliosis. *Spine* 2003;28:2397-2406.

12. Pehrsson K, Larsson S, Oden A, Nachemson A: Long-term follow-up of patients with untreated scoliosis: A study of mortality, causes of death, and symptoms. *Spine* 1992;17:1091-1096.

13. Pehrsson K, Bake B, Larsson S, Nachemson A: Lung function in adult idiopathic scoliosis: a 20 year follow up. *Thorax* 1991;46:474-478.

14. Weinstein SL, Dolan LA, Spratt KF, et al: Health and function of patients with untreated idiopathic scoliosis: a 50-year natural history study. *JAMA* 2003;289:559-567.

15. Nachemson A: A long term follow-up study of non-treated scoliosis. *Acta Orthop Scand* 1968;39:466-476.

16. Nilsonne U, Lundgren KD: Long term prognosis in idiopathic scoliosis. *Acta Orthop Scand* 1968;39:456-465.

17. Kostuik JP, Bentivoglio J: The incidence of low-back pain in adult scoliosis. *Spine* 1981;6:268-273.

18. Haefeli M, Elfering A, Kilian R, et al: Nonoperative treatment for adolescent idiopathic scoliosis: a 10- to 60-year follow-up with special reference to health related quality of life. *Spine* 2006;31:355-366.

19. Andersen MO, Christensen SB, Thomsen K: Outcome at 10 years treatment for adolescent idiopathic scoliosis. *Spine* 2006;31:350-354.

20. Danielsson AJ, Romberg K, Nachemson AL: Spinal range of motion, muscle endurance, and back pain and function at least 20 years after fusion or brace treatment for adolescent idiopathic scoliosis: A case-control study. *Spine* 2006;31:275-283.

21. Lenke LG, Dobbs MB: Management of juvenile idiopathic scoliosis. *J Bone Joint Surg Am* 2007;89:55-63.

22. Warner WC Jr.: Juvenile idiopathic scoliosis, in Weinstein S (ed): *The Pediatric Spine: Principles and Practice*, ed 2. Philadelphia, PA: Lippincott Williams & Wilkins, 2001, p 330.

23. Akbarnia B: Management themes in early onset scoliosis. *J Bone Joint Surg Am* 2007;89:42-54.

24. Fernandes P, Weinstein SL: Natural history of early onset scoliosis. *J Bone Joint Surg Am* 2007;89:21-33.

25. Mehta M: The rib-vertebra angle in the early diagnosis between resolving and progressive infantile scoliosis. *J Bone Joint Surg Br* 1972;54:230-243.

26. Hedequist D, Emans J: Congenital scoliosis: A review and update. *J Pediatr Orthop* 2007;27:106-116.

27. Lonstein J: Scoliosis, in **Lovell WW, Winter RB, Morrissy RT, Weinstein SL** (ed): *Lovell and Winter's Pediatric Orthopaedics*, ed 4. Philadelphia, PA: Lippincott Williams Wilkins, 1996, vol II.

28. Murphy NA, Hoff C, Jorgensen T, et al: A national perspective of surgery in children with cerebral palsy. *Pediatr Rehabil* 2006;9:293-300.

29. Kaufmann B: Congenital intraspinal anomalies: spinal dysraphism-embrology, pathology, and treatment, in Bridwell KH, DeWald RL (ed): *The Textbook of Spinal Surgery*, ed 2. Philadelphia, PA: Lippincott-Raven, 1997, vol 1, p 366.

30. Thompson G: Neuromuscular disorders, in **Lovell WW, Winter RB, Morrissy RT, Weinstein SL** (ed): *Lovell and Winter's Pediatric Orthopaedics*, ed 4. Philadelphia, PA: Lippincott Williams & Wilkins, 1996, vol I.

31. Shook JE, Lubicky JP: Paralytic scoliosis, in Bridwell KH, DeWald RL (ed): *The Textbook of Spinal Surgery*, ed 2. Philadelphia, PA: Lippincott-Raven Publishers, 1997, vol 1.

32. Cheuk DKL, Wong V, Wraige E, et al: Surgery for scoliosis in Duchenne muscular dystrophy. Available at: http://www.mrw.interscience.wiley.com/cochrane/clsysrev/articles/CD005375/frame.html. Accessed August 28, 2007.

33. Sucato D: Spine deformity in spinal muscular atrophy. *J Bone Joint Surg Am* 2007;89:148-154.

34. Tachdjian MO: *Pediatric Orthopaedics*, ed 2. Philadelphia, PA: WB Saunders, 1999, vol 3.

35. Hu SS, Bradford DS: Spondylolysis and spondylolisthesis, in Weinstein S (ed): *The Pediatric Spine: Principles and Practice*, ed 2. Philadelphia, PA: Lippincott Williams & Wilkins, 2001, pp 433-434.

36. Ascani E, La Rosa G, Ascani C: Scheuermann kyphosis, in Weinstein S (ed): *The Pediatric Spine: Principles and Practice*, ed 2. Philadelphia, PA: Lippincott Williams & Wilkins, 2001, p 415.

37. Battie MC, Videman T: Lumbar disc degeneration: Epidemiology and genetics. *J Bone Joint Surg Am* 2006;88:3-9.

38. Gupta M: Degenerative scoliosis: Options for surgical management. *Ortho Clin North Am* 2003;34:269-279.

39. Carter OD, Haynes SG: Prevalence rates for scoliosis in U.S. adults: Results from the first National Health and Nutrition Examination Survey. *Int J Epidemiol* 1987;16:537-544.

40. Perennou D, Marcelli C, Herisson C, Simon L: Adult lumbar scoliosis: Epidemiologic aspects in a low-back pain population. *Spine* 1994;19:123-128.

41. Robin GC, Span Y, Steinberg R, et al: Scoliosis in the elderly: A follow-up study. *Spine* 1982;7:355-359.

42. Schwab F, Dubey A, Galez L, et al: Adult scoliosis: Prevalence, SF-36, and nutritional parameters in an elderly volunteer population. *Spine* 2005;30:1082-1085.

43. Manson NE, Goldberg EJ, Andersson GBJ: Sexual dimorphism in degenerative disorders of the spine. *Orthop Clin N Am* 2006;37:549-553.

44. Glassman SD, Berven S, Kostuik J, et al: Nonsurgical resource utilization in adult spinal deformity. *Spine* 2006;31:941-947.

Section 3.5: Spinal Deformity and Related Conditions Data Tables

Table 3.1: Estimated and Normalized Prevalence of Spinal Deformity and Related Conditions

	Cited Prevalence Rate (midpoint of range cited)		Normalized Prevalence Rate (per 100 persons)	Prevalence Rate (per 100,000 persons)
Congenital scoliosis [1]	1 in	1,000	0.100	100
Infantile idiopathic scoliosis [2]	0.04 in	100	0.040	40
Juvenile idiopathic scoliosis [3]	0.06 in	100	0.060	60
Adolescent idiopathic scoliosis [4]	2.5 in	100	2.500	2,500
Spina bifida [5]	4.6 in	10,000	0.046	46
Cerebral palsy [6]	0.001 in	100	0.001	1
Muscular Dystrophy [7]	1 in	3,500	0.029	29
Spondylolysis, age 6 [8]	6 in	100	6.000	6,000
Spinal muscular atrophy [9]	8 in	100,000	0.008	8
Scheuermann kyphosis [9,10]	4 in	100	4.000	4,000
Adult spinal deformity or scoliosis (age >18 yrs) [11,12,13]	11.3 in	100	11.300	11,300
Adult spinal deformity or scoliosis (age >60 yrs) [14]	68 in	100	68.000	68,000

[1] Hedequist D, Emans J: Congenital scoliosis: a review and update. Journal of Pediatric Orthopaedics 2007:27:106-116.

[2] Akbarnia B: Management themes in early onset scoliosis. J Bone Joint Surg Am 2007:89-A:42-54 (Prevalence rate computed based on cited rate for adolescent idiopathic scoliosis and proportion of total idiopathic cases that are infantile in citation.)

[3] Lenke LG, Dobbs MB: Management of juvenile idiopathic scoliosis. J Bone Joint Surg Am 2007:89-A:55-63 (Prevalence rate computed based on cited rate for adolescent idiopathic scoliosis and proportion of total idiopathic cases that are juvenile in citation.)

[4] Morais T, Bernier M, Turcotte F: Age- and sex-specific prevalence of scoliosis and the value of school screening programs. Am J Public Health Nations Health 1985:75:1377-1380.

[5] Kaufmann B: Congenital intraspinal anomalies: spinal dysraphism-embrology, pathology, and treatment, in Bridwell KH, DeWald RL (ed): The textbook of spinal surgery, ed 2. Philadelphia, PA: Lippincott-Raven Publishers, 1997, vol 1, p 366

[6] Murphy NA, Hoff C, Jorgensen T, et. al.: A national perspective of surgery in children with cerebral palsy. Pediatr Rehabil 2006:9:293-300 (Note: rate was computed based on census population and cited number of cases)

[7] Thompson G: Neuromuscular disorders, in Lovell WW, Winter RB, Morrissy RT, Weinstein SL (ed): Lovell and Winter's pediatric orthopaedics, ed 4. Philadelphia, PA: Lippincott Williams and Wilkins, 1996, vol I.

[8] Hu SS, Bradford DS: Spondylolysis and spondylolisthesis, in Weinstein S (ed): The pediatric spine: principles and practice, ed 2. Philadelphia, PA: Lippincott Williams & Wilkins, 2001, pp 433-434

[9] Sucato D: Spine deformity in spinal muscular atrophy. Journal of Bone and Joint Surgery American 2007:89:148-154

[10] Ascani E, La Rosa G, Ascani C Scheuermann kyphosis, in Weinstein S (ed): The pediatric spine: principles and practice, ed 2. Philadelphia, PA: Lippincott Williams & Wilkins, 2001, p 415

[11] Battie MC, Videman T: Lumbar disc degeneration: epidemiology and genetics. J Bone Joint Surg Am 2006:88:3-9

[12] Carter OD, Haynes SG: Prevalence rates for scoliosis in U.S. adults: results from the first National Health and Nutrition Examination Survey. Int J Epidemiol 1987:16:537-544

[13] Gupta M: Degenerative scoliosis: options for surgical management. Ortho Clin N Am 2003:2003:269-279

[14] Schwab F, Dubey A, Galez L, et al.: Adult scoliosis: prevalence, SF-36, and nutritional parameters in an elderly volunteer population. Spine 2005:30:1082-1085

Table 3.2: Prevalence of Adolescent Idiopathic Scoliosis

Cobb Angle	Female-to-Male Ratio	Prevalence (%)
>10	1.4-2.0 : 1	2.0%-3.0%
>20	5.4 : 1	0.3%-0.5%
>30	10 : 1	0.1%-0.3%
>40	Not applicable	<0.1%

Source: Reprinted with permission from Weinstein SL. Adolescent idiopathic scoliosis: Prevalence and natural history. Instr Course Lect 198838:115–126.

Table 3.3: Health Care Resource Usage with Spinal Deformity and Related Conditions Diagnosis by Gender and Age, United States 2004

	Total Occurrences (in 000s)[1]								
		Gender			Age (in years)				Average Age at Diagnosis
	Total	Male	Female	<18	18-44	45-64	65-74	75 & over	
Spinal Deformity & Related Conditions									
Hospital Discharges [2]	134	32	102	16	28	24	17	50	57.1
Hospital Emergency Departments [3]*	13	11	3	*	*	*	*	*	24.2
Hospital Outpatient Departments [4]	187	79	107	122	17	21	4	21	26.9
Physician Office Visits [5]*	930	191	739	519	27	129	8	247	36.2
All Spinal Deformity & Related Conditions Diagnoses	1,264	313	951	657	72	174	29	318	
Spinal Deformity & Related Conditions									
Hospital Discharges [2]	11%	24%	76%	11.9%	20.9%	17.9%	12.0%	37.3%	
Hospital Emergency Departments [3]*	1%	79%	21%	*	*	*	*	*	
Hospital Outpatient Departments [4]	15%	42%	57%	66.0%	9.1%	11.2%	2.1%	11.2%	
Physician Office Visits [5]*	74%	21%	79%	55.8%	2.9%	13.9%	0.9%	26.6%	
All Spinal Deformity & Related Conditions Diagnoses	100%	25%	75%	52.0%	5.7%	13.8%	3.0%	25.2%	

* Estimate does not meet standards for reliability

[1] Multiple occurrences per patient possible

[2] Source: Agency for Healthcare Research and Quality, Healthcare Cost and Utilization Project, Nationwide Inpatient Sample, 2004

[3] Source: National Center for Health Statistics, National Hospital Ambulatory Medical Care Survey, Hospital Emergency, 2004

[4] Source: National Center for Health Statistics, National Hospital Ambulatory Medical Care Survey, Outpatient, 2004

[5] Source: National Center for Health Statistics, National Ambulatory Medical Care Survey, 2004

Table 3.4: Hospitalization and Mean Hospital Cost [1] for Idiopathic Scoliosis by Gender and Age, United States 2004

	All Diagnoses	Proportion by Age and Gender Group	Proportion All Spinal Deformity Diagnoses of Total Group	Mean Hospital Charge	Mean Hospital Length of Stay	Estimated Total Cost (in millions)	Proportion Estimated Cost by Age Group
Hospital Discharges with Scoliosis Diagnosis (All Diagnoses, All Cases)							
				(n=130,765)	(n=134,482)		
TOTAL	134,538			$ 33,927	5.5	$ 4,564.5	
Male	32,345	24%					
Female	101,991	76%					
<18	15,888	11.8%		$ 56,197	6.2	$ 892.9	19.6%
18-44	27,737	20.6%		$ 29,202	5.2	$ 810.0	17.7%
45-64	24,165	18.0%		$ 42,179	5.2	$ 1,019.3	22.3%
65-74	17,124	12.7%		$ 39,280	5.1	$ 672.6	14.7%
75 & over	49,568	36.9%		$ 23,862	5.7	$ 1,182.8	25.9%
18 & over	118,594	88.1%				$ 3,684.7	80.7%
Hospital Discharges with Idiopathic Scoliosis Diagnosis (Dx=737.30)							
				(n=80,570)	(n=83,038)		
TOTAL	83,093		61.8%	$ 32,843	5.5	$ 2,729.0	
Male	20,327	24.5%	62.8%				
Female	62,608	75.3%	61.4%				
<18	11,606	14.0%	73.0%	$ 51,307	5.8	$ 595.5	21.8%
18-44	18,597	22.4%	67.0%	$ 28,433	5.4	$ 528.8	19.4%
45-64	16,495	19.9%	68.3%	$ 37,642	5.3	$ 620.9	22.8%
65-74	10,172	12.2%	59.4%	$ 33,940	4.8	$ 345.2	12.7%
75 & over	26,167	31.5%	52.8%	$ 24,656	5.8	$ 645.2	23.6%
18 & over	71,431	86.0%	60.2%			$ 2,140.1	78.4%

[1] Generally, total charges do not include professional fees and non-covered charges. In the rare cases where professional fees cannot be removed, they are included in the database. Emergency department charges incurred prior to admission to the hospital may be included in total charges.

Source: Agency for Healthcare Research and Quality, Healthcare Cost and Utilization Project, Nationwide Inpatient Sample, 2004

Table 3.4: Hospitalization and Mean Hospital Cost [1] for Idiopathic Scoliosis by Gender and Age, United States 2004 (continued)

	All Idiopathic Scoliosis Diagnoses	Proportion by Age and Gender Group	Proportion All Spinal Deformity Diagnoses of Total Group	Mean Charge	Mean Hospital Length of Stay	Estimated Total Cost (in millions)	Proportion Estimated Cost by Age Group
Hospital Discharges with Primary Diagnosis of Idiopathic Scoliosis (Dx1=737.30)							
				(n=7038)	(n=7582)		
TOTAL	7,583		9.1%	$ 90,772	6.1	$688.3	
Male	2,087	27.7%	10.3%				
Female	5,440	72.3%	8.7%				
<18	4,545	59.9%	39.1%	$ 82,225	5.4	$373.7	54.3%
18-44	1,119	14.8%	6.0%	$ 105,895	5.8	$118.5	17.2%
45-64	1,078	14.2%	6.5%	$ 144,510	10.3	$155.8	22.6%
65-74	502	6.6%	4.9%	$ 64,915	4.6	$32.6	4.7%
75 & over	339	4.5%	1.3%	$ 24,790	6.1	$8.4	1.2%
18 & over	3,038	40.1%	2.6%			$315.3	45.8%

Hospital Discharges with Pediatric Idiopathic Scoliosis Diagnosis (Age <18 Years)

	Idiopathic Scoliosis Diagnosis in Under 18 Population (All Diagnoses)	Proportion Idiopathic in All Spinal Deformity Diagnoses by Age Group	Primary Diagnosis (Dx1)	Proportion Primary in All Idiopathic Diagnoses by Age Group
TOTAL	11,606		4,545	39.1%
0-3	664	5.7%	*	0.0%
4-7	772	6.7%	44	1.0%
8-10	1,152	9.9%	197	4.3%
11-13	3,180	27.4%	2,069	45.5%
14-17	5,839	50.3%	2,180	48.0%

[1] Generally, total charges do not include professional fees and non-covered charges. In the rare cases where professional fees cannot be removed, they are included in the database. Emergency department charges incurred prior to admission to the hospital may be included in total charges.

Source: Agency for Healthcare Research and Quality, Healthcare Cost and Utilization Project, Nationwide Inpatient Sample, 2004

Table 3.5: Physician Office Visits for Idiopathic Scoliosis* by Gender and Age, United States 2004

Physician Office Visits for Spinal Deformity (All Diagnoses, All Cases)*

	All Diagnoses of Spinal Deformity	Proportion All Spinal Deformity by Age and Gender
TOTAL	929,610	
Male	190,685	21%
Female	738,925	80%
<18	519,015	55.8%
18-44	26,741	2.9%
45-64	128,781	13.9%
65-74	7,599	0.8%
75 & over	247,474	26.6%
18 & over	410,595	44.2%

Primary Diagnosis Idiopathic Scoliosis (Dx1=737.30)

	Primary Idiopathic Scoliosis	Proportion Primary Idiopathic Diagnosis by Age and Gender	Proportion Primary Idiopathic to All Idiopathic Diagnosis
TOTAL	352,569		69.0%
Male	111,346	31.6%	72.5%
Female	241,223	68.4%	67.5%
<18	326,996	92.7%	79.9%
18-44	*	0.0%	0.0%
45-64	*	0.0%	0.0%
65-74	*	0.0%	0.0%
75 & over	25,573	7.3%	62.3%
18 & over	25,573	7.3%	25.0%

Idiopathic Scoliosis (Dx=737.30)*

	Idiopathic Scoliosis Diagnosis	Proportion Idiopathic Diagnosis by Age and Gender	Proportion Idiopathic to All Spinal Deformity Diagnoses
TOTAL	511,155		55.0%
Male	153,578	30.0%	80.5%
Female	357,577	70.0%	48.4%
<18	409,056	80.0%	78.8%
18-44	26,741	5.2%	100.0%
45-64	26,695	5.2%	20.7%
65-74	7,599	1.5%	100.0%
75 & over	41,064	8.0%	16.6%
18 & over	102,099	20.0%	24.9%

Pediatric Idiopathic Scoliosis Diagnosis (Age <18 Years)*

	Prevalence Idiopathic Scoliosis in Under 18 Population (All Diagnoses)	Proportion Idiopathic to All Spinal Deformity Diagnoses by Age	Primary (Dx1) Diagnosis	Proportion Primary to All Idiopathic Diagnoses by Age
TOTAL	409,056		326,996	79.9%
0-3	*	0.0%	*	0.0%
4-7	9736	2.4%	*	0.0%
8-10	52,654	12.9%	52,654	16.1%
11-13	103,872	25.4%	31,548	9.6%
14-17	242,794	59.4%	242,794	74.2%

* Estimates do not meet standards for reliability. Data is included because it constitutes the majority of patient visits for spinal deformity and scoliosis in 2004.

Source: National Center for Health Statistics, National Ambulatory Medical Care Survey, 2004

Chapter 4

Arthritis and Related Conditions

In adults, arthritis is the most common cause of disability[1] and is among the leading conditions causing work limitations.[2] Over the next 25 years the number of people affected with doctor-diagnosed arthritis and the corresponding arthritis-attributable activity limitations are projected to increase by 40% in the United States.[3] Estimating the prevalence and burden of the various conditions that comprise arthritis and other rheumatic conditions (AORC) is important to understanding the current and potential impact of these conditions on health care and the public health systems. Equally important is identifying the gaps in our understanding of these measures.

Prevalence estimates presented in this chapter are based on studies[4,5] recently published by the National Arthritis Data Workgroup (NADW), a consortium of experts in epidemiology organized to provide a single source of national data on the prevalence and impact of AORC. The NADW found that for estimates of specific conditions they often had to rely on a few, small-sized studies of uncertain generalizability to the U.S. population. Until there are better data, the results of NADW reviews are the best prevalence estimates available and their application to the 2005 population provides the best estimate of the number of people affected by AORC overall and by selected rheumatic conditions.

Section 4.1: Prevalence of Arthritis and Other Rheumatic Conditions

The NADW focuses on AORC, as distinct from other highly prevalent musculoskeletal conditions such as back problems and osteoporosis. Initially, AORC was defined in terms of ICD-9-CM codes, a definition still in use for analyses of health care system data. (Table 4.1) However, due to changes in national surveys previously used to estimate prevalence of AORC, prevalence is now estimated using self-reported, doctor-diagnosed arthritis, defined as a "yes" response to the question, "Have you EVER been told by a doctor or other health professional that you have some form of arthritis, rheumatoid arthritis, gout, lupus, or fibromyalgia?"

Section 4.1.1: Prevalence of Arthritis and Other Rheumatic Conditions

Using doctor-diagnosed arthritis as the basis for analysis, the prevalence of AORC among U.S. adults aged 18 or older was 21.6%, or 46.4 million, in 2003-2005[6]. (Table 4.2 and Graph 4.1.1) Although arthritis prevalence is higher in older age groups, with half of adults aged 65 and over now affected, nearly two-thirds of the adults reporting doctor-diagnosed arthritis are younger than 65 years. More than 60% are women.

Adjusting prevalence by age, the prevalence of all types of arthritis is higher among women than men (24% versus 18%). Among race/ethnic groups, AORC is similar for non-Hispanic whites and African Americans (~22%), while lower among Hispanics (16.5%).

By 2030, the number of persons with doctor-diagnosed arthritis is projected to increase by 40% over current levels to nearly 67 million, or 25% of the adult population.[3]

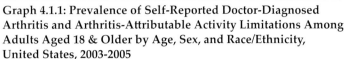

Graph 4.1.1: Prevalence of Self-Reported Doctor-Diagnosed Arthritis and Arthritis-Attributable Activity Limitations Among Adults Aged 18 & Older by Age, Sex, and Race/Ethnicity, United States, 2003-2005

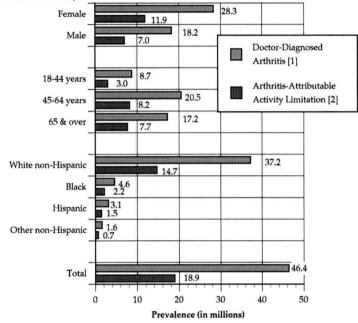

[1] Responded "Yes" when asked: Have you EVER been told by a doctor or other health professional that you have some form of arthritis, rheumatoid arthritis, gout, lupus, or fibromyalgia?

[2] Responded "Yes" when asked: Are you now limited in any way in any of your usual activities because of arthritis or joint symptoms?

Source: National Center for Health Statistics, National Health Interview Survey, 2003-2005

Section 4.1.2: Impact and Health Care Utilization for All Arthritis and Other Rheumatic Conditions

In 2003-2005, an estimated 8.8% of all adults in the United States, or nearly 19 million persons over the age of 18, had self-reported arthritis-attributable activity limitations. (Table 4.2 and Graph 4.1.1). The prevalence of activity limitations increases as people age. Among adults aged 65 years and older, 22% reported arthritis-attributable activity limitations. Activity limitations are also higher among women, but lower among Hispanics. Among all adults with doctor-diagnosed arthritis, arthritis or joint symptoms limited activities in over 40%. Arthritis-attributable activity limitations are projected to affect 9.3% of the adult population, or 25 million persons, by the year 2030.[3]

The high prevalence of arthritis and of arthritis-related activity limitations results in significant personal and societal burdens; this burden often differs by race or ethnicity.[7] For example, "arthritis and rheumatism" is the most common cause of disability in the U.S.,[1] and affected persons have a substantially lower health-related quality of life.[8] In 1997, AORC was the underlying cause of death for 9,340 persons,[9] while 19% of nursing home residents were diagnosed with AORC.[10] The estimated incremental cost of medical care expenditures and earnings losses for persons with an AORC condition was $128 billion in 2003.[11]

AORC, as a primary, or 1st, diagnosis for persons aged 18 and older accounted for 44.2 million noninjury ambulatory care visits in 2004, or 5.0% of all health care visits, and affected broad components of the health care system. (Table 4.3) Health care visits for AORC occurred in physicians offices (89%), outpatient departments (6%), and emergency departments (5%), a proportion that has changed little since 1997. (Table 4.4) By physician specialty, physician office visits in 2004 were to primary care physicians (45%), orthopaedic surgeons (36%), rheumatologists, neurologists or physical medicine and rehabilitation specialists (5%), and other providers (14%). Since 1997, the proportion of AORC patients seeing an orthopaedic surgeon has increased. Health care providers included physicians (98%), nurses (41%), and midlevel practitioners (3%), with many patients seeing multiple providers. (Table 4.4 and Graph 4.1.2)

AORC, as the primary diagnosis, accounted for 992,100 nonfederal, short stay hospitalizations in 2004, or 3.1% of all such disease-related (nondelivery) hospitalizations. In 2004, two-thirds

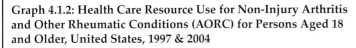

Graph 4.1.2: Health Care Resource Use for Non-Injury Arthritis and Other Rheumatic Conditions (AORC) for Persons Aged 18 and Older, United States, 1997 & 2004

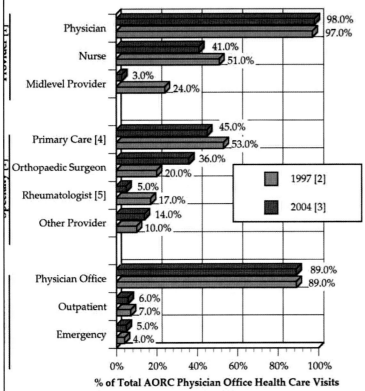

[1] Proportion of primary diagnosis of AORC visits
[2] Source: Hootman JM, Helmick CG, Schappert SM. Magnitude and characteristics of arthritis and other rheumatic conditions on ambulatory medical care visits, United States, 1997. Arthritis Rheum 2002;47:571–581
[3] Source: National Center for Health Statistics, National Ambulatory Medical Care Survey, 2004
[4] Includes family practice, family practice (geriatric medicine), sports medicine (family practice), general practice, general surgery, internal medicine, geriatric medicine (intermal medicine).
[5] Includes rheumatology, neurology, neurological surgery, physical medicine and rehabilitation.

(66%) of the primary diagnosis AORC cases involved joint arthroplasty procedures, an increasingly common treatment to restore function in arthritis diseased joints. The majority of arthroplasty procedures were for primary knee replacement (65%), with total hip replacement accounting for 29% of the procedures, and other joints 6% of procedures. AORC, as either a principal or secondary diagnosis, accounted for 4.6 million hospitalizations, or over 14% of all disease-related hospitalizations, in 2004. In addition to the above numbers, persons hospitalized with a principal diagnosis of an orthopaedic procedure, rather than an arthritis

condition, or those related to arthritis treatment complications (e.g., gastrointestinal bleeding related to NSAID use) add to the overall burden of arthritis in this country.

Section 4.2: Osteoarthritis

Osteoarthritis (OA), also known as degenerative joint disease, is the most common type of arthritis. It is characterized by progressive damage to the cartilage and other joint tissues, and frequently affects the hand, knees, and hips.

Section 4.2.1: Prevalence and Incidence of Osteoarthritis

Estimating the prevalence of OA is difficult as radiographic changes related to the presence of osteoarthritis can be seen in most persons as they age. However, these changes may not be accompanied by symptoms. Symptomatic OA, experienced as frequent pain and radiographic changes indicating osteoarthritis in the joint, is considered a better measure of important or consequential OA and is used to identify prevalence.

Longitudinal studies conducted in several communities, some as long as 40 years or more, have focused on identifying the prevalence of osteoarthritis, as well as other factors related to its causes. The longest study has been of adults aged 26 years and older living in Framingham, MA. The prevalence of symptomatic hand OA in the Framingham study is 6.8% of adults aged 26 and over; however, in older adults it is found much more frequently. Among persons aged 71 and older, OA is found in 26.2% of females and in 13.4% of males. The NADW estimated that 13.1 million adults in the United States experienced symptomatic hand OA in 2005.

The prevalence of symptomatic knee OA is about 5% of adults aged 26 years and older in the Framingham study. In another study conducted in Johnston County, NC, 17% of adults aged 45 and over were found to have symptomatic knee OA, while the 1988-1994 NHANES III survey found 12.1% of adults aged 60 years and older suffered from symptomatic knee OA. Again, older adults and females were more affected, and an estimated 9.3 million adults had symptomatic knee OA in 2005. (Table 4.5 and Graph 4.2.1)

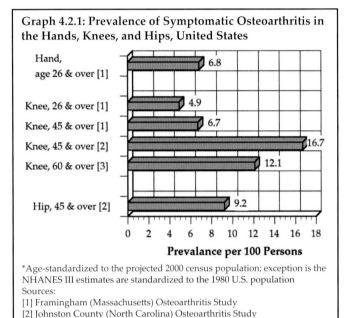

Graph 4.2.1: Prevalence of Symptomatic Osteoarthritis in the Hands, Knees, and Hips, United States

*Age-standardized to the projected 2000 census population; exception is the NHANES III estimates are standardized to the 1980 U.S. population
Sources:
[1] Framingham (Massachusetts) Osteoarthritis Study
[2] Johnston County (North Carolina) Osteoarthritis Study
[3] NHANES III, 1988-1994

The prevalence of symptomatic hip OA was 10% among adults aged 45 years and older in the Johnston County study. No prevalence estimates for symptomatic OA at multiple joints exists, but the NADW estimated that clinical OA in at least one joint, based on a physician's examination in a national survey, affected 26.9 million adults in 2005.

Section 4.2.2: Impact and Health Care Utilization for Osteoarthritis

Osteoarthritis as a primary diagnosis accounted for 11.1 million ambulatory care visits in 2004, or 25.1% of the 44.2 million non-injury visits with a primary diagnosis of AORC. (Table 4.3) Osteoarthritis as the primary diagnosis accounted for 67% of the 992,100 nonfederal, short stay hospitalizations in 2004. This estimate does not capture arthritis hospitalizations with orthopaedic procedures as the principal diagnosis or those related to arthritis treatment complications, such as gastrointestinal bleeding related to NSAID use.

Section 4.3: Rheumatoid Arthritis

Rheumatoid arthritis (RA) is a chronic autoimmune disease that causes pain, stiffness, swelling, and limitation in the motion and function of multiple joints. Though joints are the principal body parts affected by RA, inflammation can develop in other organs as well.

Section 4.3.1: Prevalence of Rheumatoid Arthritis

The only current source of data from which to estimate the prevalence of rheumatoid arthritis is a study from Rochester, MN. This study reported a prevalence of RA in 1985 of 1.07% among adults aged 35 years and older, but by 1995 this estimate had fallen to 0.85%. Twice as many women as men are affected by rheumatoid arthritis (1.06% vs. 0.61%).[4] Trends in prevalence in Rochester, MN, by age and calendar year, show increasing prevalence with older age but reflect the decreasing overall prevalence in most age groups in more recent time periods. (Table 4.6 and Graphs 4.3.1) This observation, along with the expected rapid growth in the population of Americans aged 60 years and older, suggests that RA associated morbidity, mortality, and disability are likely to increase among older adults. The NADW studies found that older adults and females are more affected, and estimated that 1.3 million adults over the age of 17 years, 0.6% of all adults, had RA in 2005.

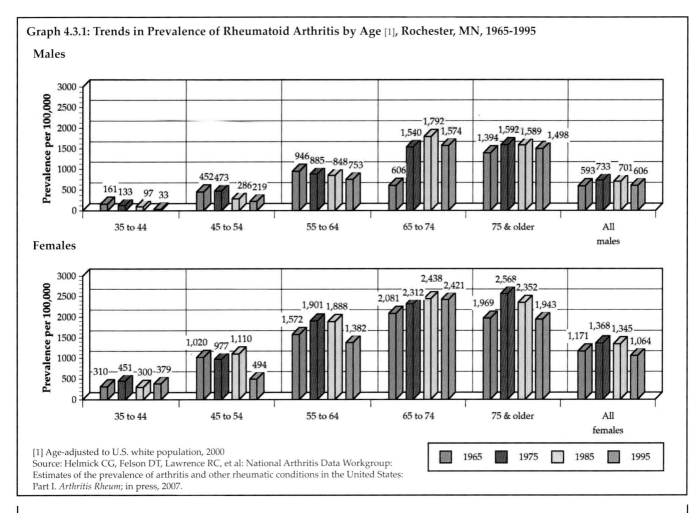

Graph 4.3.1: Trends in Prevalence of Rheumatoid Arthritis by Age [1], Rochester, MN, 1965-1995

Males

Females

[1] Age-adjusted to U.S. white population, 2000
Source: Helmick CG, Felson DT, Lawrence RC, et al: National Arthritis Data Workgroup:
Estimates of the prevalence of arthritis and other rheumatic conditions in the United States:
Part I. *Arthritis Rheum*; in press, 2007.

■ 1965　■ 1975　□ 1985　▨ 1995

Section 4.3.2: Impact and Health Care Utilization for Rheumatoid Arthritis

Rheumatoid arthritis as a primary diagnosis accounted for 1.1 million ambulatory care visits in 2004, representing 2.4% of the 44.2 million non-injury visits with a primary diagnosis of AORC. (Table 4.3) As the primary diagnosis, RA accounted for about 18,000, or 2%, of the 922,100 nonfederal, short stay hospitalizations for AORC in 2004. This estimate does not capture arthritis hospitalizations with orthopaedic procedures as the principal diagnosis or those related to arthritis treatment complications, such as gastrointestinal bleeding related to NSAID use.

Section 4.4: Other Forms of Arthritis

AORC, as a group of conditions, includes more than 100 kinds of arthritis and rheumatic diseases, most of which last a lifetime. Although prevalence numbers for these individual conditions do not begin to approach those of osteoarthritis and rheumatoid arthritis, these conditions are as disabling, and often more so, than medical conditions found in higher numbers. Because these conditions are less common and affect fewer numbers of patients, research to treat or prevent them has fallen behind that of other conditions. Only a few of these conditions are described below, but many more need to be brought to awareness and supported with research funding.

Section 4.4.1: Juvenile Arthritis

Juvenile arthritis appears in a variety of types, with the most common form being juvenile rheumatoid arthritis. All types cause joint inflammation, begin before the age of 16, and are often associated with symptoms and complications that are different from those in adults. Although some types of juvenile arthritis resolve over time and with maturity, damage to young joints can remain throughout a lifetime.

The prevalence of juvenile arthritis in children is very difficult to estimate because of the variety of the diseases and their subtypes.[12] The NADW reported a novel approach using pediatric ambulatory care visits[4, 13] to estimate that 294,000 (95% CI[i] 188,000-400,000) children aged 0 to 17 were affected by the broadly defined "arthritis or other rheumatic conditions" annually for the years 2001 to 2004. The same study estimates these children made 827,000 ambulatory care visits per year during the same time period.

Section 4.4.2: Gout and Other Crystal Arthropathies

Gout is a painful, episodic, recurrent, and sometimes chronic and disabling form of arthritis that has been recognized since ancient times. Symptoms typically consist of intense episodes of painful swelling in single joints, most often in the feet and especially in the big toe. The underlying metabolic cause is an excess of serum uric acid that results in the deposition of crystal in joints and elsewhere.

The self-reported prevalence of gout in a 12-month period prior to the interview has increased over time, reaching 0.94% of all adults aged 18 years and older in 1996.[5] Prevalence increases with age, is higher in men than women at all ages, and is higher in African Americans than

[i] Confidence interval

whites aged 45 years and older. Lifetime self-reported prevalence was 2.6% of adults aged 20 and older between the years 1988-1994, with 8% in adults aged 70 to 79 years reporting they have suffered from gout at some point in their lives. The NADW estimates 3.0 million adults aged 18 years and older had gout in the previous 12 months in 2005, while 6.1 million adults had experienced gout during their lifetime. Prevalence numbers may be overestimated as they are based on self-reported data rather than clinical examination.

Gout and other crystal arthropathies as a primary diagnosis accounted for 730,500 ambulatory care visits in 2004, or 1.7% of the 44.2 million non-injury visits with a primary diagnosis of AORC. (Table 4.3) Gout and other crystal arthropathies as the principal diagnosis accounted for 1.5% of the 992,100 nonfederal, short stay hospitalizations in 2004.

Section 4.4.3: Connective Tissue Diseases

Section 4.4.3a: Systemic Lupus Erythematosus

Systemic lupus erythematosus, also called SLE or lupus, is an autoimmune disorder that can affect the skin, joints, kidneys, lungs, nervous system, and other organs of the body. The most common symptoms include skin rashes and arthritis, often accompanied by fatigue and fever. The clinical course of SLE varies from mild to severe, and typically involves alternating periods of remission and relapse.

Estimates of the prevalence of SLE vary considerably because it is difficult to diagnose and because few good surveys have been done. The NADW used data from the San Francisco study[4,14] and estimates that definite and suspected SLE together affects 322,000 persons, with women affected far more than men, and African

Americans far more than whites. Diffuse diseases of connective tissue, mainly SLE, as a primary diagnosis accounted for 621,000 ambulatory care visits in 2004, or 1.4% of the 44.2 million non-injury visits with a primary diagnosis of AORC. (Table 4.3) Diffuse diseases of connective tissue, mainly SLE, as the principal diagnosis accounted for 1.3% of the 992,100 nonfederal, short stay hospitalizations in 2004.

Section 4.4.3b: Systemic Sclerosis (SSc, scleroderma)

Diffuse systemic sclerosis (SSc) is an autoimmune disease that causes thickening and hardening of the skin. It can also affect the lungs, the heart, gastrointestinal tract, and other internal organs. A population-based study in southeast Michigan estimates the prevalence of SSc to be 27.6 cases per 100,000 population, translating to 49,000 adults nationally, with women affected far more frequently than men and African Americans slightly more than whites in 2005.[4]

Section 4.4.3c: Primary Sjögren's Syndrome

Sjögren's syndrome is an autoimmune, inflammatory disease that most often affects the tear and saliva glands, leading to dry eyes and mouth. "Primary" Sjögren's syndrome occurs in people with no other rheumatologic disease. "Secondary" Sjögren's syndrome occurs in people also diagnosed with another rheumatologic disease, most often SLE and rheumatoid arthritis. The NADW reports the prevalence of primary Sjögren's syndrome to range from 0.19% to 1.39% of the adult population, affecting from 0.4 to 3.1 million adults in 2005.[4]

Section 4.4.4: Other Rheumatic Conditions

Section 4.4.4a: Fibromyalgia

Fibromyalgia is a clinical syndrome defined by chronic widespread muscular pain, fatigue and tenderness of unknown cause. Primary fibromyalgia occurs in people with no other rheumatologic disease. Secondary fibromyalgia occurs in people who are diagnosed with another rheumatologic disease, most often SLE and rheumatoid arthritis.

The NADW used a 1993 Wichita, Kansas, study and estimates about 5.0 million adults aged 18 years and older had primary fibromyalgia in 2005. Prevalence is much higher among women than among men (3.4% vs. 0.5%).[5] A primary diagnosis of "myalgia and myositis, unspecified", a very crude surrogate for primary fibromyalgia, accounted for 2.8 million ambulatory care visits in 2004, or 6.3% of the 44.2 million non-injury visits with a primary diagnosis of AORC. (Table 4.3) "Myalgia and myositis, unspecified" as the principal diagnosis accounted for less than 1% of the 922,100 nonfederal, short stay hospitalizations in 2004.

Section 4.4.4b: Polymyalgia Rheumatica and Giant Cell (temporal) Arteritis

Polymyalgia rheumatica (PMR) typically causes a symmetrical and rapidly developing aching and stiffness around the upper arms, neck, lower back and thighs among persons aged 50 and older. It is closely related to giant cell arteritis (GCA), an inflammation of blood vessels. The most commonly involved blood vessels are the arteries of the scalp and head. The NADW used the only population-based study of PMR and GCA, conducted in Olmsted County, Minnesota, to estimate that among persons 50 years of age or older in the U.S., PMR affected 711,000 (0.74%) and GCA affected 228,000 (0.28%) in 2005.[5] In both of these conditions, prevalence is higher in women than men, and increases dramatically with age.

Section 4.4.4c: Spondylarthropathies

Spondylarthropathies are a family of diseases that include ankylosing spondylitis (AS), reactive arthritis (formerly known as Reiter's syndrome), psoriatic arthritis, enteropathic arthritis (associated with ulcerative colitis or Crohn's disease), juvenile spondylarthropathy, and undifferentiated spondylarthropathy, which encompasses disorders expressing elements of, but failing to fulfill, criteria for the above diseases.

The NADW estimates the prevalence of spondylarthropathies to range roughly from 0.35% to 1.31% of the population aged 25 and older, affecting between 639,000 and 2,417,000 adults. Spondylosis/spondylitis and allied disorders as a primary diagnosis accounted for 1.5 million ambulatory care visits in 2004, or 3.5% of the 44.2 million non-injury visits with a primary diagnosis of AORC. (Tables 4.3a and 4.3b) Spondylosis/spondylitis and allied disorders as the primary diagnosis accounted for 10% of the 992,100 nonfederal, short stay hospitalizations in 2004.

Section 4.4.5: Joint Symptoms and Joint Pain

Longitudinal prevalence numbers for joint pain are not available; however, as noted in Chapter 1, Burden of Musculoskeletal Diseases Overview, chronic joint pain, pain experienced for at least 3 months, was self-reported by 58.9 million persons aged 18 and older in 2005.[15] Chronic joint pain is experienced by persons of all ages, with nearly one-third (29%) of adults under the age of 44 reporting chronic joint pain, and close to one-half (43%) between the ages of 45 and 64 reporting it. In 2004, an estimated 10.3 million ambulatory

care visits, or 23.3% of the 44.2 million non-injury visits with a primary diagnosis of AORC were for joint pain. (Tables 4.3a and 4.3b) Joint pain as the principal diagnosis accounted for 4.5% of the 992,100 nonfederal, short stay hospitalizations in 2004.

Section 4.5: Treatments and Prevention of Arthritis

In recent years, a greater variety of medications have been used to address pain and disability associated with arthritis and other rheumatic conditions. For pain, acetaminophen has remained a primary treatment. For conditions thought to involve inflammation, generic non-steroidal anti-inflammatory drugs (NSAIDs) remain in widespread use. More specific NSAIDs, the Cox-2 inhibitors, have also been developed, although concerns about heart disease as a side effect have limited their use. For specific types of inflammatory arthritis, disease modifying anti-rheumatic drugs (DMARDs) are being used earlier in the course of disease and more widely to try to prevent joint damage and disability. A major improvement in the treatment of rheumatoid arthritis and other types of inflammatory arthritis has been the introduction of expensive, but effective, biological agents, such as tumor necrosis factor-alpha (TNF-α) inhibitors, which often work well where other DMARDs have failed.

Primary prevention, the preventing of an occurrence of AORC, remains a sought-after but elusive goal. Risk factors are not well understood for most of the conditions, and studies are needed to identify these before preventive measures can be developed. Secondary prevention, which is early diagnosis and treatment to help prevent joint damage, is a goal for those with rheumatoid arthritis and other inflammatory types of arthritis. Tertiary prevention, or the prevention of complications for those with AORC, is being pursued through the use of medications and other recommended interventions, such as self-management of the disease, education, physical activity, and weight loss. Cures at specific joint sites may come about through joint replacement surgery.

Section 4.6: Arthroplasty and Total Joint Procedures

Total joint arthroplasty remains the definitive treatment for advanced, symptomatic joint destruction regardless of the underlying cause. Arthroplasty procedures have been developed for a multitude of joints, including hips, knees, shoulders, ankles, elbows, wrists and smaller joints of the hand and foot. The most frequently replaced joints are the knee and hip, followed by the shoulder. The frequency of arthroplasty procedures involving the hand and foot, such as carpal metacarpal arthroplasty, is difficult to estimate because these procedures are often performed on an outpatient basis. Outpatient surgical data are not captured as reliably as inpatient procedures.

Section 4.6.1: Anatomic Distribution of Joint Arthroplasty

In 2004, hip and knee replacements, including revision replacement procedures, accounted for

95% of the 1.07 million arthroplasty procedures performed. (Table 4.7 and Graph 4.6.1) Shoulder procedures accounted for another 4%, with all other joint replacement procedures representing only 1% of the total arthroplasty procedures performed. As previously noted, hand and foot arthroplasties are often performed on an outpatient basis and may be undercounted.

Section 4.6.2: Underlying Diagnoses

Total hip and primary knee replacements are done almost exclusively due to an underlying diagnosis of osteoarthritis (82% and 97%, respectively). (Table 4.8) A small proportion of patients having primary knee replacement have an underlying diagnosis of rheumatoid arthritis or other disorders. Among patients having primary total hip replacement, 5% are due to fracture and 7% to other disorders, such as avascular necrosis, a disease resulting from the temporary or permanent loss of the blood supply to the bone. Two percent (2%) of hip replacements are due to rheumatoid arthritis. Partial total hip replacement, generally a hemiarthoplasty, in which the prosthesis is placed in the femur but not in the acetabulum, is performed principally for hip fracture (83% of cases).

Section 4.6.3: Age and Gender Distribution of Arthroplasty Procedures

Females undergo 62% of all total joint replacement procedures. (Table 4.7) The most striking difference in procedure rates between males and females are in partial hip replacement, 71% of which are performed on females. This difference reflects the much greater incidence of osteoporotic hip fracture in females than occurs in males. Females also undergo total knee replacement almost twice as frequently as males. This difference likely reflects the greater prevalence of knee osteoarthritis in females than in males, which in turn likely reflects

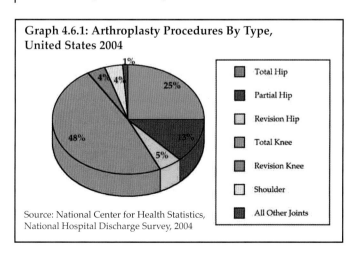

Graph 4.6.1: Arthroplasty Procedures By Type, United States 2004

- Total Hip
- Partial Hip
- Revision Hip
- Total Knee
- Revision Knee
- Shoulder
- All Other Joints

Source: National Center for Health Statistics, National Hospital Discharge Survey, 2004

disproportionate distributions of risk factors. In particular, females have higher prevalence of obesity, which has been identified as a risk factor in osteoarthritis of the knee.

Age distributions of joint arthroplasty procedures are predictable on the basis of the underlying diagnosis. The mean age of patients at the time various arthroplasty procedures are performed has remained fairly constant since 1991 at around 66 to 68 years of age. The exception, partial hip replacements, are performed on patients approximately a decade older due to the incidence of hip fracture in the elderly population. (Table 4.9) Three-fourths (75%) of partial hip replacements are performed in patients older than 74 years and 36% are performed on patients older than 85. Primary and revision total hip and knee arthroplasty procedures are distributed across the adult age strata, but about 60% of each of these procedures are performed on patients aged 65 and older.

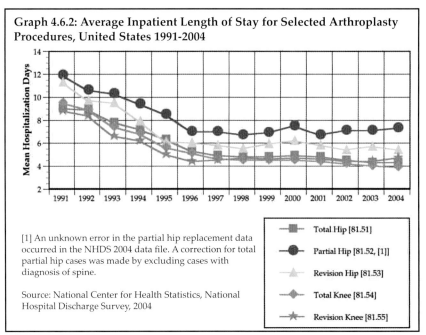

Graph 4.6.2: Average Inpatient Length of Stay for Selected Arthroplasty Procedures, United States 1991-2004

[1] An unknown error in the partial hip replacement data occurred in the NHDS 2004 data file. A correction for total partial hip cases was made by excluding cases with diagnosis of spine.

Source: National Center for Health Statistics, National Hospital Discharge Survey, 2004

- Total Hip [81.51]
- Partial Hip [81.52, [1]]
- Revision Hip [81.53]
- Total Knee [81.54]
- Revision Knee [81.55]

Section 4.6.4: Hospitalization for Arthroplasty Procedures

The length of the average hospital stay following total joint procedures has declined by 50% since 1991, although the reductions appear to be reaching a plateau over the last several years. (Table 4.10 and Graph 4.6.2) The length of stay for partial hip replacement remains considerably higher than those for elective total hip and knee replacement, reflecting the older age and more frail medical status of the hip fracture population. Additionally, surgery is not always done on the day of admission for hip fracture patients, as it generally is for the elective total joint arthroplasty population. Patients undergoing revision hip and knee replacements remain as inpatients for a full

day more, on average, than patients undergoing the primary procedure. This observation is consistent with the greater level of complexity of revision than of primary elective procedures.

Length of stay provides only part of the story of inpatient utilization following total joint arthroplasty. Rates of discharge to home (routine), short-term/skilled nursing/intermediate care, or other discharge sites varies with the national database analyzed and the age of the population. Overall, rates of routine discharge to home are lower in the Nationwide Inpatient Survey (NIS) than are shown in the National Hospital Discharge Survey (NHDS). Using the most optimum picture (NHDS), nearly one-half of joint arthroplasty recipients (44%) who are aged 65 and over are discharged to rehabilitation and nursing facilities for an additional period of inpatient recovery and rehabilitation. (Table 4.11 and Graph 4.6.3) This rate compares to 26% of all hospital inpatient discharges of patients aged 65 and older to another care facility. Even more striking is the 72% of partial hip replacement recipients discharged to long or short-term care facilities for further care, reflecting the frailty of this population.

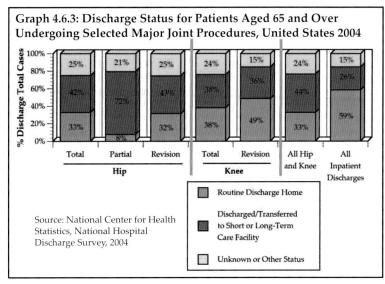

Graph 4.6.3: Discharge Status for Patients Aged 65 and Over Undergoing Selected Major Joint Procedures, United States 2004

Source: National Center for Health Statistics, National Hospital Discharge Survey, 2004

Thus, hospital length of stay by itself substantially underestimates the totality of health system care, especially for the hip fracture population.

Section 4.6.5: Trends in Recent Utilization of Joint Arthroplasty Procedures

From 1991 to 2004, the annual number of total knee replacements increased by almost 3-fold, while the annual number of total hip replacements doubled. (Table 4.12 and Graph 4.6.4) Revision joint arthroplasty procedures for total knee replacement in 2004 were 220% to 235% of the 1991 level. Partial hip joint replacements

saw the slowest increase, up 133% of 1991 levels. These increases in joint arthroplasty utilization are far more dramatic than would be expected from overall population growth and from the increase in the proportion of the population that is elderly.[16] As joint replacement procedures become safer and more durable, the range of symptoms for which joint replacement is successful is broadening. Total hip and knee replacement are now suggested to younger and more active patients on the one hand, and older and more frail patients on the other. The more modest increase in partial hip replacements, a procedure reflective of the epidemiology of age-related hip fracture rather than of physiological changes, supports this hypothesis of total replacement in younger, active patients.

The slower increase in the rate of revisions than in primary procedures likely reflects the temporal lag between primary and revision procedures, which generally occurs with a wearing out of the original replacement device. One would expect that the rate of increase in revisions will reflect the increased rate in primaries after 10 to 15 years.

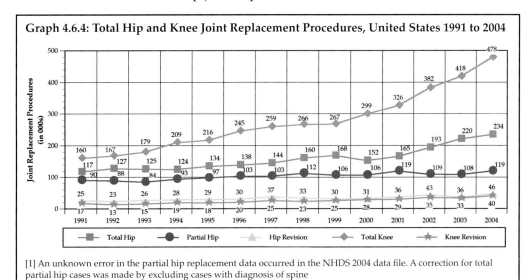

Graph 4.6.4: Total Hip and Knee Joint Replacement Procedures, United States 1991 to 2004

[1] An unknown error in the partial hip replacement data occurred in the NHDS 2004 data file. A correction for total partial hip cases was made by excluding cases with diagnosis of spine
Source: National Center for Health Statistics, National Hospital Discharge Survey, 2004

The mean hospitalization cost of hip and knee joint replacement procedures, excluding charges not routinely billed by the hospital such as physician and prescription costs, increased from 1998 to 2004 by an average 70%, with partial hip replacements (76%) and knee revision

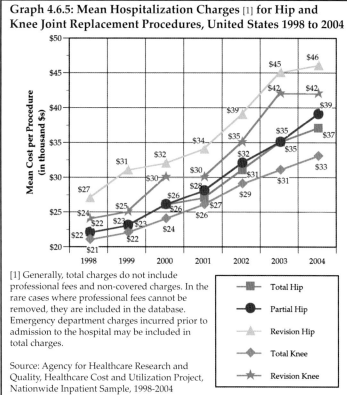

Graph 4.6.5: Mean Hospitalization Charges [1] for Hip and Knee Joint Replacement Procedures, United States 1998 to 2004

[1] Generally, total charges do not include professional fees and non-covered charges. In the rare cases where professional fees cannot be removed, they are included in the database. Emergency department charges incurred prior to admission to the hospital may be included in total charges.

Source: Agency for Healthcare Research and Quality, Healthcare Cost and Utilization Project, Nationwide Inpatient Sample, 1998-2004

procedures (78%) showing the highest level of increase. (Table 4.13 and Graph 4.6.5) Total knee replacements, with a mean increase of 56% in cost, showed the lowest level of per procedure cost increase. In spite of this, due to the rapid

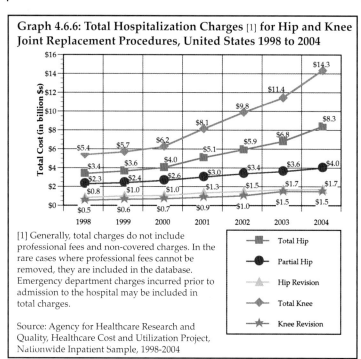

Graph 4.6.6: Total Hospitalization Charges [1] for Hip and Knee Joint Replacement Procedures, United States 1998 to 2004

[1] Generally, total charges do not include professional fees and non-covered charges. In the rare cases where professional fees cannot be removed, they are included in the database. Emergency department charges incurred prior to admission to the hospital may be included in total charges.

Source: Agency for Healthcare Research and Quality, Healthcare Cost and Utilization Project, Nationwide Inpatient Sample, 1998-2004

increase in the number of total knee procedures performed, the total estimated cost of performing total knee replacement procedures jumped from $5.36 billion in 1998 to $14.26 billion in 2004, an increase of 166%. (Table 4.13 and Graph 4.6.6) The total hospitalization cost of hip and knee joint replacements in 2004 was approximately $30 billion. Joint replacement procedures are proven to be one of the most successful procedures available today. In the vast majority of cases, the procedure significantly improves quality of life and the patient's ability to continue work, activities of daily living, and recreational activities. Continued research to improve the longevity of implants with younger, more active patients will reduce the overall burden of arthritis and damaged joints on future generations.

Section 4.6.6: Forecasting Future Utilization of Joint Arthroplasty Procedures

Kurtz and colleagues have performed sophisticated modeling of projected growth in hip and knee replacement procedures.[17] These investigators included in their estimates the growth in the overall population and in the proportion of elderly, as well as recent age and sex specific increases in arthroplasty rates. The results are striking. The investigators estimate that by 2030 there will be over 570,000 primary total hip replacements performed annually in the U.S. and nearly 3.5 million primary total knee replacements. (Table 4.14 and Graph 4.6.7) Although the rate of revision procedures is expected to slowly decline, revisions are projected to remain at a rate of 17% to 18% of primary hip replacements and around 8% of primary knee replacements. (Table 4.14 and Graph 4.6.8) Such staggering growth will have profound consequences for manpower needs, operating room capacity, and health care costs. In 2007 dollars, this volume of total joint

Graph 4.6.7: Projected Number of Primary Total Hip and Knee Arthroplasties, United States 2005-2030

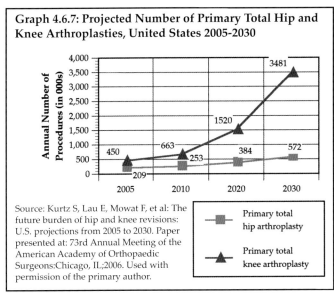

Source: Kurtz S, Lau E, Mowat F, et al: The future burden of hip and knee revisions: U.S. projections from 2005 to 2030. Paper presented at: 73rd Annual Meeting of the American Academy of Orthopaedic Surgeons:Chicago, IL;2006. Used with permission of the primary author.

Graph 4.6.8: Projected Number of Revision Total Hip and Knee Arthroplasties, United States 2005-2030

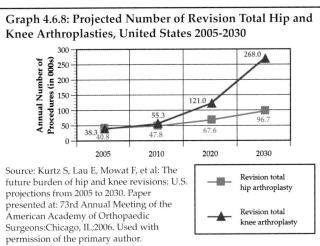

Source: Kurtz S, Lau E, Mowat F, et al: The future burden of hip and knee revisions: U.S. projections from 2005 to 2030. Paper presented at: 73rd Annual Meeting of the American Academy of Orthopaedic Surgeons:Chicago, IL;2006. Used with permission of the primary author.

replacement would generate costs exceeding $100 billion, or 1% of the gross domestic product (GDP). It is critical that the orthopaedic profession anticipate these profound needs for total knee and hip replacement services over the next generation.

Section 4.7: Economic Cost of Arthritis and Related Conditions

The estimated annual cost for medical care of arthritis and joint pain for patients with any diagnosis in 2004 was $281.5 billion, an average of $7,500 for each of the 37.6 million persons who reported having arthritis or joint pain. (Chapter 9:

Health Care Utilization and Economic Cost of Musculoskeletal Diseases) Of this total, $37.3 billion is estimated to be incremental cost that can be directly attributed to arthritis and joint pain, and not a combination of arthritis and other medical conditions. A breakdown of the $281.5 billion cost due to arthritis and joint pain shows 32% for ambulatory care, 32% for emergency room or inpatient care, 23% for prescription drugs, and 13% for other expenses. The cost of arthritis and joint pain, in 2004 dollars, rose from $184.3 billion in 1996 to the $281.5 billion in 2004, an increase of 53%. The increasing cost of prescription drugs accounts for the largest percentage of this total cost increase, rising from 15% of total cost to 23% over the 9 year period.

The indirect cost of earnings losses for persons aged 18 to 64 years with a work history due to three major AORC conditions totals $54.3 billion per year. This includes an estimated $15.2 billion due to gout, $22 billion as a result of osteoarthritis and allied disorders, and $17.1 billion resulting from rheumatoid arthritis.

1. Centers for Disease Control (CDC): Prevalence of disabilities and associated health conditions among adults-United States, 1999. *MMWR Morb Mortal Wkly Rep* 2001;50:120-125.

2. Stoddard S, Jans L, Ripple J, Kraus L: Chartbook on work and disability in the United States, 1998, in *An InfoUse Report*. Washington DC: U.S. National Institute on Disability and Rehabilitation Research, 1998.

3. Hootman JM, Helmick CG: Projections of US prevalence of arthritis and associated activity limitations. *Arthritis Rheum* 2006;54:226-229.

4. Helmick CG, Felson DT, Lawrence, RC, et al: Estimates of the prevalence of arthritis and other rheumatic conditions in the United States: part I. *Arthritis Rheum* 2007;in press.

5. Helmick CG, Felson DT, Lawrence, RC, et al: Estimates of the prevalence of arthritis and other rheumatic conditions in the United States: part II. *Arthritis Rheum* 2007;in press.

6. Hootman J, Bolen J, Helmick C, Langmaid G: Prevalence of doctor-diagnosed arthritis and arthritis-attributable activity limitation-United States, 2003-2005. *MMWR Morb Mortal Wkly Rep* 2006;55:1089-1092.

7. Bolen J, Sniezek J, Theis K, et al: Racial and ethnic differences in the prevalence and impact of doctor-diagnosed arthritis-United States, 2002. *MMWR Morb Mortal Wkly Rep* 2005;54:119-123.

8. Mili F, Helmick CG, Moriarty DG: Health related quality of life among adults reporting arthritis: Analysis of data from the Behavioral Risk Factor Surveillance System,US, 1996-99. *J Rheumatol* 2003;30:160-166.

9. Sacks JJ, Helmick CG, Langmaid G: Deaths from arthritis and other rheumatic conditions, United States, 1979-1998. *J Rheumatol* 2004;31:1823-1828.

10. Abell JE, Hootman JM, Helmick CG: Prevalence and impact of arthritis among nursing home residents. *Ann Rheum Dis* 2004;63:591-594.

11. Yelin E, Murphy L, Cisternas MG, et al: Medical care expenditures and earnings losses among persons with arthritis and other rheumatic conditions in 2003 and comparisons with 1997. *Arthritis Rheum* 2007;56:1397-1407.

12. Manners PJ, Bower C: Worldwide prevalence of juvenile arthritis - Why does it vary so much? *J Rheumatol* 2002;29:1520-1530.

13. Sacks JJ, Helmick CG, Luo Y-H, et al: Prevalence of and annual ambulatory health care visits for pediatric arthritis and other rheumatologic conditions, United States, 2001-2004. *Arthritis Rheum* 2007;57(8):1439-1445.

14. Fessel W: Systemic lupus erythematosus in the community: incidence, prevalence, outcome and first symptoms: The high prevalence in black women. *Arch Intern Med* 1974;134:1027-1035.

15. National Center for Health Statistics: National Health Interview Survey, Adult Sample Level File, 2005.

16. Praemer A, Furner S, Rice DP: *Musculoskeletal Conditions in the United States,* ed 2. Rosemont, IL: American Academy of Orthopaedic Surgeons, 1999, p 182.

17. Source: Kurtz S, Lau E, Mowat F, et al: The future burden of hip and knee revisions: U.S. projections from 2005 to 2030. Paper presented at: 73rd Annual Meeting of the American Academy of Orthopaedic Surgeons:Chicago, IL;2006.

Section 4.8: Arthritis and Related Conditions Data Tables

Table 4.1: Diagnostic Categories ICD-9-CM Codes for Arthritis and Other Rheumatic Conditions (AORC)

Osteoarthritis and allied disorders
715-Osteoarthritis and allied disorders
Rheumatoid arthritis
Gout and other crystal arthropathies
274-Gout
712-Crystal arthropathies
Joint pain, effusion and other unspecified joint disorders
716.1, .3-.6-.9 - Other unspecified arthropathies
719.0, .4-.9-Other and unspecified joint disorders
Spondylarthropathies
720-AS/inflammatory spondylopathies
721-Spondylosis and allied disorders
99.3-Reiter's Disease
696.0-Psoriatic arthopathy
Systemic Lupus Erythematosus (SLE)
710.0-Systemic lupus erythematosus
Systemic Sclerosis (SSC, scleroderma)
710.1-Systemic sclerosis
Fibromyalgia
729.1-Myalgia and myositis unspecified
Sjögren's syndrome
710.2-Sicca syndrome (also called Sjögren's syndrome)
Polymyalgia rheumaticus (PMR) and Giant cell
(termpol) arteritis (GCA)
725-Polymyalgia rheumatica
446.5-Polyarteritis nodosa and allied conditions
Other specified rheumatic conditions
Difuse connective tissue disease
710-Diffuse connective tissue disease [excl 710.0-.2]
Carpal tunnel syndrome
354.0-Carpal tunnel syndrome

Other specified rheumatic conditions (continued)
Other AORC
711-Arthritis associated with infections
713-Arthropathy associated w/disorders
classified elsewhere
716.0, .2, .8-Specified arthropathies
719.2, .3-Specified joint disorders
95.6-Syphilis of muscle
95.7-Syphilis of synovium/tendon/bursa
98.5-Gonococcal infection of joint
136.1-Behcet's syndrome
277.2-Other disorders purine/pyrimidine metabolism
287.0-Allergic purpura
344.6-Cauda equina syndrome
353.0-Brachial plexus/thoracic outlet lesions
355.5-Tarsal tunnel syndrome
357.1-Polyneuropathy in collagen vascular disease
390-Rheumatic fever w/o heart disease
391-Rheumatic fever w/heart disease
437.4-Cerebral arteritis
443.0-Raynaud's syndrome
446-Polyarteritis nodosa and allied conditions
[excl 446.5]
447.6-Arteritis, unspecified
Soft tissue disorders (excluding back)
726-Peripheral enthesopathies and allied disorders
727-Other disorders of synovium/tendon/bursa
728.0-.3, .6–.9-Disorders of muscle/ligament/fascia
729.0-Rheumatism, unspecified and fibrositis
[excl 729.1]
729.4-Fascitis, unspecified

Source: Centers for Disease Control and Prevention, Arthritis Program, National Arthritis Data Workgroup. Available at: http://www.cdc.gov/arthritis/data_statistics/arthritis_codes_2004.pdf. Accessed: August 16, 2007

Table 4.2: Prevalence of Self-Reported Doctor-Diagnoses Arthritis and Arthritis-Attributable Activity Limitations Among Adults Age 18 & Older by Age, Sex, and Race/Ethnicity, United States, 2003-2005

| | Arthritis and Arthritis-Attributable Activity Limitation Prevalence | | | | | | Proportion with Arthritis-Attributable Activity Limitation Among Those with Doctor-Diagnosed Arthritis | |
| | Doctor-Diagnosed Arthritis [1] | | | Arthritis-Attributable Activity Limitation [2] | | | | |
	Unadjusted Prevalence (in millions)	% Age Unadjusted	% Age-Adjusted*	Unadjusted Prevalence (in millions)	% Age Unadjusted	% Age-Adjusted*	% Age Unadjusted	% Age-Adjusted*
Gender								
Male	18.2	17.6%	18.1%	7.0	6.8%	7.0%	38.8%	36.6%
Female	28.3	25.4%	24.4%	11.9	10.7%	10.3%	42.3%	39.0%
Age								
18-44 years	8.7	7.9%	na	3.0	2.7%	na	34.6%	na
45-64 years	20.5	29.3%	na	8.2	11.8%	na	40.3%	na
65 & Over	17.2	50.0%	na	7.7	22.4%	na	44.9%	na
Race/Ethnicity								
White, non-Hispanic	37.2	24.3%	22.6%	14.7	9.6%	8.9%	39.5%	36.4%
Black, non-Hispanic	4.6	19.2%	21.4%	2.2	9.2%	10.3%	47.8%	44.3%
Hispanic	3.1	11.4%	16.5%	1.5	5.4%	8.2%	47.6%	45.2%
Other non-Hispanic	1.6	14.7%	17.3%	0.7	6.0%	7.2%	41.1%	40.5%
Total	46.4	21.6%	21.5%	18.9	8.8%	8.8%	40.9%	38.1%

* Age adjusted to the projected 2000 population age 18 years or older by three age groups: 18-44, 45-64 and 65 & over

[1] Responded "Yes" when asked: Have you EVER been told by a doctor or other health professional that you have some form of arthritis, rheumatoid arthritis, gout, lupus, or fibromyalgia?

[2] Responded "Yes" when asked: Are you now limited in any way in any of your usual activities because of arthritis or joint symptoms?

Source: National Center for Health Statistics, National Health Interview Survey, 2003-2005

Table 4.3a: Impact and Health Care Utilization for Select Arthritis and Other Rheumatic Conditions for Adults Aged 18 & Older, United States, 2004

All Diagnosis

Visits (in 000s)

AORC Condition [1]	Inpatient Hospitalization [2]	Ambulatory Care Services Physician Visits [3]	ER Visits [4]	Outpatient Visits [5]	Total Ambulatory Care
Osteoarthritis	2,225.6	17,425.7	206.0	1,233.7	18,659.4
Rheumatoid Arthritis	343.7	1,823.5	41.3 *	169.5	1,993.0
Gout and Other Crystal Arthropathies	421.0	1,583.3	221.7	102.9	1,686.2
Systemic Lupus Erythematosus (SLE)	141.7	770.3 *	35.3 *	76.2	846.5
Systemic Sclerosis (SSc, scleroderma)	0.0	0.0	0.0	0.0	0.0
Primary Sjögren's Syndrome	22.7	578.2 *	0.0	13.5 *	591.7
Fibromyalgia	221.8	4,222.7	473.2	392.4	4,615.1
Polymyalgia Rheumatica and Giant Cell Arteritis	90.8	568.7 *	9.4 *	14.6 *	583.3
Spondylarthropathies	377.9	3,103.2	40.2 *	145.6	3,248.8
Joint Pain	713.5	16,013.9	1,590.1	1,453.5	17,467.4
All Other Arthritis and Other Rheumatic Conditions	588.3	21,248.8	913.6	1,512.3	22,761.1
Total AORC Diagnoses	4,572.5	61,847.8	3,320.6	4,589.1	66,436.9
All Visits	31,950.0	739,398.6	83,074.3	62,991.3	885,464.2

Primary (1st) Diagnosis

Visits (in 000s)

AORC Condition [1]	Inpatient Hospitalization [2]	Ambulatory Care Services Physician Visits [3]	ER Visits [4]	Outpatient Visits [5]	Total Ambulatory Care
Osteoarthritis	662.2	10,448.4	101.4 *	611.5	11,059.9
Rheumatoid Arthritis	17.5	957.7 *	25.3 *	123.2	1,080.9
Gout and Other Crystal Arthropathies	15.2	695.3 *	159.0	35.2 *	730.5
Systemic Lupus Erythematosus (SLE)	12.9	570.2 *	18.3 *	50.8	621.0
Systemic Sclerosis (SSc, scleroderma)	0.0	0.0	0.0	0.0	0.0
Primary Sjögren's Syndrome	0.5 *	317.2 *	0.0	7.2 *	324.4
Fibromyalgia	8.3	2,591.2	338.6	195.2	2,786.4
Polymyalgia Rheumatica and Giant Cell Arteritis	5.2	424.7 *	3.7 *	7.6 *	432.3
Spondylarthropathies	99.7	1,485.1	9.5 *	56.8	1,541.9
Joint Pain	44.9	9,391.2	1,053.6	891.1	10,282.3
All Other Arthritis and Other Rheumatic Conditions	126.5	14,338.5	596.1	977.2	15,315.7
% Total AORC Diagnoses to All Diagnoses	992.1	41,195.1	2,304.8	2,955.9	44,151.0
% of Ambulatory Visits	31,950.0	739,398.6	83,074.3	62,991.3	885,464.2

* Estimate does not meet standards for reliability

[1] ICD-9-CM diagnosis codes for AORC listed in appendix

[2] Source: Agency for Healthcare Research and Quality, Healthcare Cost and Utilization Project, Nationwide Inpatient Sample, 2004

[3] Source: National Center for Health Statistics, National Ambulatory Medical Care Survey, 2004

[4] Source: National Center for Health Statistics, National Hospital Ambulatory Medical Care Survey, Hospital Emergency, 2004

[5] Source: National Center for Health Statistics, National Hospital Ambulatory Medical Care Survey, Outpatient Centers, 2004

NOTE: This table and all related graphs created by the Burden of Musculoskeletal Disease project analyst.

Table 4.3b: Proportion of Total AORC Visits for Select Arthritis and Other Rheumatic Conditions for Adults Aged 18 & Older, United States 2004

All Diagnosis

Visits (in 000s)

Ambulatory Care Services

AORC Condition [1]	Inpatient Hospitalization [2]	Physician Visits [3]	ER Visits [4]	Outpatient Visits [5]	Total Ambulatory Care
Osteoarthritis	48.7%	28.2%	6.2%	26.9%	28.1%
Rheumatoid Arthritis	7.5%	2.9%	1.2%	3.7%	3.0%
Gout and Other Crystal Arthropathies	9.2%	2.6%	6.7%	2.2%	2.5%
Systemic Lupus Erythematosus (SLE)	3.1%	1.2%	1.1%	1.7%	1.3%
Systemic Sclerosis (SSc, scleroderma)	0.0%	0.0%	0.0%	0.0%	0.0%
Primary Sjögren's Syndrome	0.5%	0.9%	0.0%	0.3%	0.9%
Fibromyalgia	4.9%	6.8%	14.3%	8.6%	6.9%
Polymyalgia Rheumatica and Giant Cell Arteritis	2.0%	0.9%	0.3%	0.3%	0.9%
Spondylarthropathies	8.3%	5.0%	1.2%	3.2%	4.9%
Joint Pain	15.6%	25.9%	47.9%	31.7%	26.3%
All Other Arthritis and Other Rheumatic Conditions	12.9%	34.4%	27.5%	33.0%	34.3%
Total AORC Diagnoses	14.3%	8.4%	4.0%	7.3%	7.5%
All Visits		88.7%	4.8%	6.6%	

Primary (1st) Diagnosis

Visits (in 000s)

Ambulatory Care Services

AORC Condition [1]	Inpatient Hospitalization [2]	Physician Visits [3]	ER Visits [4]	Outpatient Visits [5]	Total Ambulatory Care
Osteoarthritis	66.7%	25.4%	4.4%	20.7%	25.1%
Rheumatoid Arthritis	1.8%	2.3%	1.1%	4.2%	2.4%
Gout and Other Crystal Arthropathies	1.5%	1.7%	6.9%	1.2%	1.7%
Systemic Lupus Erythematosus (SLE)	1.3%	1.4%	0.8%	1.7%	1.4%
Systemic Sclerosis (SSc, scleroderma)	0.0%	0.0%	0.0%	0.0%	0.0%
Primary Sjögren's Syndrome	0.1%	0.8%	0.0%	0.2%	0.7%
Fibromyalgia	0.8%	6.3%	14.7%	6.6%	6.3%
Polymyalgia Rheumatica and Giant Cell Arteritis	0.5%	1.0%	0.2%	0.3%	1.0%
Spondylarthropathies	10.0%	3.6%	0.4%	1.9%	3.5%
Joint Pain	4.5%	22.8%	45.7%	30.1%	23.3%
All Other Arthritis and Other Rheumatic Conditions	12.8%	34.8%	25.9%	33.1%	34.7%
% Total AORC Diagnoses to All Diagnoses	3.1%	5.6%	2.8%	4.7%	5.0%
% of Ambulatory Visits		88.7%	5.0%	6.4%	

* Estimate does not meet standards for reliability

[1] ICD-9-CM diagnosis codes for AORC listed in appendix

[2] Source: Agency for Healthcare Research and Quality, Healthcare Cost and Utilization Project, Nationwide Inpatient Sample, 2004

[3] Source: National Center for Health Statistics, National Ambulatory Medical Care Survey, 2004

[4] Source: National Center for Health Statistics, National Hospital Ambulatory Medical Care Survey, Hospital Emergency, 2004

[5] Source: National Center for Health Statistics, National Hospital Ambulatory Medical Care Survey, Outpatient Centers, 2004

NOTE: This table and all related graphs created by the Burden of Musculoskeletal Disease project analyst.

Table 4.4: Ambulatory Care Resource Use for Non-Injury Arthritis and Other Rheumatic Conditions (AORC) for Persons Aged 18 and Older, United States, 1997 and 2004

Proportion of All Primary (1st) Diagnosis of AORC, United States 1997

Physician Office Visits

Ambulatory Care Resource		Physician Specialty		Health Care Provider	
Physician Office	89%	Primary Care Physician	53%	Physician	97%
Outpatient Department	7%	Orthopaedic Surgeon	20%	Nurse	51%
Emergency Department	4%	Rheumatologist	17%	Midlevel Provider	24%
		Other Provider	10%		
Total Visits for AORC	36.5 million			AORC as % All Health Care Visits	3.8%

Source: Hootman JM, Helmick CG, Schappert SM. Magnitude and characteristics of arthritis and other rheumatic conditions on ambulatory medical care visits, United States, 1997. Arthritis Rheum 200247:571–81

Proportion of All Primary (1st) Diagnosis of AORC, United States 2004

Physician Office Visits [1]

Ambulatory Care Resource		Physician Specialty		Health Care Provider Visits	
Physician Office [1]	89%	Primary Care Physician [4]	45%	Physician	98%
Outpatient Department [2]	6%	Orthopaedic Surgeon	36%	Nurse [6]	41%
Emergency Department [3]	5%	Rheumatologist, Neurologist, PM&R [5]	5%	Midlevel Provider [7]	3%
		Other Provider	14%	Other Provider	8%
Total Visits for AORC	41.2 million			AORC as % All Health Care Visits	5.6%

[1] Source: National Center for Health Statistics, National Ambulatory Medical Care Survey, 2004

[2] Source: National Center for Health Statistics, National Hospital Ambulatory Care Survey, Outpatient Centers, 2004

[3] Source: National Center for Health Statistics, National Hospital Ambulatory Care Survey, Hospital Emergency, 2004

[4] Includes family practice, family practice (geriatric medicine), sports medicine (family practice), general practice, general surgery, internal medicine, geriatric medicine (internal medicine).

[5] Includes rheumatology, neurology, neurological surgery, physical medicine and rehabilitation.

[6] Includes registered nurse, licensed practical nurse, and medical/nursing assistant.

[7] Includes physician assistant and nurse practitioner/midwife

Table 4.5: Prevalence of Symptomatic Osteoarthritis in the Hands, Knees and Hips, United States, Various Studies

	Age	Source	Symptomatic Osteoarthritis Prevalence per 100 Persons*		
			Male	Female	Total
Hands	26 & over	[1]	3.8	9.2	6.8
Knees	26 & over	[1]	4.6	4.9	4.9
	45 & over	[1]	5.9	7.2	6.7
	45 & over	[2]	13.5	18.7	16.7
	60 & over	[3]	10.0	13.6	12.1
Hips	45 & over	[2]	8.7	9.3	9.2

*Age-standardized to the projected 2000 census population exception is the NHANES III estimates are standardized to the 1980 U.S. population

[1] Framingham (Massachusetts) Osteoarthritis Study

[2] Johnston County (North Carolina) Osteoarthritis Study

[3] NHANES III, 1988-1994

Table 4.6: Trends in Prevalence of Rheumatoid Arthritis by Sex and Age [1], Rochester, MN, 1965-1995

FEMALES — Prevalence (in 100,000s)

Age-group	1965	1975	1985	1995
35-44	310	451	300	379
45-54	1,020	977	1,110	494
55-64	1,572	1,901	1,888	1,382
65-74	2,081	2,312	2,438	2,421
75+	1,969	2,568	2,352	1,943
All Females	1,171	1,368	1,345	1,064

MALES — Prevalence (in 100,000s)

Age-group	1965	1975	1985	1995
35-44	161	133	97	33
45-54	452	473	286	219
55-64	946	885	848	753
65-74	606	1,540	1,792	1,574
75+	1,394	1,592	1,589	1,498
All Males	593	733	701	606

[1] Age-adjusted to U.S. White population, 2000

Source: Helmick CG, Felson DT, Lawrence RC, et. al. National Arthritis Data Workgroup: Estimates of the prevalence of arthritis and other rheumatic conditions in the United States: Part I. *Arthritis & Rheumatism*; 2007 in press.

Table 4.7 Arthroplasty Procedures By Type by Gender, United States 2004

	Male		Female		All Persons	
	Number of Procedures	% of Total Procedures	Number of Procedures	% of Total Procedures	Number of Procedures	% of Total Procedures
All Hip Replacement Procedures [1,7]	203,212	39.7%	308,656	60.3%	511,868	54.1%
Total Hip Replacement (81.51)	98,266	42.2%	134,591	57.8%	232,857	24.6%
Partial Hip Replacement (81.52)	35,188	29.4%	84,500	70.6%	119,688	12.7%
Revision Hip Replacement (91.53	19,418	42.5%	26,271	57.5%	45,689	4.8%
All Knee Replacement Procedures [2]	175,131	34.7%	329,569	65.3%	504,700	53.3%
Total Knee Replacement (81.54)	157,310	34.6%	297,342	65.4%	454,652	48.1%
Revision Knee Replacement (81.55)	11,564	29.5%	27,636	70.5%	39,200	4.1%
All Shoulder Replacement Procedures [3]	19,667	46.9%	22,309	53.2%	41,934	4.4%
All Other Joint Replacement Procedures [4]	5,003	41.5%	7,052	58.5%	12,055	1.3%
All Joint Replacement Procedures [5]	402,213	37.6%	667,502	62.4%	1,069,715	100.0%

[1] Includes ICD-9-CM procedure codes for total, partial, revision, and hip repair procedures

[2] Includes ICD-9-CM procedure codes for total, revision, and knee repair procedures

[3] Includes ICD-9-CM procedure codes for primary and revision shoulder arthroplasty

[4] Includes ICD-9-CM procedure codes finger, wrist, hand, elbow, toe, foot, ankle, and lower extremity

[5] Includes ICD-9-CM procedure codes for all above procedures.

[6] Total procedures may include cases with multiple procedures.

[7] An unknown error in the partial hip replacement data occurred in the NHDS 2004 data file. A correction for total partial hip cases was made by excluding cases with diagnosis of spine (720.xx-724.xx, 737.xx, 756.xx, 805.xx, 806.xx)

Source: National Center for Health Statistics, National Hospital Discharge Survey, 2004

Table 4.8: Principal Diagnoses Associated with Hip and Knee Joint Replacement, United States 2004

	Proportion of Total Replacement Procedures		
	Total Hip Replacement [1]	Partial Hip Replacement [2,4]	Primary Knee Replacement [3]
Osteoarthritis, Primary and Secondary	82.5%	1.4%	96.8%
Rheumatoid Arthritis	1.6%		0.8%
Other or Unspecified Arthropathy	0.8%	0.3%	0.0%
Fracture of Neck of Femur, Femur or Lower Leg, Including Pathological Fracture	4.9%	82.8%	
Other Diseases of Bone and Cartilage	7.4%	0.2%	0.2%
Complication of Internal Orthopedic Device, Implant, and Graft	1.3%	4.1%	
All Other	1.5%	11.2%	2.2%
Total Procedures	232,857	119,688	454,652

[1] ICD-9-CM procedure code 8151.   [2] ICD-9-CM procedure code 8152.   [3] ICD-9-CM procedure code 8154.

[4] An unknown error in the partial hip replacement data occurred in the NHDS 2004 data file. A correction for total partial hip cases was made by excluding cases with diagnosis of spine (720.xx-724.xx, 737.xx, 756.xx, 805.xx, 806.xx)

Source: National Center for Health Statistics, National Hospital Discharge Survey, 2004

Table 4.9: Arthroplasty Procedures By Type by Mean Age, United States 1991-2004

Mean Age of Joint Replacement Patients

	Total Hip Replacement [1]	Partial Hip Replacement [2,6]	Revision Hip Replacement [3]	Total Knee Replacement [4]	Revision Knee Replacement [5]
1991	67.1	78.3	64.8	68.5	68.5
1992	67.0	76.7	68.1	69.6	68.7
1993	66.5	79.6	66.4	69.2	67.2
1994	66.6	79.7	63.6	69.1	68.5
1995	67.0	79.4	66.6	68.3	67.6
1996	67.6	78.6	65.9	69.4	67.8
1997	66.9	79.7	66.9	68.3	69.9
1998	67.7	79.5	68.9	68.4	70.3
1999	66.1	80.4	68.5	68.4	69.6
2000	65.6	78.9	66.2	68.3	67.7
2001	66.6	80.4	65.1	67.9	67.9
2002	66.7	79.9	68.4	67.6	69.7
2003	65.4	80.0	65.5	67.1	63.5
2004	65.9	74.8	68.4	67.2	67.0
14-Year Average	66.6	79.0	66.7	68.4	68.1

[1] ICD-9-CM procedure code 81.51.

[2] ICD-9-CM procedure code 81.52.

[3] ICD-9-CM procedure code 81.53

[4] ICD-9-CM procedure code 81.54.

[5] ICD-9-CM procedure code 81.55

[6] An unknown error in the partial hip replacement data occurred in the NHDS 2004 data file. A correction for total partial hip cases was made by excluding cases with diagnosis of spine (720.xx-724.xx, 737.xx, 756.xx, 805.xx, 806.xx). The resulting age drop may be due to this error.

Source: National Center for Health Statistics, National Hospital Discharge Survey, 1991-2004

Table 4.10: Average Inpatient Length of Stay for Selected Arthroplasty Procedures, United States 1991-2004

Mean Days of Hospitalization for Procedure

	Total Hip Replacement [81.51]	Partial Hip Replacement [81.52, 1]	Revision of Hip Replacement [81.53]	Total Knee Replacement [81.54]	Revision of Knee Replacement [81.55]
1991	9.0	11.9	11.3	9.5	8.8
1992	8.9	10.6	9.7	8.9	8.4
1993	7.8	10.3	9.5	7.4	6.6
1994	7.2	9.4	7.9	6.8	6.2
1995	6.3	8.5	6.1	5.6	5.0
1996	5.3	7.0	6.0	5.1	4.4
1997	4.9	7.0	5.8	4.6	4.5
1998	4.8	6.7	5.5	4.5	4.7
1999	4.8	6.9	5.9	4.5	4.6
2000	4.9	7.5	6.2	4.5	4.7
2001	4.8	6.7	5.8	4.4	4.6
2002	4.5	7.1	5.4	4.2	4.4
2003	4.3	7.1	5.7	4.0	4.4
2004	4.3	7.3	5.4	3.9	4.7

[1] An unknown errr in the partial hip replacement data occurred in the NHDS 2004 data file. A correction for total partial hip cases was made by excluding cases with diagnosis of spine (720.xx-724.xx, 737.xx, 756.xx, 805.xx, 806.xx)

Source: National Center for Health Statistics, National Hospital Discharge Survey, 2004

Table 4.11: Discharge Status for Patients Aged 18 and Over and 65 and Over Undergoing Selected Major Joint Procedures, Comparison of Two National Health Care Hospital Discharge Surveys, United States 2004

Aged 18 Years and Older

NHDS Survey [1]	Proportion of Total Replacement Patients						All Inpatient Discharges
	Total Hip [3]	Partial Hip [4,8]	Revision Hip [5]	Total Knee [6]	Revision Knee [7]	All Hip and Knee	
Routine Discharge Home	45.5%	13.2%	38.0%	47.5%	49.4%	47.0%	75.0%
Discharged/ Transferred to Short-Term/Skilled Nursing/ Intermediate Care	32.6%	65.8%	39.2%	30.8%	34.6%	32.7%	0.1%
Unknown/ Other Discharge Status	21.9%	21.0%	22.8%	21.7%	16.0%	20.3%	10.6%
Total Cases	232,857	114,576	45,068	454,382	39,155	1,007,553	31,711,934
NIS Survey [2]							
Routine Discharge Home	20.6%	5.3%	19.3%	23.2%	22.6%	20.8%	69.9%
Discharged/ Transferred to Short-Term/Skilled Nursing/ Intermediate Care	50.4%	86.2%	49.3%	46.7%	41.7%	52.0%	16.8%
Unknown/ Other Discharge Status	29.1%	8.4%	31.5%	31.1%	35.8%	27.2%	13.3%
Total Cases	226,484	104,802	37,848	434,222	35,108	845,500	31,950,026

Aged 65 Years and Older

NHDS Survey [1]	Proportion of Total Replacement Patients						All Inpatient Discharges
	Total Hip [3]	Partial Hip [4,8]	Revision Hip [5]	Total Knee [6]	Revision Knee [7]	All Hip and Knee	
Routine Discharge Home	33.1%	7.8%	31.6%	38.2%	48.6%	32.8%	58.5%
Discharged/ Transferred to Short-Term/Skilled Nursing/ Intermediate Care	41.9%	71.7%	43.0%	37.8%	36.0%	43.6%	26.1%
Unknown/ Other Discharge Status	24.9%	20.5%	25.4%	24.1%	15.4%	23.6%	15.4%
Total Cases	135,400	99,125	32,182	280,118	24,859	599,541	13,170,557
NIS Survey [2]							
Routine Discharge Home	12.6%	3.9%	13.4%	17.5%	16.6%	13.7%	50.2%
Discharged/ Transferred to Short-Term/Skilled Nursing/ Intermediate Care	66.8%	89.0%	62.4%	57.7%	52.1%	65.4%	30.1%
Unknown/ Other Discharge Status	20.6%	7.1%	24.2%	24.8%	31.4%	20.9%	19.7%
Total Cases	127,930	95,569	23,289	269,069	20,764	536,040	13,090,185

[1] Source: National Center for Health Statistics, National Hospital Discharge Survey, 2004

[2] Source: National Center for Health Statistics, Nationwide Inpatient Sample, 2004

[3] ICD-9-CM procedure code 81.51   [4] ICD-9-CM procedure code 81.52

[5] ICD-9-CM procedure code 81.53   [6] ICD-9-CM procedure code 81.54

[7] ICD-9-CM procedure code 81.55

[8] An unknown error in the partial hip replacement data occurred in the NHDS 2004 data file. A correction for total partial hip cases was made by excluding cases with diagnosis of spine (720.xx-724.xx, 737.xx, 756.xx, 805.xx, 806.xx).

Table 4.12: Joint Replacement Procedures in the United States, 1991-2004

National Hospital Discharge Survey

Joint Replacement Procedures (in 000s)

Description	ICD-9 CM Code	1991	1992	1993	1994	1995	1996	1997	1998	1999	2000	2001	2002	2003	2004
Total Hip Replacement	81.51	117.0	127.0	125.0	124.0	134.0	138.0	144.0	160.0	168.0	152.0	165.5	193.0	220.1	234.0
Partial Hip Replacement [1]	81.52	90.0	88.0	84.0	93.0	97.0	103.0	103.0	112.0	106.0	106.0	118.5	108.8	108.0	119.7
Revision of Hip Replacement	81.53	25.0	23.0	26.0	28.0	29.0	30.0	37.0	33.0	30.0	31.0		36.1	42.7	35.6	46.0
Total Knee Replacement	81.54	160.0	167.0	179.0	209.0	216.0	245.0	259.0	266.0	267.0	299.0	325.6	381.3	418.3	478.0
Revision of Knee Replacement	81.55	17.0	13.0	15.0	19.0	18.0	20.0	25.0	23.0	25.0	28.0	29.4	35.1	33.1	40.0
TOTAL Hip and Knee Replacement/Revision Procedures		409.0	418.0	429.0	473.0	494.0	536.0	568.0	594.0	596.0	616.0	675.1	760.8	815.1	917.7

[1] An unknown error in the partial hip replacement data occurred in the NHDS 2004 data file. A correction for total partial hip cases was made by excluding cases with diagnosis of spine (720.xx-724.xx, 737.xx, 756.xx, 805.xx, 806.xx)

Source: National Center for Health Statistics, National Hospital Discharge Survey, 1991-2004

Nationwide Inpatient Sample

Joint Replacement Procedures (in 000s)

Description	ICD-9 CM Code	1991	1992	1993	1994	1995	1996	1997	1998	1999	2000	2001	2002	2003	2004
Total Hip Replacement	81.51	135.7	139.9	144.1	148.2	152.6	157.0	161.6	166.7	171.7	176.1	181.5	187.7	194.3	227.5
Partial Hip Replacement	81.52	96.3	97.9	99.5	100.8	102.2	103.5	104.7	105.8	106.8	107.4	108.7	109.9	111.2	105.1
Revision of Hip Replacement	81.53	27.5	28.3	29.1	29.9	30.8	31.7	32.5	33.5	34.4	35.2	36.2	37.2	38.3	37.9
Total Knee Replacement	81.54	192.2	203.6	215.5	227.9	241.1	255.1	270.0	286.6	304.0	321.8	342.0	365.3	391.1	435.5
Revision of Knee Replacement	81.55	16.5	17.5	18.5	19.5	20.7	21.9	23.2	24.6	26.1	27.6	29.3	31.2	33.4	36.2
TOTAL Hip and Knee Replacement/Revision Procedures		468.2	487.2	506.7	526.3	547.4	569.2	592.0	617.2	643.0	668.1	697.7	731.3	768.3	842.2

Source: Agency for Healthcare Research and Quality, Healthcare Cost and Utilization Project, Nationwide Inpatient Sample, 1991-2004

Table 4.13: Mean and Total Hospitalization Charges [1] for Hip and Knee Joint Replacement Procedures, United States, 1998-2004

Average (Mean) Charges Per Hospitalization (rounded to nearest 000)							
	1998	**1999**	**2000**	**2001**	**2002**	**2003**	**2004**
Total Hip Replacement [2]	$22,000	$23,000	$26,000	$27,000	$31,000	$35,000	$37,000
Partial Hip Replacement [3]	$22,000	$23,000	$26,000	$28,000	$32,000	$35,000	$39,000
Revision Hip Replacement [4]	$27,000	$31,000	$32,000	$34,000	$39,000	$45,000	$46,000
Total Knee Replacement [5]	$21,000	$22,000	$24,000	$26,000	$29,000	$31,000	$33,000
Revision Knee Replacement [6]	$24,000	$25,000	$30,000	$30,000	$35,000	$42,000	$42,000

Total Hospitalization Charges for Joint Replacements (in billions)							
	1998	**1999**	**2000**	**2001**	**2002**	**2003**	**2004**
Total Hip Replacement [2]	$3.37	$3.64	$4.00	$5.07	$5.91	$6.77	$8.34
Partial Hip Replacement [3]	$2.27	$2.39	$2.63	$2.98	$3.35	$3.58	$3.97
Revision Hip Replacement [4]	$0.83	$0.99	$1.04	$1.32	$1.47	$1.66	$1.69
Total Knee Replacement [5]	$5.36	$5.67	$6.22	$8.06	$9.82	$11.38	$14.26
Revision Knee Replacement [6]	$0.54	$0.63	$0.70	$0.85	$1.01	$1.47	$1.48
Total Hip and Knee Replacement Cost	$12.37	$13.32	$14.59	$18.29	$21.57	$24.86	$29.74

[1] Generally, total charges do not include professional fees and non-covered charges. In the rare cases where professional fees cannot be removed, they are included in the database. Emergency department charges incurred prior to admission to the hospital may be included in total charges.

[2] ICD-9-CM procedure code 81.51   [3] ICD-9-CM procedure code 81.52   [4] ICD-9-CM procedure code 81.53
[5] ICD-9-CM procedure code 81.54   [6] ICD-9-CM procedure code 81.55

Source: Agency for Healthcare Research and Quality, Healthcare Cost and Utilization Project, Nationwide Inpatient Sample, 1998-2004

Table 4.14: Projected Number of Hip and Knee Arthroplasties, United States 2005-2030

	Annual Number of Procedures (in 000s)							
	2005		**2010**		**2020**		**2030**	
	Variable Rate [1]	**Constant Rate** [2]	**Variable Rate** [1]	**Constant Rate** [2]	**Variable Rate** [1]	**Constant Rate** [2]	**Variable Rate** [1]	**Constant Rate** [2]
Primary Total Hip Arthroplasty	209	179	253	194	384	236	572	277
Primary Total Knee Arthroplasty	450	301	663	329	1,520	415	3,481	488
Revision Total Hip Arthroplasty	40.8	36.0	47.8	38.9	67.6	47.2	96.7	56.6
Revision Total Knee Arthroplasty	38.3	25.9	55.3	28.1	121.0	35.1	268.0	41.7

[1] Projection based on arthroplasty rate increase due to aging of population and changes in the rate of joint replacement surgery.

[2] Projection based on the historical rate of procedures found in the Nationwide Inpatient Sample, 1990 to 2003.

Source: Kurtz S, Lau E, Mowat F, et al: The future burden of hip and knee revisions: U.S. projections from 2005 to 2030. Paper presented at: 73rd Annual Meeting of the American Academy of Orthopaedic Surgeons:Chicago, IL2006. Used with permission of the primary author.

Chapter 5

Osteoporosis and Bone Health

Osteoporosis has been called the "silent disease" because it typically progresses without symptoms until a fracture occurs.[1] Osteoporosis is age-related and characterized by low bone mass due to the loss of bone in the aging process. Bones are easier to break even from falls at low heights, such as standing, or during the course of simple daily activities. In 2002, an estimated 44 million persons over the age of 50 in the United States were at risk for fracture due to osteoporosis or low bone mass. By 2020, if current trends continue and effective treatments are not found and widely implemented, it is estimated that over 61 million persons will be at risk.[1]

The economic burden of inpatient, outpatient and long-term care of incident osteoporotic fractures in the U.S. was estimated at nearly $17 billion in 2005; cumulative cost over the next 2 decades are estimated to be $474 billion.[2] In addition to dollar cost, osteoporosis-related fractures bring a burden of pain and disability, resulting in time lost from work or the inability to perform activities of daily living.

Section 5.1: Osteoporosis and Low Bone Mass

Osteoporosis is a disease characterized by low bone mass and deterioration of bone structure that causes bone fragility and increases the risk of fracture. Gradual loss of bone with aging is normal; however, that loss may be accelerated by factors such as menopause, serious health conditions or their treatment, and lifestyle factors such as inadequate diet, lack of exercise, smoking, or excessive alcohol consumption.

Although often considered a disease primarily of females, within the past decade it has become apparent that osteoporosis is not solely a women's disease. It affects an estimated 2 million men in the United States, particularly older men. In men, as in women, the low bone mineral density characteristic of osteoporosis is associated with an increased risk of bone fracture. Fracture most commonly affects the hip and lumbar vertebrae, but the radius, tibia, and ribs also may be affected. Rates of fracture-related morbidity and mortality are significant in all older persons, but are substantially higher in men than in women.

The presentation and cause of osteoporosis differ between men and women in several important ways. For example, the condition manifests later in life in men, probably because men initially have a greater bone mass. Moreover, unlike among women, for nearly half of men with osteoporosis an underlying cause can be identified. Among the causes of osteoporosis in men are corticosteroid therapy for arthritis or asthma, hypogonadism in patients being treated for cancer of the prostate with androgen-withdrawal therapy, consumption of large amounts of alcohol, hyperthyroidism, and vitamin D deficiency

Currently, the diagnosis of osteoporosis is defined by the World Health Organization (WHO), and is based on the results of dual energy x-ray absorptiometry (DXA) testing, which evaluates the bone mineral density (BMD) present at several sites. WHO defines osteoporosis as a BMD value more than 2.5 standard deviations (SD) below the average value for a young, healthy woman (a T-score of <-2.5 SD).[3] Osteopenia, or low bone mass, is defined as -1.0 to -2.5 SD, or 10% to 30%, below the normal bone mass.[4]

Section 5.1.1: Osteoporosis Disease Classifications Defined

For purposes of this chapter, osteoporosis-related conditions will be presented using three broad categories, based on ICD-9-CM diagnosis codes. (Table 5.1) *Primary osteoporosis* includes only persons who have a diagnosis of osteoporosis. It is found primarily among elderly persons, with postmenopausal women affected at the highest rates. The reasons why some persons develop osteoporosis while others do not is unclear; however, estrogen deficiency has been identified by the U.S. Department of Health and Human Services, Office of the Surgeon General, as a primary cause in both men and women.[4]

Low energy fractures, formerly referred to as fragility fractures, occur from an event such as a fall from a standing height or less (versus a high energy cause such as a vehicular accident). In general, the lower the BMD, the higher risk of a low energy fracture. However, the reasons why some women and men with low BMD do not experience low energy fractures in circumstances similar to those who do are not well understood.

Secondary osteoporosis occurs when another condition or treatment causes erosion of bone health. Causes of secondary osteoporosis include certain diseases, such as hyperthyroidism or celiac disease, and certain medications, especially glucocorticoids. In addition, some lifestyle habits, such as low activity levels, diets with low calcium intake, and smoking are believed to contribute to the development of osteoporosis. In 2004, 6.1 million persons aged 45 and over in the United States were diagnosed with a condition that can contribute to the development of osteoporosis.

In recent years, knowledge about osteoporosis risk factors, diagnostic criteria, and treatment options has advanced rapidly.[1,5] Research into treatments and preventive measures is flourishing. Clinical trials have shown that suppression of bone turnover markers, an indication of a slowing of bone loss, can be achieved in as little as 3 months of using prescription therapies, reducing the risk for low energy fractures.[6] However, it is also known that many patients diagnosed with osteoporosis do not follow the treatment regime, often due to medication side effects, and that not all patients respond to current therapies. Perhaps most important, current data demonstrate that the majority of patients who suffer a low energy fracture and are subsequently among those at highest risk for repeat fracture typically are not evaluated for osteoporosis, much less treated.

Section 5.1.2: Prevalence of Osteoporosis

Estimates of the prevalence of osteoporosis and low bone mass are based on the best available scientific information from leading researchers. There are no definitive sources of information on the numbers of persons with osteoporosis or at risk for low energy fractures, as this is truly a "silent disorder." Estimates of prevalence among white females are generally believed to be more reliable because this group has been studied the most due to their high fracture rate. The incidence or prevalence among males and racial groups is even more difficult to estimate as there are no definitions of what constitutes osteoporosis and low bone mass in these groups as there are with white women. However, the incidence of osteoporosis and low bone mass among these groups is believed to be higher than previously estimated. The leading national study that provides data upon which to make these estimates is the National Health and Nutrition Examination Study (NHANES), a self-reported study that includes questions related to diagnosis and treatment of osteoporosis, fractures, and cause of fracture. Data from the NHANES surveys for the years 1999-2000, 2001-2002, and 2003-2004 were merged and analyzed for this report to provide estimated prevalence.

The National Osteoporosis Foundation (NOF) estimated there were 29.5 million women and 11.7 million men in the United States with osteoporosis or low bone mass in 2002. Asian and non-Hispanic white women are affected about equally, and at higher proportions than Hispanic and non-Hispanic black women. The prevalence of osteoporosis and low bone mass among males was substantially lower, but followed the same general racial patterns.[1]

Data in the NHANES study indicate that over the 10-year interval between 1988-1994 and 1999-2004, based on self-reported conditions, the prevalence of osteoporosis in both females and males aged 65 and over more than doubled. (Table 5.2 and Graph 5.1.1) The rapid increase in the prevalence of osteoporosis diagnosis is likely due to the

extensive educational and awareness efforts aimed at both the general public and health care professionals, as well as increased testing of bone mass in older women. During that same time frame, females of this age group reported a slight decline in the rate of hip fractures, while males

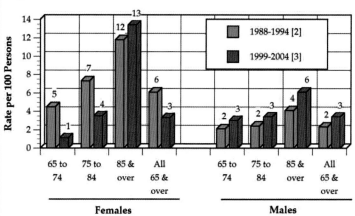

Graph 5.1.2: Self-Reported Rate of Hip Fracture [1] for Persons Aged 65 and Over, United States 1988-1994 and 1999-2004

[1] Has a doctor ever told you that you had broken or fractured your hip?
[2] Source: Praemer A, Furner S, Rice DP; *Musculoskeletal Conditions in the United States.* Rosemont, IL;American Academy of Orthopaedic Surgeons;1999;p 42.
[3] Source: National Center for Health Statistics. National Health and Nutrition Examination Survey Data, 1999-2004

aged 65 and over reported an increased rate of hip fracture. (Graph 5.1.2) A similar decline in hip fracture rates was found by a team of Dartmouth researchers in examination of Medicare databases.[4] Although reasons for this shift are unknown, greater awareness of osteoporosis and fracture potential, increased testing, and the impact of recent treatments in females may be contributing factors. Awareness of osteoporosis among men is less prevalent. They are less likely to be evaluated early for osteoporosis, even in the face of serious, contributing medical conditions.

On average, for each year between 1999 and 2004, 20 million people over the age of 45 reported they were told by their doctor they had osteoporosis or had sustained a fracture of the hip, spine, or wrist, the most common locations of fractures associated with

Graph 5.1.1: Self-Reported Rate of Osteoporosis [1] for Persons Aged 65 and Over, United States 1988-1994 and 1999-2004

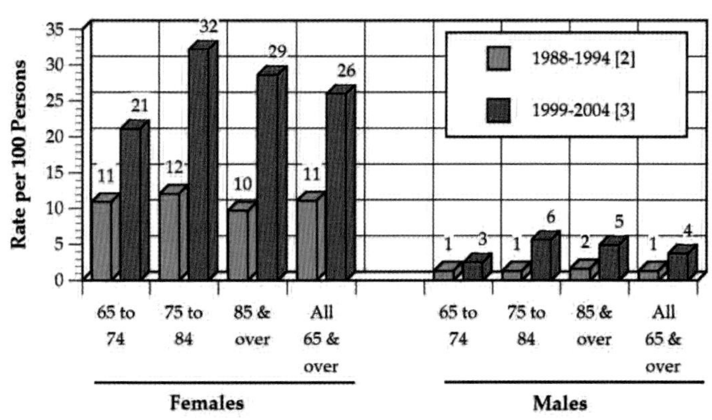

[1] Has a doctor ever told you that you had osteoporosis, sometimes called thin or brittle bones?
[2] Source: Praemer A, Furner S, Rice DP. *Musculoskeletal Conditions in the United States,* ed 2. Rosemont, IL: American Academy of Orthopaedic Surgeons;1999.
[3] Source: National Center for Health Statistics, National Health and Nutrition Examination Survey Data, 1999-2004

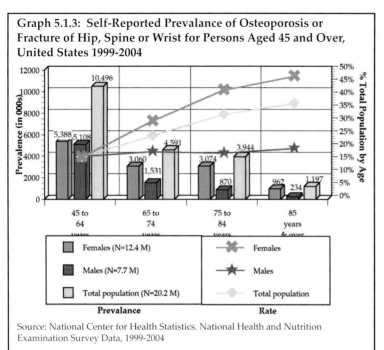

Graph 5.1.3: Self-Reported Prevalance of Osteoporosis or Fracture of Hip, Spine or Wrist for Persons Aged 45 and Over, United States 1999-2004

Source: National Center for Health Statistics. National Health and Nutrition Examination Survey Data, 1999-2004

Thirty-six percent (36%) of females, compared to 48% of males, reporting an osteoporosis condition were under the age of 65 years. (Table 5.3) The reason for this variation is not known.

Rates of treatment for osteoporosis reported between 1999 and 2004 were slightly higher for females than for males; however, the differences narrowed in individuals between the ages of 65 and 84. (Table 5.3 and Graph 5.1.4) The data suggest that if patients recognize they have osteoporosis, the likelihood they will receive treatment rises, an indication that education about screening or testing for osteoporosis is an important factor in ensuring better long term outcomes.

osteoporosis. (Table 5.3 and Graph 5.1.3) These self-reports were primarily among women in all age groups; the sole exception was persons aged 45 to 64, among whom the self-reports were nearly evenly divided between the females and males (51% to 49%, respectively.) Among those 85 years of age or older, 80% self-reporting a diagnosis of osteoporosis or fracture were female, most likely reflecting the longevity of females and their preponderance in this age group.

The higher proportions of women in older age groups reporting a diagnosis of osteoporosis and/or low energy fractures may also be due to the fact that, as the population ages, the incidence of both of these conditions rises steadily among women, while that of males remains relatively steady. Between the ages of 45 and 64, approximately 16% of both females and males report they have been told by a doctor they have osteoporosis or have had a fracture of the hip, spine, or wrist. By the age of 85 or older, 48% of females report osteoporosis and/or a fracture, while only 20% of males in this age group do so.

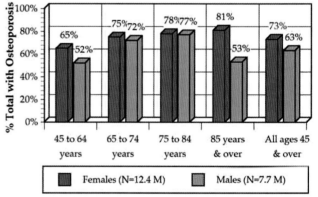

Graph 5.1.4: Self-Reported Treatment for Osteoporosis [1] by Gender for Persons Aged 45 and Over, United States 1999-2004

[1] Replied "Yes" when asked if ever been told by a doctor that you had osteoporosis and had been treated for osteoporosis.
Source: National Center for Health Statistics. National Health and Nutrition Examination Survey Data, 1999-2004

Section 5.2: Health Care Resource Utilization for Osteoporosis and Low Energy Fractures

Section 5.2.1: Patient Visits, 2004

In 2004, 6.2 million persons aged 45 and over with a diagnosis of primary osteoporosis utilized

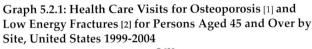

Graph 5.2.1: Health Care Visits for Osteoporosis [1] **and Low Energy Fractures** [2] **for Persons Aged 45 and Over by Site, United States 1999-2004**

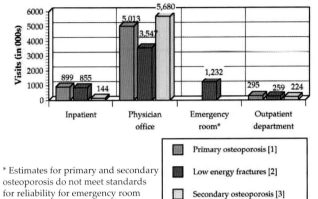

* Estimates for primary and secondary osteoporosis do not meet standards for reliability for emergency room visits.
[1] Osteoporosis and related condition ICD-9-CM codes shown in Section 5.5
[2] Treatment for fractures, excluding those with high energy causes (i.e., vehicular [auto, air, water] accidents, war injuries)
[3] Diagnosis of another medical condition that may lead to or contribute to the development of osteoporosis
Sources: National Center for Health Statistics, National Inpatient Survey, National Ambulatory Medical Care Survey, and National Hospital Ambulatory Medical Care Survey, 2004

health care resources; an additional 5.7 million persons of this age with low energy fractures also utilized health care resources. (Table 5.1) An additional 6.1 million persons aged 45 and over were diagnosed with a condition that can contribute to the development of osteoporosis, and were therefore at risk for secondary osteoporosis. An additional 1.4 million persons of this age sustained a vertebral fracture with a spinal cord injury; however, all 1.4 million of these patients received their spinal cord injury as a result of a high energy impact (i.e., motor vehicle accident). (Table 5.4)

Health care utilization by persons aged 45 and over with a diagnosis of primary osteoporosis and low energy fractures involves primarily physician office visits. In 2004, 80% of patients aged 45 and over with primary osteoporosis were diagnosed in a physician's office, while 62% of patients over the age of 45 with a low energy fracture were treated in a physician's office. (Graph 5.2.1)

Persons aged 45 and over hospitalized with a diagnosis of primary osteoporosis or a low energy fracture accounted for 5% of all inpatient admissions in 2004, representing 704,300 incidents. In addition, 1.23 million low energy fractures of persons aged 45 and over were treated in emergency rooms, 21% of all cases treated. (Table 5.4)

Ninety percent (90%) of individuals aged 45 and over diagnosed with primary osteoporosis in an inpatient setting in 2004 were females. (Table 5.5) Among individuals age 45 and over, low energy fractures occured in females at a fairly constant 3:1 ratio to males. (Tables 5.5 and 5.6 and Graph 5.2.2) The sole exception is vertebral/pelvic fractures, for which the female:male ratio was 2:1.

With the exception of inpatient hospitalization for primary osteoporosis or a low energy fracture, males aged 45 or over did not use health care resources in sufficient numbers to reach statistical reliability in the overall prevalence in the databases. However, the age of males treated as inpatients or in the emergency room for a low energy fracture is shown for comparative purposes. (Tables 5.5 and 5.6)

Graph 5.2.2: Low Energy Fracture [1] **Treatment for Persons Aged 45 and Over by Sex and Site, United States 2004**

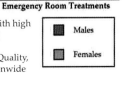

[1] Treatment for fractures, excluding those with high energy causes (i.e., vehicular [auto, air, water] accidents, war injuries)
Source: Agency for Healthcare Research and Quality, Healthcare Cost and Utilization Project, Nationwide Inpatient Sample, 2004

Section 5.2.2: Age at Time of Osteoporosis Diagnosis or Low Energy Fracture Incident, 2004

Although osteoporosis may occur in younger patients, it is primarily a condition of older adults. Among patients 45 years of age or older, the mean age at time of diagnosis of osteoporosis in a physician's office in 2004 was 71.4 years. One-fourth of these diagnoses (26%) were for females between the ages of 45 and 64. (Graph 5.2.3) Due to the very small number of males, this age is primarily representative of females.

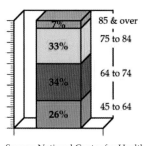

Graph 5.2.3: Age Distribution for Osteoporosis Diagnosis in Physician's Office for Persons Aged 45 and Over, United States 2004

Source: National Center for Health Statistics, National Ambulatory Medical Care Survey, 2004

The mean age of females aged 45 or over receiving a diagnosis of primary osteoporosis in an inpatient setting was 77.6 years, with 66% of the diagnosed patients aged 75 or over. However, 13% of the diagnoses occurred in females between the ages of 45 and 64, with the remaining 21% aged 65 to 74. Males aged 45 or over received a diagnosis of primary osteoporosis at a slightly younger mean age of 75.3 years. A higher proportion of males (19%) than females (13%) between the ages of 45 and 64 had a diagnosis of osteoporosis. (Table 5.5)

Low energy fractures also occur more frequently in the elderly, particularly among females. Among patients 45 years of age and older and treated for a hip fracture, 79% treated in an inpatient setting and 85% treated in an emergency department were females aged 75 years or older. However, wrist fractures treated in emergency departments were more commonly seen in younger women between the ages of 45 and 64 (50%). Among females aged 45 to 64, only 15% of all low energy fractures treated in an

inpatient setting were females, while 40% seen in an emergency department were females of this age. (Graph 5.2.4)

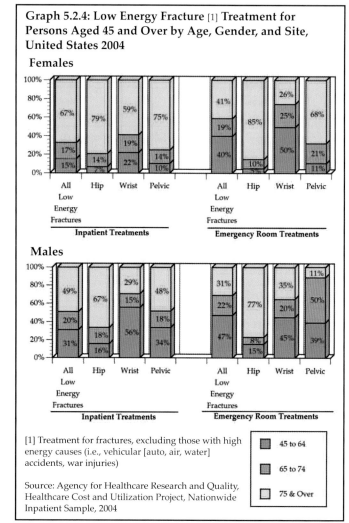

Graph 5.2.4: Low Energy Fracture [1] Treatment for Persons Aged 45 and Over by Age, Gender, and Site, United States 2004

[1] Treatment for fractures, excluding those with high energy causes (i.e., vehicular [auto, air, water] accidents, war injuries)

Source: Agency for Healthcare Research and Quality, Healthcare Cost and Utilization Project, Nationwide Inpatient Sample, 2004

With the exception of hip fractures, males aged 45 and over are more likely to have a low energy fracture at a younger age than are women. This could be due to exposure to more physical activity or settings in which low energy impacts more frequently occur. Overall, 31% of low energy fractures treated in an inpatient setting and 47% treated in emergency departments were males aged 45 to 64 in 2004. (Graph 5.2.4)

In 2004, the proportion of low energy fractures in persons aged 45 and over who also are diagnosed with osteoporosis as a potential contributing

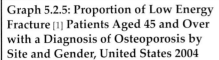

Graph 5.2.5: Proportion of Low Energy Fracture [1] Patients Aged 45 and Over with a Diagnosis of Osteoporosis by Site and Gender, United States 2004

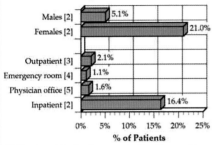

[1] Treatment for fractures, excluding those with high energy causes (i.e., vehicular [auto, air, water] accidents, war injuries)
[2] Source: Agency for Healthcare Research and Quality, Healthcare Cost and Utilization Project, Nationwide Inpatient Sample, 2004
[3] Source: National Center for Health Statistics, National Hospital Ambulatory Medical Care Survey, Outpatient Centers, 2004
[4] Source: National Center for Health Statistics, National Hospital Ambulatory Medical Care Survey, Hospital Emergency, 2004
[5] Source: National Center for Health Statistics, National Ambulatory Medical Care Survey, 2004

cause was very low. Among all patients aged 45 and older with a low energy fracture seen in a physician's office, an emergency room, or an outpatient setting in 2004, fewer than 2% were also diagnosed with osteoporosis. Even in an inpatient setting, only 16% of low energy fracture patients also had an osteoporosis diagnosis, an indication that osteoporosis is under-diagnosed even when patients are admitted to a hospital. Females with a low energy fracture were four times as likely as males with a fracture to be diagnosed with osteoporosis. The failure to recognize osteoporosis as a possible contributing cause of the fracture increases the possibility of future fractures in this already at risk population. (Tables 5.4 and 5.5 and Graph 5.2.5)

Section 5.2.3: Short/Long-Term Care for Low Energy Fracture Patients

Regardless of the age at which a low energy fracture occurs, both females and males are more likely to be transferred to a short, intermediate, or long-term skilled nursing care setting upon their release from inpatient care than are persons without a fracture. The older the patient, the greater the likelihood that such a transfer will be necessary. Among non-fracture female patients, approximately 24% are released to additional care settings, while approximately 38% of non-fracture patients aged 75 and over are released to another care setting. By contrast, among all female hip fracture patients, the proportions are 83% and 86% for all patients and those aged 75 and over, respectively. Even female patients with a wrist fracture are more likely to be released to additional care, with 45% of all patients with this type of fracture going to another care setting, and 60% of those aged 75 and over doing so. The rates for males released to an additional care setting are slightly lower, but still substantially higher than for patients with no fracture. (Table 5.7 and Graph 5.2.6) The cost of additional care for patients with low energy fractures has not been quantified due to lack of available data.

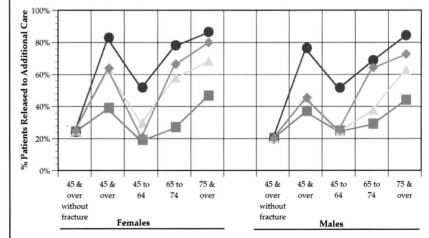

Graph 5.2.6: Hospital Discharge to Short/Intermediate/Skilled Nursing Care for Persons Aged 45 and Over by Age and Sex for Persons with Osteoporosis, Low Energy Fractures [1] and without a Fracture, United States 2004

[1] Treatment for fractures, excluding those with high energy causes (i.e., vehicular [auto, air, water] accidents, war injuries)
Source: Agency for Healthcare Research and Quality, Healthcare Cost and Utilization Project, Nationwide Inpatient Sample, 2004

Section 5.2.4: Nursing Home Population and Risks of the Fragile Elderly

After an elderly person has sustained a fall resulting in fracture, his or her ability to live independently is reduced due to pain and limitations in activity. These patients are also at risk of additional falls and consequent fractures. These patients require additional care and resources. Among persons in the nursing home population in 2004, 7,640 (< 1% of total admissions) were diagnosed with osteoporosis at the time of their admission; the majority were aged 75 and older. (Table 5.8) A substantially larger number, more than 118,000 (8% of admissions), had sustained a low energy fracture at the time of admission, most likely due to osteoporosis and fragile bones. Females accounted for more than 82% of the nursing home admittances due to fracture; 92% of the nursing home admittances were aged 75 years of age or older at the time of the fracture. Hip fractures are the most common type of fracture that places older persons in a nursing home, accounting for 44% of admittances due to fracture. However, pelvic, upper and lower limb, ankle or foot, and stress fractures are also a common cause of placement in a nursing home for persons aged 75 and older.

At the time of interview in 2004, nearly 40,200 nursing home residents aged 65 and older had sustained a new fracture since being admitted. The majority of these were females (74%); more than one-half (58%) were 85 years of age or older. Nearly 522,000 nursing home residents aged 65 and older, or two in five, reported reported a fall within the past 6 months. Of those falling, 2%, or 27,600, sustained a hip fracture within the past 6 months, and 33,900 (3%) another type of fracture.

As the number of U.S. persons over the age of 75 increases in the next few decades, the burden placed on nursing home care due to fragile bones will increase. Reducing the incidence and severity of osteoporosis will be critical to maintaining the health of the aging population, as well as reducing health care costs.

Section 5.3: Falls and Low Energy Fractures

Falls are the leading cause of injury, including mortality and non-fatal injuries, for persons aged 65 and older in the United States and a leading cause of hospitalization among persons of all ages. In 2000, falls accounted for 46% of all hospitalizations from injuries; 309 out of every 100,000 persons suffering a fall were hospitalized.[7] In 2002, 12% of unintentional injury deaths resulted from falls and 1.6 million nonfatal injuries from falls were treated at hospital emergency departments throughout the United States.[8]

Fractures are the primary cause of hospitalization or death following a fall, particularly among individuals aged 65 and over. Osteoporosis is a leading underlying cause of low energy fractures after a fall, especially among the elderly. One in two women and one in four men over aged 50 will have an osteoporosis-related fracture in her or his remaining lifetime.[9]

Self-reported fracture rates for hip, wrist, and spine, from 1999 to 2004, indicate an increasing rate of fracture among females as the population ages, particularly among individuals aged 85 and older. Among males, relatively stable rates of spine fracture occurred between the ages of 45 and older, while wrist fracture rates decreased with age and hip fracture rates increased. (Table 5.9 and Graph 5.3.1) Overall, 12% of fractures reported for persons aged 45 and over were hip fractures; 19% were spine fractures; and 69% were wrist fractures.

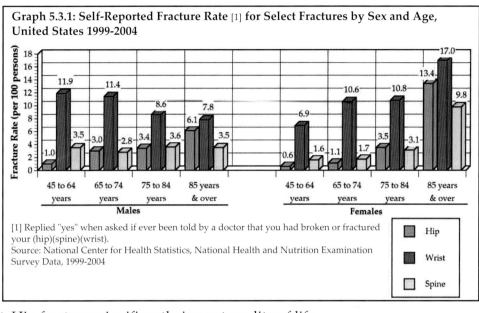

Graph 5.3.1: Self-Reported Fracture Rate [1] for Select Fractures by Sex and Age, United States 1999-2004

[1] Replied "yes" when asked if ever been told by a doctor that you had broken or fractured your (hip)(spine)(wrist).
Source: National Center for Health Statistics, National Health and Nutrition Examination Survey Data, 1999-2004

obtain prevalence than incidence. Often they are diagnosed when the patient complains of chronic back pain as the result of compression or stress on the weakened spine.[4] Even without acute symptoms, vertebral compression fractures can impact significantly on quality of life, affecting the ability to walk, balance, and sometimes cause upper back, neck or abdominal pain. The presence of existing vertebral fractures are generally considered a predictor for future fracture risk of the spine, wrist and hip.

Among all females aged 45 and over, falls were responsible for nearly all wrist fractures, as well as for the majority of hip fractures, treated between 1999 and 2004. Males follow a similar pattern, although falls account for a slightly lower proportion of fractures among men. Roughly half of spine fractures are caused by falls, with other causes, including automobile accidents, accounting for the remainder. The older the patient, the more likely that a fall is the cause of a fracture. (Table 5.9 and Graph 5.3.2)

The mean age at time of first fracture of the wrist caused by a fall for all females aged 45 and over reporting a wrist fracture was 62.9 years. The mean age at first fracture of the spine was 70.6 years; for first hip fracture it was 74.8 years. Wrist and spine fractures are more common among younger females, while hip fracture rates increase significantly among females aged 85 and older. Among males, the mean age of first wrist fracture is 60.2 years, reflecting the higher rate of fracture in younger males than in older males. The mean

Hip fractures significantly impact quality of life, and are invariably associated with chronic pain, reduced mobility, disability, and an increasing degree of dependence.[10] The mortality rate in the first 12 months after hip fracture is 20%, and is higher in males than females.[9] Some studies suggest that mortality may be higher, with a 30% rate following hip fracture surgery noted.[11] Current estimates are that one in four hip fractures occur in males, and recent research indicates that men will have a different course of recovery than women, with higher rates of disability as well as mortality.[12,13] Fifty percent of persons experiencing a hip fracture will be unable to walk without assistance, and 25% will require long term care.[14]

There is no generally accepted definition of a spine fracture, also referred to as compression fractures, resulting in a wide variation of overall prevalence estimates.[15] Only about one in four spinal fractures are diagnosed as a result of falls. The most widely accepted definition of suspected spine fractures in use today is a 20% loss of height from early adulthood, hence compressing the vertebral column. Since many of these fractures occur without acute symptoms and patients are rarely admitted to the hospital, it is easier to

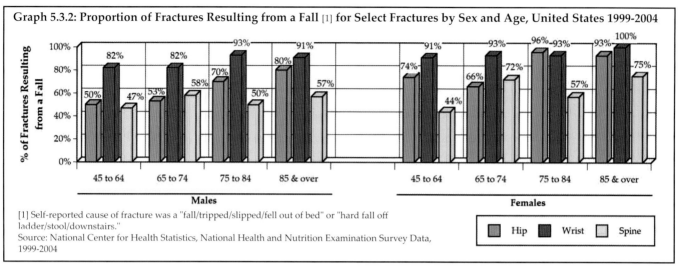

Graph 5.3.2: Proportion of Fractures Resulting from a Fall [1] for Select Fractures by Sex and Age, United States 1999-2004

[1] Self-reported cause of fracture was a "fall/tripped/slipped/fell out of bed" or "hard fall off ladder/stool/downstairs."
Source: National Center for Health Statistics, National Health and Nutrition Examination Survey Data, 1999-2004

age of first hip fracture among males, at 69.2 years, is nearly 5 years younger than among females. Spine fractures due to a fall also occur at a younger age, 60.2 years, among males. As the population ages, the age at which they report

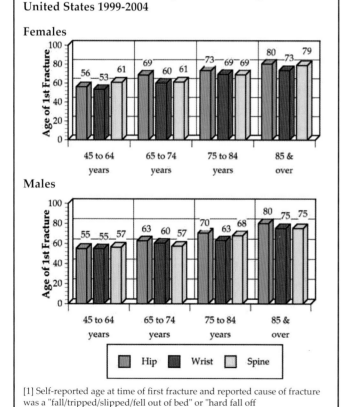

Graph 5.3.3: Mean Age of 1st Fracture When Cause is a Fall [1] for Select Fractures by Gender and Age, United States 1999-2004

[1] Self-reported age at time of first fracture and reported cause of fracture was a "fall/tripped/slipped/fell out of bed" or "hard fall off ladder/stool/downstairs."
Source: National Center for Health Statistics.,National Health and Nutrition Examination Survey Data, 1999-2004

their first fracture also rises. (Table 5.9 and Graph 5.3.3)

The mean number of lifetime fractures of all sites reported by all persons in the NHANES for the years 1999 to 2004 was slightly over one; however, some persons reported multiple fractures. For example, in the 2003-2004 NHANES, the most recent year of data available, some respondents reported 2 lifetime hip fractures, up to 6 lifetime wrist fractures, and up to 10 lifetime spine fractures.[16]

Section 5.3.1: Inpatient Treatment for Low Energy Fractures, 2004

In 2004, slightly more than 704,000 persons over age 45 were discharged from the hospital after sustaining a low energy fracture. More than one-third of the inpatient fractures were hip fractures (43% for females and 39% for males). Vertebrae/pelvic fractures comprised about one-fifth (19% and 22% for females and males, respectively). The remaining fracture sites accounted for 10% or less of all fractures treated in inpatient facilities. In the same year, more than 1.2 million fractures to persons aged 45 and older were treated in emergency rooms. Fractures of the wrist or hand accounted for the largest proportion of these low energy fractures in both females and males,

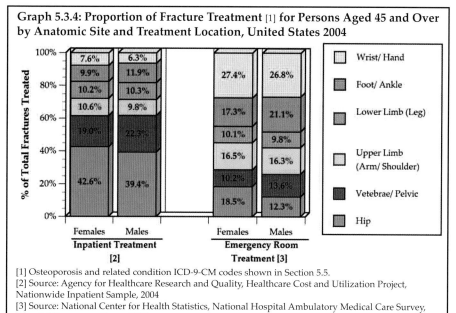

Graph 5.3.4: Proportion of Fracture Treatment [1] for Persons Aged 45 and Over by Anatomic Site and Treatment Location, United States 2004

Legend:
- Wrist/ Hand
- Foot/ Ankle
- Lower Limb (Leg)
- Upper Limb (Arm/ Shoulder)
- Vetebrae/ Pelvic
- Hip

[1] Osteoporosis and related condition ICD-9-CM codes shown in Section 5.5.
[2] Source: Agency for Healthcare Research and Quality, Healthcare Cost and Utilization Project, Nationwide Inpatient Sample, 2004
[3] Source: National Center for Health Statistics, National Hospital Ambulatory Medical Care Survey, Hospital Emergency Room, 2004

The mean length of inpatient stay for persons aged 45 and older with a low energy fracture in 2004 was 6.1 days, or 13% longer than the mean stay of 5.4 days for patients without a fracture injury. The mean cost per inpatient stay for persons aged 45 and older with a low energy fracture in 2004 was $28,077, a cost that was 8% greater than that of patients with similar demographics but without a fracture. The estimated cost in 2004 of treating low energy fractures in patients aged 45 and older who were hospitalized as a result of the fracture was $24.2 billion. (Table 5.11)

accounting for 27% of total fractures incurred by both genders. This was followed by fractures of the foot and ankle and upper limb (arm/shoulder) fractures. (Table 5.10 and Graph 5.3.4)

Section 5.4: Cost and Burden of Osteoporosis and Low Energy Fractures, 2004

The mean length of inpatient stay for persons aged 45 and older with a diagnosis of osteoporosis (but not a fracture) in 2004 was 5.3 days, or 2% shorter than the mean stay of 5.4 days for patients without an osteoporosis diagnosis. The mean cost per inpatient stay for persons aged 45 and older with an osteoporosis diagnosis in 2004 was $21,209, which was 19% less than that of patients with similar demographics but without an osteoporosis diagnosis. The estimated cost in 2004 of treating patients aged 45 and older who were hospitalized and had a diagnosis of osteoporosis was $19.1 billion. (Table 5.11) It is unlikely the osteoporosis diagnosis was the primary diagnosis for which the patients were hospitalized.

The burden of osteoporosis is already high, and it is growing. The costs associated with this disease are also increasing in both men and women and in all ethnic groups. These data provide strong support for the initiation of societywide prevention measures, including early and regular screening for bone health, as well as for greater emphasis on the diagnosis of individuals at risk for osteoporosis and identification of new strategies to improve treatment and treatment adherence in high risk groups.

1. National Osteoporosis Foundation (NOF): *America's Bone Health: The State of Osteoporosis and Low Bone Mass in Our Nation.* Washington DC: National Osteoporosis Foundation, 2002.

2. Burge RT, Dawson-Hughes B, Solomon DH, et al: Incidence and economic burden of osteoporosis-related fractures in the United States, 2005-2025. *J Bone Miner Res* 2007;22:465-475.

3. World Health Organization (WHO): *WHO Scientific Group on the Assessment of Osteoporosis at Primary Health Care Level.* Brussels, Belgium: WHO Press, Geneva, Switzerland, 2004.

4. US Department of Health and Human Services (USDHHS): *Bone Health and Osteoporosis: A Report of the Surgeon General*. Rockville, MD: U.S. Government Printing Office, Office of the Surgeon General, 2004, p 107.

5. Baim S, Biegel R, Binkley NC: Medicare and private reimbursement of osteoporosis diagnosis and treatment, in *Osteoporosis Clinical Updates*. Washington DC: National Osteoporosis Foundation, 2006, vol 7, pp 1-8.

6. Bonnick SL, Shulman L: Monitoring osteoporosis therapy: bone mineral density, bone turnover markers, or both? *Am J Med* 2006;119:25S-31S.

7. Finkelstein EA, Corso PS, Miller TR: *The Incidence and Economic Burden of Injuries in the United States.* New York, NY: Oxford University Press, Inc., 2006, p 187.

8. National Safety Council (NSC): *Injury Facts, 2005-2006 Edition*. Itasca, IL: National Safety Council, 2006.

9. National Osteoporosis Foundation (NOF): National Osteoporosis Foundation Fast Facts. Available at: http://www.nof.org/osteoporosis/diseasefacts.htm. Accessed September 19, 2007.

10. International Osteoporosis Foundation (IOF): Facts and statistics about osteoporosis and its impact, in, 2007. Available at: http://www.iofbonehealth.org/facts-and-statistics.html. Accessed September 19, 2007.

11. Moran CG, Wenn RT, Sikand M, Taylor AM: Early mortality after hip fracture: is delay before surgery important? *J Bone Joint Surg Am* 2005;87:483-489.

12. Orwig DL, Chan J, Magaziner J: Hip fracture and its consequences: differences between men and women. *Orthop Clin North Am* 2006;37:611-622.

13. Hawkes WG, Wehren L, Orwig D, et al: Gender differences in functioning after hip fracture. *J Gerontol A Biol Sci Med Sci* 2006;61:495-499.

14. Riggs BL, Melton LJ: The worldwide problem of osteoporosis: insights afforded by epidemiology. *Bone* 1995;17:505S-511S.

15. Genant HK, Jergas M: Assessment of prevalent and incident vertebral fractures in osteoporosis research. *Osteoporos Int* 2003;14:S43-S55.

16. National Center for Health Statistics (NCHS): *National Health and Nutrition Examination Survey 2003-2004: Documentation, Codebook, and Frequencies*. Hyattsville, MD: Centers for Disease Control, 2006, p 34.

Section 5.5: Osteoporosis and Bone Health Data Tables

For purposes of this study, osteoporosis has been categorized into the three classifications. *Primary osteoporosis* is a diagnosis of osteoporosis. *Low energy fracture* is one caused by an event such as a fall from a standing height. (A high energy fracture, by contrast, is caused by involvement in a motor vehicle accident.) *Secondary osteoporosis* is the presence of another condition or treatment that may cause eroding of bone health and osteoporosis. Codes included in these three osteoporosis categories are as shown in Table 5.1.

Table 5.1: Osteoporosis and Bone Health: Analysis Codes

CODE	ICD-9-CM CODE DESCRIPTION	CODE	ICD-9-CM CODE DESCRIPTION
OSTEOPOROSIS			
73300	Osteoporosis NOS	73303	Disuse Osteoporosis
73301	Senile Osteoporosis	73309	Osteoporosis NEC
73302	Idiopathic Osteoporosis		

LOW ENERGY FRACTURES		**Wrist and Hand Fracture**	
Vertebral and Pelvic Fractures			
80500	Vertebral Fracture (Closed)	81300	Wrist Fracture (Closed)-Radius and Ulna Upper End
80501	Vertebral Fracture (Closed)	81301	Wrist Fracture (Closed)-Radius and Ulna Upper End
80502	Vertebral Fracture (Closed)	81302	Wrist Fracture (Closed)-Radius and Ulna Upper End
80503	Vertebral Fracture (Closed)	81303	Wrist Fracture (Closed)-Radius and Ulna Upper End
80504	Vertebral Fracture (Closed)	81304	Wrist Fracture (Closed)-Radius and Ulna Upper End
80505	Vertebral Fracture (Closed)	81305	Wrist Fracture (Closed)-Radius and Ulna Upper End
80506	Vertebral Fracture (Closed)	81306	Wrist Fracture (Closed)-Radius and Ulna Upper End
80507	Vertebral Fracture (Closed)	81307	Wrist Fracture (Closed)-Radius and Ulna Upper End
80508	Vertebral Fracture (Closed)	81308	Wrist Fracture (Closed)-Radius and Ulna Upper End
80520	Vertebral Fracture (Closed)-Thoracic	81320	Wrist/forearm Fracture (Closed)-Radius and Ulna Shaft
80540	Vertebral Fracture (Closed)-Lumbar	81321	Wrist/forearm Fracture (Closed)-Radius and Ulna Shaft
80560	Pelvic Fracture (Closed)-Sacrum and Coccyx	81322	Wrist/forearm Fracture (Closed)-Radius and Ulna Shaft
80580	Vertebral Fracture (Closed)-Unspecified	81323	Wrist/forearm Fracture (Closed)-Radius and Ulna Shaft
80800	Pelvic Fracture (Closed)-Acetabulum	81340	Wrist/forearm Fracture (Closed)-Radius and Ulna Lower End
80820	Pelvic Fracture (Closed)-Pubis	81341	Wrist/forearm Fracture (Closed)-Radius and Ulna Lower End
80841	Pelvic Fracture (Closed)-Ilium	81342	Wrist/forearm Fracture (Closed)-Radius and Ulna Lower End
80842	Pelvic Fracture (Closed)-Ischium	81343	Wrist/forearm Fracture (Closed)-Radius and Ulna Lower End
80843	Pelvic Fracture (Closed)-Multiple	81344	Wrist/forearm Fracture (Closed)-Radius and Ulna Lower End
80849	Pelvic Fracture (Closed)-Other	81345	Wrist/forearm Fracture (Closed)-Radius and Ulna Lower End
80880	Pelvic Fracture (Closed)-Uunspecified	81380	Wrist/forearm Fracture (Closed)-Radius and Ulna Unspecified
		81381	Wrist/forearm Fracture (Closed)-Radius and Ulna Unspecified
Upper Limb Fracture (Shoulder and Arm)		81382	Wrist/forearm Fracture (Closed)-Radius and Ulna Unspecified
81000	Upper limb Fracture (Closed)-Clavicle (Shoulder)	81383	Wrist/forearm Fracture (Closed)-Radius and Ulna Unspecified
81001	Upper limb Fracture (Closed)-Clavicle (Shoulder)	81400	Wrist Fracture (Closed)-Carpal Bones
81002	Upper limb Fracture (Closed)-Clavicle (Shoulder)	81401	Wrist Fracture (Closed)-Carpal Bones
81003	Upper limb Fracture (Closed)-Clavicle (Shoulder)	81402	Wrist Fracture (Closed)-Carpal Bones
81100	Upper limb Fracture (Closed)-Scapula (Shoulder)	81403	Wrist Fracture (Closed)-Carpal Bones
81101	Upper limb Fracture (Closed)-Scapula (Shoulder)	81404	Wrist Fracture (Closed)-Carpal Bones
81102	Upper limb Fracture (Closed)-Scapula (Shoulder)	81405	Wrist Fracture (Closed)-Carpal Bones
81103	Upper limb Fracture (Closed)-Scapula (Shoulder)	81406	Wrist Fracture (Closed)-Carpal Bones
81109	Upper limb Fracture (Closed)-Scapula (Shoulder)	81407	Wrist Fracture (Closed)-Carpal Bones
81200	Upper limb Fracture (Closed)-Humerus Upper End	81408	Wrist Fracture (Closed)-Carpal Bones
81201	Upper limb Fracture (Closed)-Humerus Upper End	81409	Wrist Fracture (Closed)-Carpal Bones
81202	Upper limb Fracture (Closed)-Humerus Upper End	81500	Hand Fracture (Closed)-Metacarpal Bones
81203	Upper limb Fracture (Closed)-Humerus Upper End	81501	Hand Fracture (Closed)-Metacarpal Bones
81209	Upper limb Fracture (Closed)-Humerus Upper End	81502	Hand Fracture (Closed)-Metacarpal Bones
81220	Upper limb Fracture (Closed)-Humerus Upper End	81503	Hand Fracture (Closed)-Metacarpal Bones
81221	Upper limb Fracture (Closed)-Humerus Upper End	81504	Hand Fracture (Closed)-Metacarpal Bones
81240	Upper limb Fracture (Closed)-Humerus Upper End	81509	Hand Fracture (Closed)-Metacarpal Bones
81241	Upper limb Fracture (Closed)-Humerus Upper End		
81242	Upper limb Fracture (Closed)-Humerus Upper End		
81243	Upper limb Fracture (Closed)-Humerus Upper End		
81244	Upper limb Fracture (Closed)-Humerus Upper End	Table 5.1 continued next page.	
81249	Upper limb Fracture (Closed)-Humerus Upper End		

Table 5.1: Osteoporosis and Bone Health: Analysis Codes (continued)

CODE   ICD-9-CM CODE DESCRIPTION

Ankle and Foot Fracture

CODE	Description
82400	Ankle Fracture (Closed)-Medial Malleolus
82420	Ankle Fracture (Closed)-Lateral Malleolus
82440	Ankle Fracture (Closed)-Bimalleolar
82460	Ankle Fracture (Closed)-Trimalleolar
82480	Ankle Fracture (Closed)-Unspecified
82500	Foot Fracture (Closed)- Calcaneus
82520	Foot Fracture (Closed)-Unspecified (Instep)
82521	Foot Fracture (Closed)-Astragalus
82522	Foot Fracture (Closed)-Navicular (Scaphoid)
82523	Foot Fracture (Closed)-Cuboid
82524	Foot Fracture (Closed)-Cuneiform
82525	Foot Fracture (Closed)-Metatarsal Bone(s)
82529	Foot Fracture (Closed)-Other (Tarsal with Metatarsal)

Stress and Pathological Fractures

CODE	Description
73310	Unspecified Pathological Fracture
73311	Pathological Fracture-Humerus
73312	Pathological Fracture-Wrist
73313	Pathological Fracture-Vertebrae
73314	Pathological Fracture-Femur Neck
73315	Pathological Fracture-Other Femur
73316	Pathological Fracture-Tibia/Fibula
73319	Other Specified Pathological Fracture
73393	Stress Fracture of Tibia or Fibula
73394	Stress Fracture of the Metatarsals
73395	Stress Fracture of Other Bone

Exclude all cases with E-code of:

E800-E807	Railway
E810-E819	Motor Vehicle Traffic
E820-E825	Motor Vehicle Nontraffic
E826-E829	Other Road Vehicles
E830-E838	Water
E840-E845	Air and Space
E846-E848	Other Vehicle Accidents Not Elsewhere Clssified
E990-E999	Operations of War

CODE   ICD-9-CM CODE DESCRIPTION

Hip Fracture

CODE	Description
82000	Hip Fracture (Closed)-Neck of Femur
82001	Hip Fracture (Closed)-Neck of Femur
82002	Hip Fracture (Closed)-Neck of Femur
82003	Hip Fracture (Closed)-Neck of Femur
82009	Hip Fracture (Closed)-Neck of Femur
82020	Hip Fracture (Closed)-Neck of Femur
82021	Hip Fracture (Closed)-Neck of Femur
82022	Hip Fracture (Closed)-Neck of Femur
82080	Hip Fracture (Closed)-Neck of Femur

Lower Limb, Excluding Foot and Ankle

CODE	Description
82100	Lower Limb Fracture (Closed Only)-Thigh/Upper Leg
82101	Lower Limb Fracture (Closed Only)-Thigh/Upper Leg
82120	Lower Limb Fracture (Closed)-Lower End Femur Unspecified
82121	Lower Limb Fracture (Closed)-Lower End Femur Condoyle
82122	Lower Limb Fracture (Closed)-Lower End Femur Eepiphysis
82123	Lower Limb Fracture (Closed)-Lower End Femur Supracondylar
82129	Lower Limb Fracture (Closed)-Lower End Femur Multiple Fractures
82200	Lower Limb Fracture (Closed Only)-Patella
82300	Lower Limb Fracture (Closed Only)-Tibia and Fibula
82301	Lower Limb Fracture (Closed Only)-Tibia and Fibula
82302	Lower Limb Fracture (Closed Only)-Tibia and Fibula
82320	Lower Limb Fracture (Closed Only)-Tibia and Fibula Shaft
82321	Lower Limb Fracture (Closed Only)-Tibia and Fibula Shaft
82322	Lower Limb Fracture (Closed Only)-Tibia and Fibula Shaft
82380	Lower Limb Fracture (Closed Only)-Tibia and Fibula Unspecified
82381	Lower Limb Fracture (Closed Only)-Tibia and Fibula Unspecified
82382	Lower Limb Fracture (Closed Only)-Tibia and Fibula Unspecified

Table 5.1 continued next page.

Table 5.1: Osteoporosis and Bone Health: Analysis Codes (continued)

CODE	ICD-9-CM CODE DESCRIPTION	CODE	ICD-9-CM CODE DESCRIPTION

SECONDARY OSTEOPOROSIS

Diagnosis That May Lead to Osteoporosis

CODE	Description	CODE	Description
24290	Thyrotox NOS-No Crisis	25720	Testicular Hypofunction NEC
24291	Thyrotox NOS-with Crisis	25930	Ectopic Hormone Secondary NEC
25200	Hyperparathyroidism NOS	25990	Endocrine Disorder NOS
25201	Primary Hyperparathyroid	26820	Osteomalacia NOS
25202	Secondary Hyperparathyroid-Nonrenal	26890	Vitamin D Deficiency NOS
25208	Hyperparathyroidism NEC	58800	Renal Osteodystrophy
25500	Cushing's Syndrome	58881	Secondary Hyperparathyroid-Renal
25530	Corticoadren Overact NEC	62720	Female Climacteric State
25620	Postablativ Ovarian Failure	62740	Artificial Menopause States
25631	Premature Menopause	62780	Menopausal Disorder NEC
25639	Other Ovarian Failure	62790	Menopausal Disorder NOS
25710	Postblat Testic Hypofun		

Vertebral Fractures with Spinal Cord Injury

CODE	Description	CODE	Description
80600	C1-C4 Fracture-Closed/Cord Injury NOS	80626	T7-T12 Fracture-Closed/Complete Lesion of Cord
80601	C1-C4 Fracture-Closed/Complete Lesion of Cord	80627	T7-T12 Fracture-Closed/Anterior Cord Syndrome
80602	C1-C4 Fracture-Closed/Anterior Cord Syndrome	80628	T7-T12 Fracture-Closed/Central Cord Syndrome
80603	C1-C4 Fracture-Closed/Central Cord Syndrome	80629	T7-T12 Fracture-Closed/Cord Injury NEC
80604	C1-C4 Fracture-Closed/Cord Injury NEC	80630	T1-T6 Fracture-Open/Cord Injury NOS
80605	C5-C7 Fracture-Closed/Cord Injury NOS	80631	T1-T6 Fracture-Open/Complete Lesion of Cord
80606	C5-C7 Fracture-Closed/Complete Lesion of Cord	80632	T1-T6 Fracture-Open/Anterior Cord Syndrome
80607	C5-C7 Fracture-Closed/Anterior Cord Syndrome	80633	T1-T6 Fracture-Open/Central Cord Syndrome
80608	C5-C7 Fracture-Closed/Central Cord Syndrome	80634	T1-T6 Fracture-Open/Cord Injury NEC
80609	C5-C7 Fracture-Closed/Cord Injury NEC	80635	T7-T12 Fracture-Open/Cord Injury NOS
80610	C1-C4 Fracture-Open/Cord Injury NOS	80636	T7-T12 Fracture-Open/Complete Lesion of Cord
80611	C1-C4 Fracture-Open/Complete Lesion of Cord	80637	T7-T12 Fracture-Open/Anterior Cord Syndrome
80612	C1-C4 Fracture-Open/Anterior Cord Syndrome	80638	T7-T12 Fracture-Open/Central Cord Syndrome
80613	C1-C4 Fracture-Open/Central Cord Syndrome	80639	T7-T12 Fracture-Open/Cord Injury NEC
80614	C1-C4 Fracture-Open/Cord Injury NEC	80640	Closed Lumbar Fracture with Cord Injury
80615	C5-C7 Fracture-Open/Cord Injury NOS	80650	Open Lumbar Fracture with Cord Injury
80616	C5-C7 Fracture-Open/Complete Lesion of Cord	80660	Fracture Sacrum-Closed/Cord Injury NOS
80617	C5-C7 Fracture-Open/Anterior Cord Syndrome	80661	Fracture Sacrum-Closed/Cauda Equina Lesion
80618	C5-C7 Fracture-Open/Central Cord Syndrome	80662	Fracture Sacrum-Closed/Cauda Injury NEC
80619	C5-C7 Fracture-Open/Cord Injury NEC	80669	Fracture Sacrum-Closed/Cord Injury NEC
80620	T1-T6 Fracture-Closed/Cord Injury NOS	80670	Fracture Sacrum-Closed/Cord Injury NOS
80621	T1-T6 Fracture-Closed/Complete Lesion of Cord	80671	Fracture Sacrum-Closed/Cauda Equina Lesion
80622	T1-T6 Fracture-Closed/Anterior Cord Syndrome	80672	Fracture Sacrum-Closed/Cauda Injury NEC
80623	T1-T6 Fracture-Closed/Central Cord Syndrome	80679	Fracture Sacrum-Open/Cord Injury NEC
80624	T1-T6 Fracture-Closed/Cord Injury NEC	80680	Vertebrae Fracture NOS-Closed with Cord Injury
80625	T7-T12 Fracture-Closed/Cord Injury NOS	80690	Vertebrae Fracture NOS-Open with Cord Injury

Table 5.2: Self-Reported Rate of Osteoporosis and Hip Fracture for Persons Aged 65 and Over, United States 1988-1994 and 1999-2004

	Prevalence (Rate per 100 Persons)					
	Osteoporosis [1]		Hip Fracture [2]		Either Condition	
	1988-1994 [3]	1999-2004 [4]	1988-1994 [3]	1999-2004 [4]	1988-1994 [3]	1999-2004 [4]
Females						
65 to 74 years	10.9	21.1	4.5	1.1	14.2	21.8
75 to 84 years	12.1	32.2	7.3	3.5	17.7	34.0
85 years & over	9.7	28.6	11.8	13.4	19.1	32.7
All females 65 years & over	11.1	26.0	6.1	3.3	15.8	27.5
Males						
65 to 74 years	1.3	2.5	2.1	3.0	3.3	5.5
75 to 84 years	1.3	5.6	2.4	3.4	3.0	8.8
85 years & over	1.6	4.9	4.1	6.1	5.4	9.4
All males 65 years & over	1.3	3.7	2.3	3.4	3.5	6.9
Total						
65 to 74 years	6.7	12.6	3.4	2.0	10.0	14.3
75 to 84 years	8.0	21.8	5.4	3.5	13.4	24.1
85 years & over	7.0	19.8	9.4	10.7	16.4	24.1
All persons 65 years & over	7.0	16.5	4.5	3.3	10.7	18.7

[1] Has a doctor ever told you that you had osteoporosis, sometimes called thin or brittle bones?

[2] Has a doctor ever told you that you had broken or fractured your hip?

[3] Source: Praemer A, Furner S, Rice DP. Musculoskeletal Conditions in the United States. Rosemont, IL. 1999, American Academy of Orthopaedic Surgeons.

[4] Source: National Center for Health Statistics. National Health and Nutrition Examination Survey Data, 1999-2004

Table 5.3: Self-Reported Prevalence of Osteoporosis, Osteoporosis Treatment or Related Fracture [1] for Persons Aged 45 and Over, United State 1999-2004

Age Group	Prevalence (in 000s)			Occurrence by Sex		Distribution by Age		Prevalence Rate (% of population in age group)		
	Females	Males	Total Population	Females	Males	Females	Males	Females	Males	Total Population
Ever been told had osteoporosis?										
45-64	2,822	487	3,309	85.3%	14.7%	35.7%	47.7%	8.4%	1.6%	5.1%
65-74	2,145	214	2,359	90.9%	9.1%	27.2%	20.9%	21.2%	2.5%	12.6%
75-84	2,353	262	2,615	90.0%	10.0%	29.8%	25.6%	32.2%	5.6%	21.8%
85+	578	59	637	90.7%	9.3%	7.3%	5.8%	28.6%	4.9%	19.8%
Total Aged 45 & Over	7,898	1,022	8,919	88.6%	11.5%	100.0%	100.0%	14.8%	2.2%	9.0%
Ever been treated for osteoporosis? (if responded "YES" to osteoporosis)										
45-64	1,847	254	2,101	87.9%	12.1%	32.1%	39.5%	65.5%	52.2%	63.5%
65-74	1,603	155	1,759	91.1%	8.8%	27.8%	24.1%	74.8%	772.6%	74.6%
75-84	1,839	203	2,042	90.1%	9.9%	31.9%	31.6%	78.2%	77.5%	78.1%
85+	467	31	497	94.0%	6.2%	8.1%	4.8%	80.7%	52.4%	78.1%
Total Aged 45 & Over	5,756	643	6,399	90.0%	10.0%	100.0%	100.0%	72.9%	63.0%	71.7%
Ever been told had broken or fractured your hip?										
45-64	197	321	519	38.0%	61.8%	23.3%	39.4%	0.6%	1.0%	0.8%
65-74	116	267	372	31.2%	71.8%	13.7%	32.8%	1.1%	3.0%	2.0%
75-84	259	162	421	61.5%	38.5%	30.7%	19.9%	3.5%	3.4%	3.5%
85+	272	73	346	78.6%	21.1%	32.2%	9.0%	13.4%	6.1%	10.7%
Total Aged 45 & Over	844	814	1,658	50.9%	49.1%	100.0%	101.1%	1.6%	1.8%	1.7%
Ever been told had broken or fractured your spine?										
45-64	531	1,083	1,614	32.9%	67.1%	46.9%	70.3%	1.6%	3.5%	2.5%
65-74	174	245	418	41.6%	58.6%	15.4%	15.9%	1.7%	2.8%	2.2%
75-84	229	172	401	57.1%	42.9%	20.2%	11.2%	3.1%	3.6%	3.3%
85+	198	42	240	82.5%	17.5%	17.5%	2.7%	9.8%	3.5%	7.4%
Total Aged 45 & Over	1,132	1,541	2,673	42.3%	57.7%	100.0%	100.1%	2.1%	3.4%	2.7%
Ever been told had broken or fractured your wrist?										
45-64	2,333	3,707	6,340	36.8%	58.5%	51.3%	71.4%	6.9%	11.9%	9.3%
65-74	1,080	983	2,063	52.4%	47.6%	23.7%	18.9%	10.6%	11.4%	11.0%
75-84	792	407	1,198	66.1%	34.0%	17.4%	7.8%	10.8%	8.6%	10.0%
85+	345	93	438	78.8%	21.2%	7.6%	1.8%	17.0%	7.8%	13.6%
Total Aged 45 & Over	4,549	5,190	9,739	46.7%	53.3%	100.0%	100.0%	8.5%	11.4%	9.9%
Ever been told had osteoporosis, been treated for osteoporosis, or had broken or fractured hip, spine or wrist?										
45-64	5,388	5,108	10,496	51.3%	48.7%	43.2%	66.0%	16.0%	16.5%	16.2%
65-74	3,060	1,531	4,591	66.7%	33.3%	24.5%	19.8%	30.1%	17.8%	24.5%
75-84	3,074	870	3,944	77.9%	22.1%	24.6%	11.2%	42.1%	18.4%	32.8%
85+	962	234	1,197	80.4%	19.5%	7.7%	3.0%	47.5%	19.6%	37.1%
Total Aged 45 & Over	12,484	7,743	20,228	61.7%	38.3%	100.0%	100.0%	23.4%	17.0%	20.5%

[1] Replied "Yes" when asked if ever been told by a doctor that you had osteoporosis, been treated for osteoporosis, or had broken or fractured your (hip)(spine)(wrist).

Source: National Center for Health Statistics. National Health and Nutrition Examination Survey Data, 1999-2004

Table 5.4: Health Care Visits for Osteoporosis and Related Conditions [1] for Persons Aged 45 and Older by Site, United States 2004

	Visits (in 000s)				
	Inpatient Hospitalization [4]	Physician Visits [5]	Emergency Room Encounters [6]	Outpatient Visits [7]	Total All Health Care Resources
Primary Osteoporosis or Low Bone Density	899.2	5,013.2	*	294.9	6,248.5
% of Total Visits	14.4%	80.2%	0.7%	4.7%	
Low Energy Fracture [2]					
Hip	313.5	*	211.9	*	929.5
Wrist/Hand	54.4	*	342.5	82.9	1,318.7
Vertebrae/Pelvic	150.2	*	139.3	*	652.2
Upper Limb (Arm/Shoulder)	78.2	*	206.8	*	683.2
Lower Limb (Leg)	77.1	*	125.8	*	931.0
Foot/Ankle	78.7	926.5	230.2	69.3	1,304.7
All Low Energy Fractures	704.3	3,546.5	1,231.5	258.6	5,740.9
% of Total Visits	12.3%	61.8%	21.5%	4.5%	
% of Low Energy Fracture Patients with Osteoporosis Diagonsis	16.4%	1.6%	1.1%	2.1%	
Secondary Osteoporosis Diagnosis [3]					
Contributing Condition	143.7	5,679.7	*	224.1	6,053.8
Vertebral Fracture w/Spinal Cord Injury	0.0	*	*	0.0	1,430.6

* Estimate does not meet standards for reliability.

[1] Osteoporosis and related condition ICD-9-CM codes shown in the Table 5.1.

[2] Treatment for fractures, excluding those with high energy causes (i.e., vehicular [auto, air, water] accidents, war injuries)

[3] Diagnosis of another medical condition that may lead to or contribute to the development of osteoporosis

[4] Source: Agency for Healthcare Research and Quality, Healthcare Cost and Utilization Project, Nationwide Inpatient Sample, 2004

[5] Source: National Center for Health Statistics, National Ambulatory Medical Care Survey, 2004

[6] Source: National Center for Health Statistics, National Hospital Ambulatory Medical Care Survey, Hospital Emergency, 2004

[7] Source: National Center for Health Statistics, National Hospital Ambulatory Medical Care Survey, Outpatient Centers, 2004

Table 5.5: Inpatient Resource Utilization for Osteoporosis and Related Conditions [1] for Persons Age 45 and Older by Age and Sex, United States 2004

FEMALES	% by Age Group			Total Aged 45 & Older (in 000s)	Mean Age (in years)	DISTRIBUTION BY GENDER		Total Inpatient Hospitali-zations (in 000s)
	45-64	65-74	75 & Older			Females	Males	
Primary Osteoporosis	12.6%	21.1%	66.3%	809.7	77.6	90.1%	9.9%	899.2
Low Energy Fracture [2]								
Hip	6.7%	14.1%	79.2%	227.6	81.2	72.6%	27.4%	313.5
Wrist/Hand	22.1%	19.1%	58.8%	40.6	74.8	74.6%	25.4%	54.4
Vertebrae/Pelvic	10.4%	14.5%	75.1%	101.6	79.4	67.6%	32.4%	150.2
Upper Limb (Arm/Shoulder)	16.6%	20.9%	62.5%	56.8	76.6	72.7%	27.3%	78.2
Lower Limb (Leg)	29.5%	21.9%	48.6%	54.7	72.5	70.9%	29.1%	77.1
Foot/Ankle	44.4%	20.2%	35.4%	52.8	67.6	67.0%	33.0%	78.7
All Low Energy Fractures	15.6%	16.7%	67.7%	499.2	77.7	77.3%	22.7%	704.3
Low Energy Fracture with Osteoporosis Diagnosis				105.0		105.0	10.5	115.5
% Low Energy Fracture Patients with Osteoporosis Diagnosis	8.8%	19.4%	24.0%	21.0%		21.0%	5.1%	16.4%
Secondary Osteoporosis Diagnosis [3]								
Contributing Condition	43.2%	21.4%	35.5%	104.7	67.8	72.9%	27.1%	143.7
Vertebral Fracture w/Spinal Cord Injury	0.0%	0.0%	0.0%	0.0	na	0.0%	0.0%	0.0
MALES								
Primary Osteoporosis	18.8%	22.1%	59.1%	89.5	75.3			
Low Energy Fracture [2]								
Hip	15.7%	17.8%	66.5%	85.9	77.2			
Wrist/Hand	55.7%	15.0%	29.2%	13.8	64.5			
Vertebrae/Pelvic	33.6%	18.1%	48.2%	48.7	70.9			
Upper Limb (Arm/Shoulder)	41.4%	20.0%	38.6%	21.4	68.5			
Lower Limb (Leg)	54.2%	20.5%	25.3%	22.4	64.4			
Foot/Ankle	59.4%	22.1%	18.5%	25.9	61.8			
All Low Energy Fractures	32.8%	18.7%	48.5%	204.3	71.4			
Low Energy Fracture with Osteoporosis Diagnosis				10.5				
% Low Energy Fracture Patients with Osteoporosis Diagnosis	2.7%	3.2%	7.6%	5.1%				
Secondary Osteoporosis Diagnosis [3]								
Contributing Condition	45.8%	26.1%	28.0%	39.0	66.2			
Vertebral Fracture w/Spinal Cord Injury	0.0%	0.0%	0.0%	0.0	na			

[1] Osteoporosis and related condition ICD-9-CM codes shown in the Table 5.1.

[2] Treatment for fractures, excluding those with high energy causes (i.e., vehicular [auto, air, water] accidents, war injuries).

[3] Diagnosis of another medical condition that may lead to or contribute to the development of osteoporosis.

Source: Agency for Healthcare Research and Quality, Healthcare Cost and Utilization Project, Nationwide Inpatient Sample, 2004

Table 5.6: Hospital Emergency Room Resource Utilization for Low Energy Fractures [1] for Persons Aged 45 and Older by Age and Sex, United States 2004

FEMALES	45-64	65-74	75 & Older	Total 45 & Older (in 000s)	Mean Age (in years)	Females	Males	Total Emergency Room Treatments (in 000s)
Low Energy Fracture [2]								
Hip	4.9%	10.0%	85.1%	172.3	83.0	81.3%	18.7%	211.9
Wrist/Hand	49.5%	24.8%	25.7%	255.7	65.6	74.7%	25.3%	342.5
Vertebrae/Pelvic	10.5%	21.4%	68.1%	95.3	78.0	68.4%	31.6%	139.3
Upper Limb (Arm/ Shoulder)	31.0%	29.6%	39.3%	154.0	71.0	74.5%	25.5%	206.8
Lower Limb (Leg)	49.4%	14.1%	36.5%	94.1	67.1	74.8%	25.2%	125.8
Foot/Ankle	79.3%	11.1%	9.6%	161.9	57.4	70.3%	29.7%	230.2
All Low Energy Fractures	40.0%	19.2%	40.9%	920.4	69.5	74.7%	25.3%	1,231.5
MALES								
Low Energy Fracture [2]								
Hip	15.2%	7.8%	77.0%	39.6	77.0			
Wrist/Hand	44.8%	20.0%	35.2%	86.7	68.4			
Vertebrae/Pelvic	39.0%	49.7%	11.4%	44.0	64.0			
Upper Limb (Arm/ Shoulder)	16.9%	33.9%	49.2%	52.8	73.3			
Lower Limb (Leg)	80.1%	5.0%	14.9%	31.7	57.9			
Foot/Ankle	81.8%	11.5%	6.6%	68.3	54.9			
All Low Energy Fractures	48.1%	22.4%	29.5%	311.1	65.3			

* Estimate does not meet standards for reliability.

[1] Osteoporosis and related condition ICD-9-CM codes shown in the Table 5.1.

[2] Treatment for fractures, excluding those with high energy causes (i.e., vehicular [auto, air, water] accidents, war injuries).

Source: National Center for Health Statistics, National Hospital Ambulatory Medical Care Survey, Hospital Emergency Room, 2004

Table 5.7: Hospital Discharge to Short/Intermediate/Skilled Nursing Care for Persons with Osteoporosis and Related Conditions [1] Aged 45 and Older by Age and Sex, United States 2004

	% of Total WITH Condition				% of Total WITHOUT Condition			
FEMALES	**45-64**	**65-74**	**75 & Older**	**All 45 & Over**	**45-64**	**65-74**	**75 & Older**	**All 45 & Over**
Primary Osteoporosis	18.6%	26.6%	46.3%	38.7%	10.8%	21.8%	37.9%	24.0%
Low Energy Fracture [2]								
Hip	51.4%	77.8%	86.1%	82.6%	10.8%	21.4%	37.0%	23.9%
Wrist/Hand	16.4%	31.8%	60.1%	45.0%	10.9%	22.1%	38.7%	24.9%
Vertebrae/Pelvic	29.3%	57.6%	68.0%	62.4%	10.9%	21.9%	38.4%	24.6%
Upper Limb (Arm/Shoulder)	20.6%	42.9%	67.2%	54.4%	10.9%	22.0%	38.6%	24.8%
Lower Limb (Leg)	35.2%	66.0%	79.6%	63.5%	10.8%	21.9%	38.6%	24.8%
Foot/Ankle	20.3%	48.3%	68.0%	42.8%	10.9%	22.0%	38.7%	24.9%
All Low Energy Fractures	**28.0%**	**60.0%**	**77.0%**	**66.5%**	**10.6%**	**20.8%**	**36.0%**	**23.1%**
MALES								
Primary Osteoporosis	24.5%	28.7%	43.6%	36.7%	12.5%	19.0%	30.8%	20.0%
Low Energy Fracture [2]								
Hip	51.2%	68.5%	84.0%	76.1%	12.4%	18.7%	30.0%	19.7%
Wrist/Hand	14.0%	37.4%	52.5%	28.8%	12.6%	19.0%	31.0%	20.2%
Vertebrae/Pelvic	24.1%	37.5%	62.3%	45.0%	12.5%	19.0%	30.8%	20.0%
Upper Limb (Arm/Shoulder)	19.8%	39.5%	60.0%	39.3%	12.6%	19.0%	30.9%	20.1%
Lower Limb (Leg)	25.1%	63.9%	72.3%	45.1%	12.5%	19.0%	30.9%	20.1%
Foot/Ankle	15.3%	32.1%	58.2%	26.9%	12.6%	19.0%	31.0%	20.2%
All Low Energy Fractures	**24.8%**	**50.8%**	**74.1%**	**53.6%**	**12.3%**	**18.5%**	**29.6%**	**19.4%**

[1] Osteoporosis and related condition ICD-9-CM codes shown in the Table 5.1.

[2] Treatment for fractures, excluding those with high energy causes (i.e., vehicular [auto, air, water] accidents, war injuries).

Source: Agency for Healthcare Research and Quality, Healthcare Cost and Utilization Project, Nationwide Inpatient Sample, 2004

Table 5.8: Osteoporosis and Related Conditions [1] in Nursing Home Population Aged 65 and Over, United States 2004

			Prevalence (in 00s)			
	65-74	75-84	85 & Over	Male	Female	Total Population
Diagnosis at Time of Admittance (based on age at time of admission)						
Primary Osteoporosis	*	21.6	49.9	*	71.0	76.4
Low Energy Fracture (All)	90.8	387.8	650.5	207.5	973.1	1,180.6
Hip	35.0	171.6	302.6	103.4	411.7	515.1
Vertebrae/Pelvic	*	49.3	106.3	*	148.5	173.1
Upper Limb (Arm, Shoulder)	*	35.1	32.9	*	66.3	77.8
Lower Limb (Leg)	25.2	98.9	135.1	47.0	235.9	282.9
Ankle/Foot	*	*	*	*	42.9	51.7
Secondary Osteoporosis Condition Present				*	*	*
Current Primary Diagnosis (based on age at time of interview)						
Primary Osteoporosis	*	33.8	104.4	*	149.8	152.5
Low Energy Fracture (All)	22.3	113.2	234.6	104.6	297.0	401.6
Hip	*	47.4	102.5	36.8	122.8	159.5
Vertebrae/Pelvic	*	*	46.7	*	52.9	73.6
Upper Limb (Arm, Shoulder)	*	*	*	*	*	*
Lower Limb (Leg)	*	29.6	47.3	*	73.0	98.8
Ankle/Foot	*	*	*	*	*	*
Secondary Osteoporosis Condition Present	*	*	*	*	*	29.0
Current Secondary Diagnosis (based on age at time of interview)						
Primary Osteoporosis	155.9	666.7	1,272.0	170.6	2,018.3	2,188.8
Secondary Osteoporosis Condition Present	42.5	164.4	297.8	68.3	479.8	548.1
Falls and Fractures (based on age at time of interview)						
Reported Fall Within Past 6 Months	*	1,849.0	2,560.0	1,498.0	3,719.0	5,217.0
Sustained Hip Fracture Within Past 180 Days	*	95.0	141.0	69.0	206.0	276.0
Sustained Other Fracture Within Past 180 Days	*	107.0	159.0	78.0	260.0	339.0
Total Nursing Home Population Aged 65 & Older, 2004	1,741.2	4,688.7	6,742.1	3,368.2	9,803.9	13,172.1

* Estimate does not meet standards for reliability.

[1] Osteoporosis and related condition ICD-9-CM codes shown in the Table 5.1.

Source: National Center for Health Statistics, National Nursing Home Survey, 2004

Table 5.9: Self-Reported Fracture (Ever) for Persons Aged 45 and Over by Age and Sex, United States 1999-2004

FEMALES

	45-64	65-74	75-84	85 & Older	45 & Over
Rate per 100 Persons					
Broken or Fractured Hip	0.6	1.1	3.5	13.4	1.6
Broken or Fractured Wrist	6.9	10.6	10.8	17.0	8.5
Broken or Fractured Spine	1.6	1.7	3.1	9.8	2.1
% of First Fractures Caused by a Fall [1]					
Broken or Fractured Hip	74%	66%	96%	93%	90%
Broken or Fractured Wrist	91%	93%	93%	100%	94%
Broken or Fractured Spine	44%	72%	57%	75%	69%
Mean Age of First Fracture Caused by a Fall (in years)					
Broken or Fractured Hip	56.0	68.5	73.1	80.2	74.8
Broken or Fractured Wrist	53.2	60.0	69.2	73.3	62.9
Broken or Fractured Spine	60.9	61.2	68.9	78.8	70.6

MALES

	45-64	65-74	75-84	85 & Older	45 & Over
Rate per 100 Persons					
Broken or Fractured Hip	1.0	3.0	3.4	6.1	1.8
Broken or Fractured Wrist	11.9	11.4	8.6	7.8	11.4
Broken or Fractured Spine	3.5	2.8	3.6	3.5	3.4
% of First Fractures Caused by a Fall [1]					
Broken or Fractured Hip	50%	53%	70%	80%	69%
Broken or Fractured Wrist	82%	82%	93%	91%	86%
Broken or Fractured Spine	47%	58%	50%	57%	64%
Mean Age of First Fracture Caused by a Fall (in years)					
Broken or Fractured Hip	55.0	62.8	70.4	80.0	69.2
Broken or Fractured Wrist	54.7	60.4	62.8	75.0	60.2
Broken or Fractured Spine	56.5	57.4	68.0	75.1	60.9

[1] Self-reported cause as a "fall/tripped/slipped/fell out of bed" or "hard fall off ladder/stool /downstairs."

Source: National Center for Health Statistics. National Health and Nutrition Examination Survey Data, 1999-2004.

Table 5.10: Low Energy Fractures [1] Treated as Inpatient or Emergency Room Visits for Persons Aged 45 and Over by Anatomic Site by Sex, United States 2004

Inpatient Treatment [2]

	Females		Males	
	Prevalence (in 000s) [4]	% of Total Fracture Sites	Prevalence (in 000s) [4]	% of Total Fracture Sites
Hip	227.6	42.6%	85.9	39.4%
Vertebrae/Pelvic	101.6	19.0%	48.7	22.3%
Upper Limb (Arm/Shoulder)	56.8	10.6%	21.4	9.8%
Lower Limb (Leg)	54.7	10.2%	22.4	10.3%
Foot/Ankle	52.8	9.9%	25.9	11.9%
Wrist/Hand	40.6	7.6%	13.8	6.3%
All Low Energy Fractures	499.2	100.0%	204.3	100.0%

Emergency Room Treatment [3]

	Females		Males	
	Prevalence (in 000s) [4]	% of Total Fracture Sites	Prevalence (in 000s) [4]	% of Total Fracture Sites
Hip	172.3	18.5%	39.6	12.3%
Vertebrae/Pelvic	95.3	10.2%	44.0	13.6%
Upper Limb (Arm/Shoulder)	154.0	16.5%	52.8	16.3%
Lower Limb (Leg)	94.1	10.1%	31.7	9.8%
Foot/Ankle	161.9	17.3%	68.3	21.1%
Wrist/Hand	255.7	27.4%	86.7	26.8%
All Low Energy Fractures	920.4	100.0%	311.1	100.0%

[1] Treatment for fractures, excluding those with high energy causes (i.e., vehicular [auto, air, water] accidents, war injuries)

[2] Source: Agency for Healthcare Research and Quality, Healthcare Cost and Utilization Project, Nationwide Inpatient Sample, 2004

[3] Source: National Center for Health Statistics, National Hospital Ambulatory Medical Care Survey, Hospital Emergency Room, 2004

[4] Multiple fractures sites per patient possible.

Source: National Center for Health Statistics. National Hospital Discharge Survey, 2004.

Table 5.11: Inpatient Cost Associated with Osteoporosis [1] and Low Energy Fractures [2] for Persons Aged 45 and Older, United States 2004

	Prevalence (in 000s)	Mean Length of Stay (in days)	Mean Cost per Patient Stay	Estimated Total Cost (in billions)
Osteoporosis Diagnosis Patients				
Osteoporosis Without Fracture	783.7	5.3	$ 20,704	$ 16.23
Osteoporosis With Fracture	115.5	5.7	$ 24,634	$ 2.85
All Osteoporosis Diagnosis	**899.2**	**5.3**	**$ 21,209**	**$ 19.07**
Non-Osteoporosis Patients	20,758.9	5.4	$ 26,264	$ 545.21
Low Energy Fracture Patients				
Hip	313.5	6.7	$ 32,310	$ 10.13
Vertebrae/Pelvic	150.2	6.6	$ 27,610	$ 4.15
Upper Limb (Arm/Shoulder)	78.2	5.2	$ 24,347	$ 1.90
Lower Limb (Leg)	77.1	6.2	$ 29,190	$ 2.25
Foot/Ankle	78.7	4.5	$ 21,618	$ 1.70
Wrist/Hand	54.4	4.9	$ 23,893	$ 1.30
All Low Energy Fractures	**704.3**	**6.1**	**$ 27,919**	**$ 19.66**
Non-Fracture Patients	20,723.3	5.4	$ 25,883	$ 536.38

[1] Osteoporosis and related condition ICD-9-CM codes shown in the Section 5.5

[2] Treatment for fractures, excluding those with high energy causes (i.e., vehicular [auto, air, water] accidents, war injuries)

Source: Agency for Healthcare Research and Quality, Healthcare Cost and Utilization Project, Nationwide Inpatient Sample, 2004

Source: National Center for Health Statistics. National Hospital Discharge Survey, 2004.

Chapter 6

Musculoskeletal Injuries

More than three of every five unintentional injuries that occur annually in the United States are to the musculoskeletal system. Although the incidence of total unintentional injuries is difficult to estimate, numerous databases and reports have shown that a consistent 60% to 67% of injuries that occur annually involve the musculoskeletal system. (Table 6.1 and Graph 6.0.1)

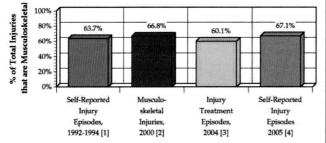

Graph 6.0.1: Musculoskeletal Injuries as Proportion of Total Injuries, United States 1992-1994, 2000, 2004, and 2005

[1] Praemer A, Furner S, Rice DP: *Musculoskeletal Conditions in the United States*, ed 2. Rosemont, IL:American Academy of Orthopaedic Surgeons, 1999, p 83.
[2] Finkelstein EA, Corso PS, Miller TR: *The Incidence and Economic Burden of Injuries in the United States*. New York, NY: Oxford University Press, 2006, p 13.
[3] National Center for Health Statistics, National Ambulatory Medical Care Survey, 2004; National Hospital Ambulatory Medical Care Survey, Emergency Room Visits, 2004; National Hospital Ambulatory Medical Visits, Outpatient Department Visits, 2004.
[4] National Center for Health Statistics, National Health Interview Survey, 2005.

Musculoskeletal injuries are injuries occurring to the neck, spine, pelvis and extremities; they include fractures, derangements, dislocations, sprains and strains, contusions, crushing injuries, open wounds, and traumatic amputations. The most common cause of musculoskeletal injuries is falls. Additional major causes of musculoskeletal injuries are sports injuries, playground accidents, motor vehicle crashes, civilian interpersonal violence, war injuries, stress injuries, over-exertion, and repetitive workplace injuries.

In 2004, more than 57.2 million episodes of treatment for musculoskeletal injuries were recorded in physician offices, emergency rooms, outpatient clinics, and hospitalizations. This compares to 95.3 million episodes of treatment for all kinds of injuries, including burns, poisoning, and drowning.

Section 6.1: Prevalence of Musculoskeletal Injuries

While the number of self-reported injury episodes has been declining since 1997 and is believed to be under-reported,[1] the distribution of types of musculoskeletal injuries is similar for both self-reported and injury treatment episodes. In 2005, persons in the civilian non-institutionalized population self-reported 20.2 million musculoskeletal injury episodes in the annual National Health Interview Survey. This compares to an annual average of 36.9 million musculoskeletal injury episodes reported in the same survey 1992-1994,[2] and to 57.2 million musculoskeletal injury treatment episodes in physician offices, emergency rooms, outpatient clinics, and hospitalizations reported in 2004. (Table 6.2) Injury treatment episodes in 2004 reflect actual injury burden more reliably than self-reported injury episodes and will define the musculoskeletal injury burden in this chapter.

Section 6.1.1: Musculoskeletal Injuries by Type

Among self-reported musculoskeletal injuries, sprains and strains were the most frequent, accounting for 38%. Fractures, representing 22% of self-reported musculoskeletal injuries, were the second most frequent. Among musculoskeletal injury treatment episodes, these two types of injuries were nearly equal, accounting for 26% and 25% of the total injury treatment episodes, respectively. Open wounds and contusions accounted for 17% and 14%, respectively, both in self-reported and injury treatment episodes, while dislocations accounted for 8% of injury treatment episodes and only 2% of self-reported injury episodes. (Table 6.3 and Graph 6.1.1)

Nearly 15.3 million fractures were treated in physician offices, emergency and outpatient clinics, and hospitals in 2004. (Table 6.4) More than 2.9 million of these occurred in young males under the age of 18, while another 2.7 million occurred in females aged 65 and over.

Sprains and strains accounted for nearly 16.3 million musculoskeletal injury treatment episodes in 2004, with 6.8 million treated in persons aged 18 to 44, the most common age in which a sprain or strain is reported and treated.

Open wounds are the third most frequently treated musculoskeletal injury, accounting for more than 10.3 million injury treatment episodes in 2004. Open wounds were treated with similar frequency in all age groups, but were more commonly treated in males (6.0 million treatment episodes) than females (4.3 million treatment episodes).

Approximately 8.4 million contusions were treated in 2004, with 2.8 million occurring in persons between the ages of 18 and 44; persons aged 65 and over experienced contusions more frequently than other age groups.

Section 6.1.2: Rate of Musculoskeletal Injuries by Age and Sex

The 2004 annual rate of all injury and of musculoskeletal injury treatment episodes was similar for males and females. (Table 6.4 and Graph 6.1.2) Overall, in 2004, persons aged 65 and

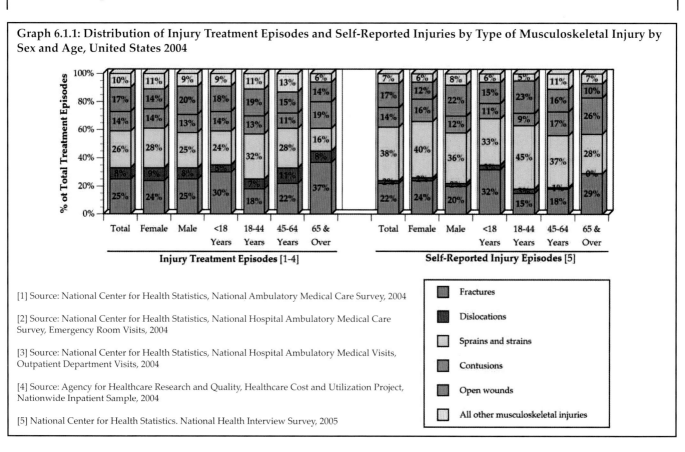

Graph 6.1.1: Distribution of Injury Treatment Episodes and Self-Reported Injuries by Type of Musculoskeletal Injury by Sex and Age, United States 2004

[1] Source: National Center for Health Statistics, National Ambulatory Medical Care Survey, 2004

[2] Source: National Center for Health Statistics, National Hospital Ambulatory Medical Care Survey, Emergency Room Visits, 2004

[3] Source: National Center for Health Statistics, National Hospital Ambulatory Medical Visits, Outpatient Department Visits, 2004

[4] Source: Agency for Healthcare Research and Quality, Healthcare Cost and Utilization Project, Nationwide Inpatient Sample, 2004

[5] National Center for Health Statistics. National Health Interview Survey, 2005

Legend:
- Fractures
- Dislocations
- Sprains and strains
- Contusions
- Open wounds
- All other musculoskeletal injuries

over were more likely to sustain any type of injury (46.3 per 100 persons) or a musculoskeletal injury (26.5 per 100 persons) than were persons of any other age group.

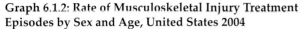
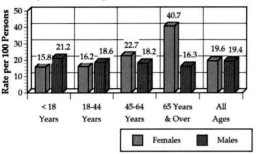

Graph 6.1.2: Rate of Musculoskeletal Injury Treatment Episodes by Sex and Age, United States 2004

Sources: National Center for Health Statistics: National Ambulatory Medical Care Survey, 2004; National Hospital Ambulatory Medical Care Survey, Emergency Room Visits, 2004; National Hospital Ambulatory Medical Visits, Outpatient Department Visits, 2004.
Agency for Healthcare Research and Quality: Healthcare Cost and Utilization Project, Nationwide Inpatient Sample, 2004.

Musculoskeletal injury rates vary between males and females by age, with the injury rate highest among males under the age of 18 (21.2 per 100 males), while females aged 65 and over have the highest musculoskeletal injury rate (40.7 per 100 females). Fractures are the most common musculoskeletal injury in both young males and older females, while sprains and strains are more common among males and females between the ages of 18 and 64.

In 2004, fractures accounted for 25% of the 57.2 million musculoskeletal injuries treated in physician offices, emergency and outpatient clinics, and hospitalizations. The overall fracture injury treatment rate in 2004 was 5.2 per 100 persons. Among males under the age of 18, the fracture injury treatment rate was 8.0 per 100 persons, while females of this age were treated for fractures at a rate of 3.8 per 100 persons. Among females aged 65 and older, fracture injury treatment rates were 17.5 per 100, while men in this age group were treated for fractures at a much lower (5.4 per 100 persons) rate. (Table 6.4)

In all injury categories, females aged 65 and older were treated at higher rates than males of the same age. Treatment for contusions was 7.8 episodes per 100 among older females, and 3.4 among older males; 6.1 for sprains and strains among females, and 3.1 among males. The only type of musculoskeletal injury to show similar rates of treatment between females and males aged 65 and over in 2004 was open wounds, with rates of 4.0 and 3.9, respectively, per 100 persons. (Table 6.4)

Among the young, aged 18 and under, males had higher rates of injury treatment for all types of injury than did females, with overall musculoskeletal treatment rates of 21.2 and 15.8 per 100 persons, respectively, among this age group. (Table 6.4)

Males between the ages of 18 and 44 were treated for musculoskeletal injuries at slightly higher rates than females in this age group, 18.6 versus 16.2 per 100 persons, respectively. Fractures and open wounds accounted for the higher treatment rates among males in this age group. Between the ages of 45 and 64, females begin to show a higher rate of musculoskeletal injury treatment than males, with 22.7 per 100 females treated, compared to 18.2 per 100 males. Fractures, dislocations, strains and strains, and contusions all showed higher treatment rates, while open wounds were still treated at a higher rate among males than females in this age group. (Table 6.4)

Section 6.1.3: Fracture Trends

The total number of fractures of the upper and lower extremities treated in physician offices, emergency departments, and hospitals, while fluctuating year to year, has remained fairly constant since 1998. (Table 6.5 and Graph 6.1.3) In 1998, 13.65 million treatment episodes for fractures of the upper and lower limbs were reported; in 2004, 12.36 million were treated.

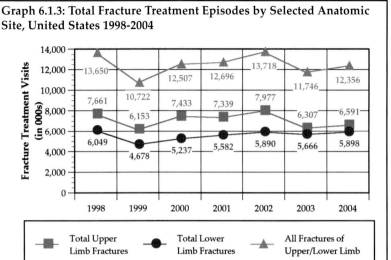

Graph 6.1.3: Total Fracture Treatment Episodes by Selected Anatomic Site, United States 1998-2004

Sources: National Center for Health Statistics, National Hospital Discharge Survey, 1998-2004; National Center for Health Statistics, National Hospital Ambulatory Medical Care Survey, Emergency Room Visits, 1998-2004; National Center for Health Statistics, National Hospital Ambulatory Medical Visits, Physician Visits, 1998-2004

Upper limb fractures account for 53% to 59% of the total fractures treated, while lower limb fractures accounted for 42% to 48% across the years. (Table 6.5a)

Wrist, hand, and finger fractures accounted for about one-half of upper limb fractures, with forearm fractures accounting for 28% to 41% of the remaining upper limb fractures. Fractures to the upper arm, or humerus, accounted for 8% or less of all reported treatment episodes for upper limb fractures. Fractures of the ankle, foot or toes accounted for more than one-half of treated lower limb fractures. The majority of fractures, 62% to 71%, were treated in a physician's office. Fewer than one in ten fractures (8% or less) were treated with inpatient hospitalization in any given year. (Table 6.5a)

Section 6.2: Location and Causes of Musculoskeletal Injuries

The most common location where musculoskeletal injury episodes occur is at home. In 2004, nearly one in two of the 21.6 million self-reported injury episodes occurred in or around the home. Musculoskeletal injury episodes that occurred in automobile or pedestrian related incidents—injuries that occurred on the streets or highways—accounted for only 9% of the reported injury episodes. An additional 9% of musculoskeletal injury episodes occurred while participating in sport activities, while 8% occurred in schools. The remaining 29% occurred in other locations, including shopping centers and restaurants. (Table 6.6 and Graph 6.2.1)

Falls were the leading cause of nonfatal unintentional injuries treated in hospital emergency departments in 2003 for all age groups. (Table 6.7 and Graph 6.2.2) Falls occurred at a rate of 27.1 per 1,000 persons and accounted for nearly 8 million of the nonfatal unintentional injuries treated in hospital emergency departments in the United States in 2003, nearly one in three (29%) of all unintentional injuries treated. Falls accounted for 63% of the nonfatal injuries treated for persons aged 65 and older.[3] (Table 6.8)

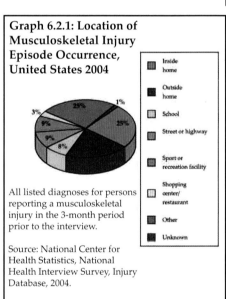

Graph 6.2.1: Location of Musculoskeletal Injury Episode Occurrence, United States 2004

Inside home
Outside home
School
Street or highway
Sport or recreation facility
Shopping center/ restaurant
Other
Unknown

All listed diagnoses for persons reporting a musculoskeletal injury in the 3-month period prior to the interview.

Source: National Center for Health Statistics, National Health Interview Survey, Injury Database, 2004.

Falls were also the leading cause of death in uninten-tional injuries for persons aged 75 and over in 2003,[3] accounting for nearly 12,000 of the 25,600 deaths due to unintentional injury in this age group. The rate of death from falls for

Graph 6.2.2: Nonfatal Unintentional Injuries Treated in Hospital Emergency Departments, United States 2003

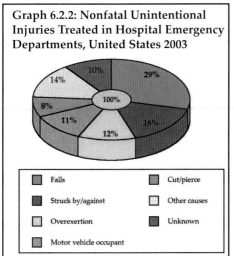

Source: National Safety Council: *Injury Facts, 2005-2006*. Itasca, IL: National Safety Council, 2006, p 13.

persons aged 75 to 84 years was 46.2 per 100,000 persons; that rate jumped to 131.8 per 100,000 among persons aged 85 years and older. (Table 6.9) In 1984, 54% of falls resulting in death occurred in the home; by 2004, the proportion had risen to 63%. (Table 6.10)

The most frequently self-reported type of injury is a sprain, strain or twist, accounting for one-third (32%) of all self-reported injury episodes in 2005. (Table 6.11) Motor vehicle incidents were the cause of more sprain, strain or twist injuries than any other reported mechanism, with one-half (49%) of persons involved in a motor vehicle incident reporting a sprain/strain injury.

Fractures occurred in more than one-third (35%) of the 273,000 accidents involving sports equipment (e.g., bikes, scooters, skateboards, skis, skates) and in 29% of the 2.5 million falls. Fractures occurred in more than one-half (53%) of the reported 39,000 incidents in which a pedestrian was struck. (Table 6.11)

Contusion or bruising injuries were reported in 16% of all accidents, with a high level occurring in incidents that involved motor vehicles, either as a passenger or as a pedestrian struck by a motor vehicle.

Section 6.3: Musculoskeletal Injury Sites

The Centers for Disease Control estimates that more than 50 million injuries occurred in 2000.[4] Traumatic brain injuries, injuries to the torso, systemwide injuries, and unspecified injuries represented nearly all the fatal injuries; however, injuries to the upper and lower extremities accounted for the greatest number of hospitalized and non-hospitalized injury episodes. (Table 6.12)

Fractures occur most frequently in the upper limb, including the hand, fingers, and arm. Of the 9.1 million fractures of the upper limb treated overall in 2004, 60% were treated in physician offices, accounting for 31% of all fractures treated in physician offices. (Table 6.13 and Graph 6.3.1) The ankle was the third most common site (13%) for fractures treated in physician offices, with the ribs/sternum, tibia and fibula (leg), and foot including toes accounting for 9% each of treated fractures.

Two-thirds (67%) of the 16.3 million sprain and strain injuries were treated in physician offices in 2004. Of these sprain and strain injuries, the back, including the sacroiliac joint, was the most common site, representing 34% of the treated injuries. Shoulder (22%) and ankle and foot injuries (20%) represented the other two most common anatomic sites for sprains and strains

Graph 6.3.1: Visits to Physicians in Office-Based Practice for Fractures at Selected Anatomic Sites, United States 2004

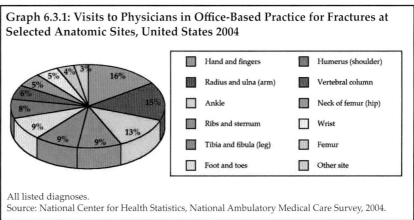

All listed diagnoses.
Source: National Center for Health Statistics, National Ambulatory Medical Care Survey, 2004.

treated in physician offices. (Table 6.13 and Graph 6.3.2)

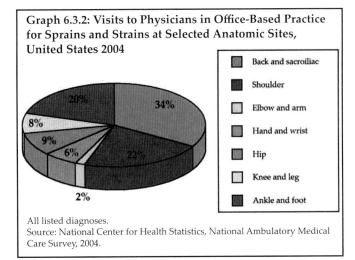

Graph 6.3.2: Visits to Physicians in Office-Based Practice for Sprains and Strains at Selected Anatomic Sites, United States 2004

Legend:
- Back and sacroiliac
- Shoulder
- Elbow and arm
- Hand and wrist
- Hip
- Knee and leg
- Ankle and foot

All listed diagnoses.
Source: National Center for Health Statistics, National Ambulatory Medical Care Survey, 2004.

A substantial majority of the 5.1 million dislocation injuries (85%) treated in 2004 were treated in physician offices. Dislocation of the knee joint represented 63% of these injuries, with the shoulder (6%) the only other anatomic site to account for more than a very small fraction of dislocations. (Table 6.13) This finding is likely an artifact of an ICD-9 coding anomaly. Isolated acute ligamentous injuries of the knee, (i.e., anterior cruciate ligament (ACL), medial collateral ligament (MCL), posterior cruciate ligament (PCL), and lateral collateral ligament (LCL) disruptions) are coded as dislocations using ICD-9 methodology, whereas equivalent injuries in other joints are coded as sprains or strains rather than dislocations. True complete dislocations of the knee joint are actually quite rare, and associated with marked morbidity.

The annual National Health Interview Survey (NHIS) provides data on self-reported injuries. In the 2004 NHIS, injuries to the ankle (11.6%) and knee (11.4%) were reported more frequently than other anatomical sites. (Table 6.14) Among persons under the age of 18, injuries to the ankle, foot, and toes were the most common. Persons aged 18 to 44 years reported injury to their ankle,

knee, and finger/thumb about equally, accounting for more than one-third of all reported musculoskeletal injuries. Persons aged 45 to 64 years reported knee injuries the most frequently. Knee, shoulder, and hip injuries were most common among persons aged 65 and over.

Section 6.4: Musculoskeletal Injury Limitations

Musculoskeletal injuries are often a cause of physical limitations in the ability to perform activities of daily living (e.g., eating, personal care, and dressing). In 2004, four out of every 100 persons reported they were currently experiencing limitations in their ability to perform daily activities as a result of a fracture or bone/joint injury. (Table 6.15 and Graph 6.4.1) Among persons aged 65 and over, the rate with limitations was nearly 11 out of 100 due to fracture or bone/joint injury. With the exception of persons aged 65 and over, males are more likely to report a limitation in ability to perform

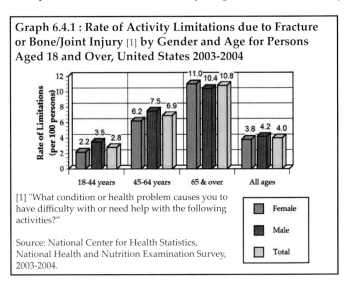

Graph 6.4.1 : Rate of Activity Limitations due to Fracture or Bone/Joint Injury [1] by Gender and Age for Persons Aged 18 and Over, United States 2003-2004

[1] "What condition or health problem causes you to have difficulty with or need help with the following activities?"

Source: National Center for Health Statistics, National Health and Nutrition Examination Survey, 2003-2004.

Legend:
- Female
- Male
- Total

activities of daily living due to fracture or other bone/joint injury than are women.

Many common chores around the house are reported as difficult to perform by persons with a musculoskeletal injury. As many as 84% of

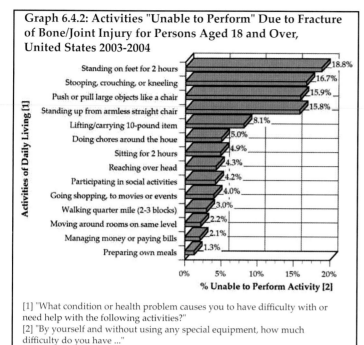

Graph 6.4.2: Activities "Unable to Perform" Due to Fracture of Bone/Joint Injury for Persons Aged 18 and Over, United States 2003-2004

[1] "What condition or health problem causes you to have difficulty with or need help with the following activities?"
[2] "By yourself and without using any special equipment, how much difficulty do you have ..."
Source: National Center for Health Statistics, National Health and Nutrition Examination Survey, 2003-2004.

persons reporting a musculoskeletal injury reported "some" to "unable to do" difficulty in performing twenty common tasks of daily living. (Table 6.16 and Graph 6.4.2) The most frequently mentioned limitation due to a fracture or bone/joint injury was "stooping, crouching or kneeling," with 84% reporting some degree of difficulty doing this. However, "standing on their feet for two hours or more" was reported by the highest percentage (19%) as "unable to perform."

In 2005, 4.4 million persons over the age of 18 reported spending a mean of 28.6 days in bed due to a fracture or bone/joint injury, resulting in a total of 127.1 million bed days. Bed days are defined as illness or injury that kept a person in bed more than one-half of a day, excluding hospitalization. An additional 10.6 million reported a mean of 29.4 bed days due to back or neck problems, for a total of 312.8 million bed days. Overall, musculoskeletal conditions, including arthritis and rheumatism, were responsible for 72% of all bed days reported for seven chronic or traumatic health conditions in the United States in 2005, with musculoskeletal injuries accounting for 13% of 2005 bed days. (Tables 6.17 and 6.19 and Graph 6.4.3)

Eleven percent (11%) of persons reporting they had been in the paid workforce over the previous 12 months also reported missing a mean of 24.8 days from work due to fractures, bone, or joint injury, for a total of 72.1 million lost work days. A missed work day is defined as absence from work due to illness or injury in the past 12 months, excluding maternity or family leave. Although other types of injuries were reported by

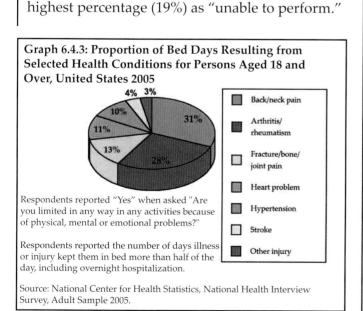

Graph 6.4.3: Proportion of Bed Days Resulting from Selected Health Conditions for Persons Aged 18 and Over, United States 2005

Respondents reported "Yes" when asked "Are you limited in any way in any activities because of physical, mental or emotional problems?"

Respondents reported the number of days illness or injury kept them in bed more than half of the day, including overnight hospitalization.

Source: National Center for Health Statistics, National Health Interview Survey, Adult Sample 2005.

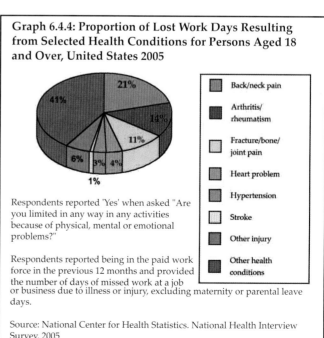

Graph 6.4.4: Proportion of Lost Work Days Resulting from Selected Health Conditions for Persons Aged 18 and Over, United States 2005

Respondents reported 'Yes' when asked "Are you limited in any way in any activities because of physical, mental or emotional problems?"

Respondents reported being in the paid work force in the previous 12 months and provided the number of days of missed work at a job or business due to illness or injury, excluding maternity or parental leave days.

Source: National Center for Health Statistics. National Health Interview Survey, 2005

only 4% of the workforce, mean lost work days were much higher at 48.7 days, for a total of 40.4 million lost work days. (Tables 6.18 and 6.19 and Graph 6.4.4)

Section 6.5: Workplace Injuries

Cumulative and repetitive motion injuries, also described as musculoskeletal disorders (MSDs), occur when the body reacts to strenuous motion (i.e., bending, climbing, crawling, reaching, twisting), overexertion, or repetitive motion. MSD injuries include sprains, strains, tears, back pain, soreness, carpal tunnel syndrome, hernia, and musculoskeletal system and connective diseases. MSD cases are more severe than the average nonfatal workplace injury or illness, typically involving an average of 2 additional days away from work.[5] In 2005, the median number of days away from work for all workplace injuries was 7 days; for MSD injuries, the median was 9 days.

In addition to MSD injuries as defined above, musculoskeletal workplace injuries include fractures, bruises/contusions, and amputations.

Section 6.5.1: Trends in Workplace Musculoskeletal Disorders

Although the rate of nonfatal occupational injuries and illnesses has decreased over the past 15 years, the relative percentage of MSD cases has fluctuated within a narrow range of 30% to 34%. (Table 6.20 and Graph 6.5.1) During this same time frame, total cases of work-related injuries and illnesses dropped from 2.33 million in 1998 to 1.23 million in 2005, a change of 47%. At the same time, MSDs declined from 784,100 to 375,500, a change of 52%.

The distribution of MSD injuries by type of injury has remained essentially constant over the past six years, as has the distribution between males (62%-64%) and females (36%-38%). (Tables 6.21 and 6.22) Slightly more than one-half (57%) of all sprain, strain, and tear injuries resulting in days away from work in 2005 were classified as an MSD injury. Although sprains, strains and tears represent about 40% of total workplace injuries and illnesses involving days away from work, they represent nearly three-fourths (72.5%) of all MSD injuries. (Graph 6.5.2) Back pain, carpal

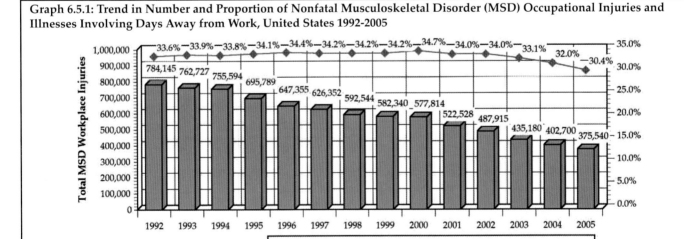

Graph 6.5.1: Trend in Number and Proportion of Nonfatal Musculoskeletal Disorder (MSD) Occupational Injuries and Illnesses Involving Days Away from Work, United States 1992-2005

Source 1998 to 2005: U.S. Department of Labor, Bureau of Labor Statistics: Case and Demographic Characteristics for Work-related Injuries and Illnesses Involving Days Away from Work. Supplemental Table 11: Number of nonfatal occupational injuries and illnesses involving days away from work by selected worker and case characteristics and musculoskeletal disorders, all United States, private industry, 2000-2005. Available at: http://www.bls.gov/iif/oshcdnew.htm#Resource%20Table%20categories%20-%202005. Accessed July 27, 2007.
Source 1992 to 1997: U.S. Department of Labor, Bureau of Labor Statistics: Worker Health Chartbook 2004. Available at: http://www2a.cdc.gov/niosh-Chartbook/imagedetail.asp?imgid=77. Accessed August 24, 2007.

The Burden of Musculoskeletal Diseases in the United States - Copyright © 2008

tunnel syndrome, tendonitis, soreness and pain (other than back pain), and a range of other conditions comprise the remaining MSD injuries. About 62% of back pain injuries and 42% of all soreness/pain injuries are classified as MSD injuries.

Graph 6.5.2: Proportion of Musculoskeletal Disorders (MSDs) by Type for Nonfatal Occupational Injuries [1] and Illnesses Involving Days Away from Work, United States 2005

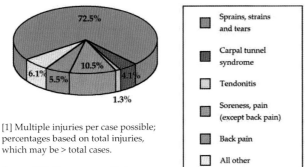

[1] Multiple injuries per case possible; percentages based on total injuries, which may be > total cases.

Source: U.S. Department of Labor, Bureau of Labor Statistics: Bureau of Case and Demographic Characteristics for Work-related Injuries and Illnesses Involving Days Away from Work. Supplemental Tables, Table 11: Number of nonfatal occupational injuries and illnesses involving days away from work by selected worker and case characteristics and musculoskeletal disorders, all United States, private industry, 2005. Available at: http://www.bls.gov/iif/oshcdnew.htm#Resource%20Table%20categories%20-%202005. Accessed July 27, 2007.

Section 6.5.2: Demographic Characteristics of MSD Workplace Injuries

Workplace injuries resulting in days away from work, both overall and for MSD injuries, are far more likely to be sustained by males than by females (2:1 ratio). This is most likely due to the differences in work environments, with males more likely employed in workplace settings with different risks and exposures. However, the ratio of full-time workers sustaining a carpal tunnel syndrome injury severe enough to result in days away from work is 2:1 for females versus males; 55% of the 2005 tendonitis injuries were incurred by females. (Table 6.23 and Graph 6.5.3)

Two-thirds or more of all workplace injuries and MSD injuries resulting in days away from work in 2005 were sustained by white workers. Carpal

Graph 6.5.3: Proportion of Musculoskeletal Disorders (MSDs) by Type for Nonfatal Occupational Injuries and Illnesses Involving Days Away from Work by Sex, United States 2005

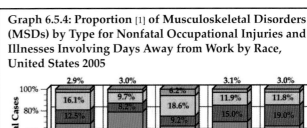

Source: U.S. Department of Labor, Bureau of Labor Statistics: Case and Demographic Characteristics for Work-related Injuries and Illnesses Involving Days Away from Work. Supplemental Tables 2005, Table 9: Number of nonfatal occupatonal injuries and illnesses involving days away from work by selected worker case characteristics and nature of injury or illness, all United States, private industry, 2005, and Table 11: Number of nonfatal occupational injuries and illnesses involving days away from work by selected worker and case characteristics and musculoskeletal disorders, all United States, private industry, 2005. Available at: http://www.bls.gov/iif/oshcdnew.htm#Resource%20Table%20categories%20-%202005. Accessed July 27, 2007.

Graph 6.5.4: Proportion [1] of Musculoskeletal Disorders (MSDs) by Type for Nonfatal Occupational Injuries and Illnesses Involving Days Away from Work by Race, United States 2005

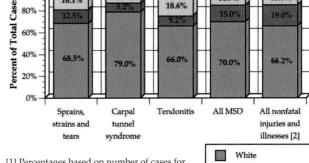

[1] Percentages based on number of cases for which race is reported.
[2] Nonfatal injuries and illnesses include the total of all nonfatal injuries and illnesses involving days away from work

Source: U.S. Department of Labor, Bureau of Labor Statistics: Case and Demographic Characteristics for Work-related Injuries and Illnesses Involving Days Away from Work. Supplemental Tables 2005, Table 9: Number of nonfatal occupatonal injuries and illnesses involving days away from work by selected worker case characteristics andnature of injury or illness, all United States, private industry, 2005, and Table 11: Number of nonfatal occupational injuries and illnesses involving days away from work by selected worker and case characteristics and musculoskeletal disorders, all United States, private industry, 2005. Available at: http://www.bls.gov/iif/oshcdnew.htm#Resource%20Table%20categories%20-%202005. Accessed July 27, 2007.

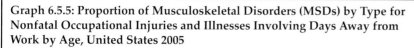

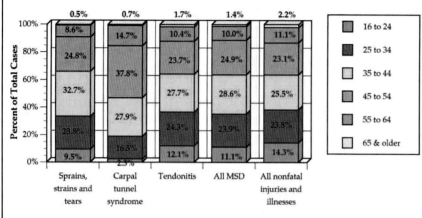

Graph 6.5.5: Proportion of Musculoskeletal Disorders (MSDs) by Type for Nonfatal Occupational Injuries and Illnesses Involving Days Away from Work by Age, United States 2005

Source: U.S. Department of Labor, Bureau of Labor Statistics: Case and Demographic Characteristics for Work-related Injuries and Illnesses Involving Days Away from Work. Supplemental Tables 2005, Table 9: Number of nonfatal occupational injuries and illnesses involving days away from work by selected worker case characteristics and nature of injury or illness, all United States, private industry, 2005, and Table 11: Number of nonfatal occupational injuries and illnesses involving days away from work by selected worker and case characteristics and musculoskeletal disorders, All United States, private industry, 2005. Available at: http://www.bls.gov/iif/oshcdnew.htm#Resource%20Table%20 categories%20-%202005. Accessed July 27, 2007.

shoulder (12%), trunk (10%), and knee (5%), together representing 91% of days away from work in 2005. (Table 6.26 and Graph 6.5.6) Carpal tunnel syndrome, an injury exclusively of the wrist, and tendonitis, which focuses primarily in the arm, wrist, hand, fingers, and shoulder, accounted for 74% and 16%, respectively, of MSD injuries resulting in days away from work in 2005. Sprains and strains occur primarily in the back and lower extremities (42% and 24%, respectively). (Table 6.26 and Graph 6.5.6)

The incidence of sprain, strain and tear injuries is much higher than any other type of injury, with a rate

tunnel syndrome injuries occur almost exclusively to whites (79%). Although Hispanics or Latinos represent only 12% of all MSD injuries, they are the second most likely race to sustain sprains/strains/tears (16%) or tendonitis (19%) injuries. (Table 6.24 and Graph 6.5.4)

Workers between the ages of 25 and 54 represent about 75% of all workplace injuries that resulted in days away from work in 2005. Injuries to workers younger than 20 years of age and older than 65 years are fairly rare, accounting for less than 1% to 6% of all injury cases, most likely due to lower representation in the workforce. Carpal tunnel syndrome is more likely to occur to workers aged 45 to 54; workers aged 35 to 44 are slightly more likely to report tendonitis. (Table 6.25 and Graph 6.5.5)

Section 6.5.3: Incidence Rates for Workplace Injuries by Type of Injury and Body Part Affected

While workplace injuries affect all parts of the anatomy, MSD workplace injuries primarily target the back (49%), upper extremities (15%),

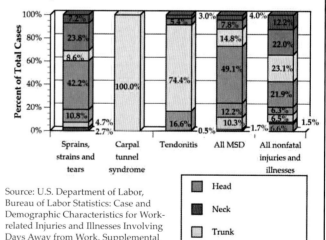

Graph 6.5.6: Proportion of Musculoskeletal Disorders (MSDs) by Type for Nonfatal Occupational Injuries and Illnesses Involving Days Away from Work by Body Part Affected, United States 2005

Source: U.S. Department of Labor, Bureau of Labor Statistics: Case and Demographic Characteristics for Work-related Injuries and Illnesses Involving Days Away from Work. Supplemental Tables 2005, Table 9: Number of nonfatal occupational injuries and illnesses involving days away from work by selected worker case characteristics and nature of injury or illness, all United States, private industry, 2005, and Table 11: Number of nonfatal occupational injuries and illnesses involving days away from work by selected worker and case characteristics and musculoskeletal disorders, All United States, private industry, 2005. Available at: http://www.bls.gov/iif/oshcdnew.htm# Resource%20Table%20categories%20-%20200. Accessed July 27, 2007.

of 55.3 injuries per 10,000 full-time workers in 2005. While not all sprain, strain and tear injuries are classified as MSD injuries, more than one-half were so classified in 2005. In addition to the sprain and strain injuries, bruises, and contusions and fractures also have high incidence rates (11.8 and 10.5, respectively, per 10,000 full-time workers). Amputations, a serious but less frequent musculoskeletal injury, occurred at a rate of 0.9 per 10,000 workers. The incidence of all MSD injuries per 10,000 workers declined by 39% between 1996 and 2005; tendonitis cases had the steepest drop (71%). This reflects the overall decline in workplace injuries seen in this time period. (Table 6.27 and Graph 6.5.7)

The incidence rate per 10,000 full-time workers in 2005 of injuries to the trunk (47.1, including the shoulder, 8.6, and back, 29.8), upper extremities (31.3), and lower extremities (29.9, including the knee, 11.1), were all high and accounted for a majority of nonfatal occupational injuries in all industries. The overall incidence of all nonfatal occupational injuries involving days away from work was 135.7 per 10,000 full-time workers. (Table 6.28)

Section 6.5.4: MSD Injuries by Occupation

MSD injuries occur in relatively equal proportion to all nonfatal workplace injuries with respect to worker occupation. (Table 6.29) However, carpal tunnel syndrome has a much higher occurrence rate in office and administrative support occupations, and a somewhat higher occurrence rate in management/business/finance and production occupations than do other types of injuries. Carpal tunnel syndrome is found in a lower proportion of service industry workers than other types of injuries. Tendonitis occurs at a higher rate among service, office, and administrative support, and production workers. Not unexpectedly, the highest incidence of workplace injuries is in the construction industry. (Table 6.29)

Section 6.5.5: Days Away from Work

In 2005, MSD injuries, as in most years since 1998, involved 2 additional days away from work when compared to all nonfatal workplace injury cases (9 days versus 7 days). (Table 6.30 and Graph 6.5.8) Both carpal tunnel syndrome (median of 27 days) and tendonitis (median of 12 days) contributed to the higher time away from work, although the number of cases for these injuries is low. The difference in median days away from work due to sprain/ strain injuries that are classified as MSD injuries and those other than MSD injuries is not available. However, fractures (median of 27 days) and amputation injuries (median 22 days), which are not included in the MSD classification, add significantly to the nonfatal workplace musculoskeletal

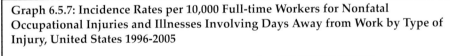
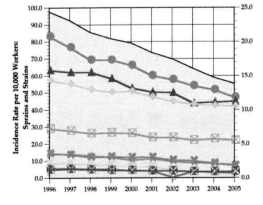
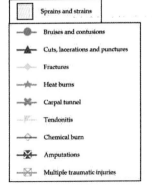

Graph 6.5.7: Incidence Rates per 10,000 Full-time Workers for Nonfatal Occupational Injuries and Illnesses Involving Days Away from Work by Type of Injury, United States 1996-2005

Source: U.S. Department of Labor, Bureau of Labor Statistics: Survey of Occupational Injuries and Illnesses. Table: Incidence rates for nonfatal occupational injuries and illnesses involving days away from work per 10,000 full-time workers for selected characteristics and major industry sector: Nature of injury or illness. Lost work time. Available at: www.bls.gov/iif/oshcdnew.htm. Accessed July 7, 2007.

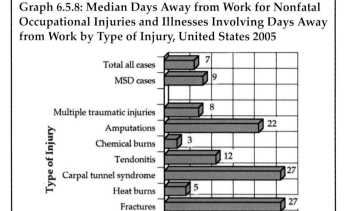

Graph 6.5.8: Median Days Away from Work for Nonfatal Occupational Injuries and Illnesses Involving Days Away from Work by Type of Injury, United States 2005

Source: U.S. Department of Labor, Bureau of Labor Statistics: Survey of Occupational Injuries and Illnesses. Table 11: Percent distribution of nonfatal occupational injuries and illnesses involving days away from work by selected injury or illness characteristics and and number of days away from work: Nature of injury or illness. Lost work time:1995-2005. Available at: www.bls.gov/iif/ oshcdnew.htm. Accessed July 7, 2007.

from work. Even through long term trends show significant reductions in the total number of worker injuries each year, the proportion that are musculoskeletal related (MSD, fractures, bruises/contusions, and amputations) continues to account for more than one-half of all worker nonfatal injury cases involving days away from work. In addition to the cost of medical care for these injuries, the cost of lost wages and the potential for long term impacts on worker productivity are enormous.

Section 6.6: Health Care Resource Utilization for Musculoskeletal Injuries

Injury treatment episodes in 2004, for purposes of this study, have been defined as the accumulative total of cases for all diagnoses treated in physician offices, emergency rooms, outpatient clinics, and hospitals, as identified in four major national health care databases. Of the 57.2 million musculoskeletal injury treatment episodes that occurred in 2004, 60% were treated in a physician's office. (Table 6.32 and Graph 6.6.1) Another one-third (31%) were treated in emergency rooms. Only 6% were treated in outpatient clinics, with 3% of persons with

injury burden. Shoulder, wrist, and knee injuries involved the highest median number of days away from work (15, 14, and 12, respectively). (Table 6.31)

Overall, musculoskeletal workplace injuries are a major concern, accounting for a large proportion of all nonfatal injuries that result in days away

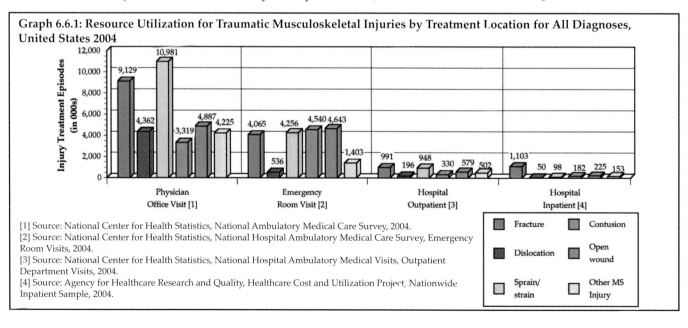

Graph 6.6.1: Resource Utilization for Traumatic Musculoskeletal Injuries by Treatment Location for All Diagnoses, United States 2004

[1] Source: National Center for Health Statistics, National Ambulatory Medical Care Survey, 2004.
[2] Source: National Center for Health Statistics, National Hospital Ambulatory Medical Care Survey, Emergency Room Visits, 2004.
[3] Source: National Center for Health Statistics, National Hospital Ambulatory Medical Visits, Outpatient Department Visits, 2004.
[4] Source: Agency for Healthcare Research and Quality, Healthcare Cost and Utilization Project, Nationwide Inpatient Sample, 2004.

musculoskeletal injuries admitted to a hospital. Persons hospitalized for a musculoskeletal injury represented 31% of all hospitalizations for an injury; musculoskeletal injuries accounted for 60% of all injury treatment episodes.

Males and females show only slight differences in where they are treated for a musculoskeletal injury. However, females were slightly more likely to be hospitalized (52% of all hospitalized injuries) or to be treated in a physician's office (54%) than are males. Males were slightly more likely to visit a hospital emergency room (52%) or hospital outpatient clinic (51%) for treatment.

The age of a person seeking treatment for a musculoskeletal injury is a factor in where treatment is given. (Table 6.33) Persons aged 65 and over are the most likely to be hospitalized for a musculoskeletal injury of any type, accounting for 47% of hospitalized musculoskeletal injury treatment episodes in 2004 but representing only 17% of all musculoskeletal injuries. Persons under the age of 18 are the least likely to be hospitalized, representing only 8% of hospitalized episodes, while accounting for 24% of all musculoskeletal injury treatment episodes. Persons aged 18 to 44 years are more likely to seek treatment in an

emergency room, while those aged 45 to 64 are more likely to seek treatment in a physician's office.

In 85% of the 2004 musculoskeletal injury treatment episodes, or 48.8 million injury episodes, the primary (1st) diagnosis was a musculoskeletal injury. (Table 6.34 and Graph 6.6.2) Among the 1.6 million persons hospitalized for a musculoskeletal injury, 65% were hospitalized with a primary (1st) diagnosis of a musculoskeletal injury. Hospitalization for a fracture is usually the primary (1st) diagnosis (77%).

Fractures and open wounds are commonly the primary (1st) diagnosis (88% and 87%, respectively) regardless of the treatment site, while sprains and strains are less frequently a primary (1st) diagnosis (49%). Persons seeking treatment in outpatient clinics or emergency rooms for injuries are the most likely to have a musculoskeletal injury as the primary (1st) diagnosis (90% and 89%, respectively).

The 1.04 million persons hospitalized for a primary (1st) diagnosis of a musculoskeletal injury in 2004 spent an average of 4.7 days in the

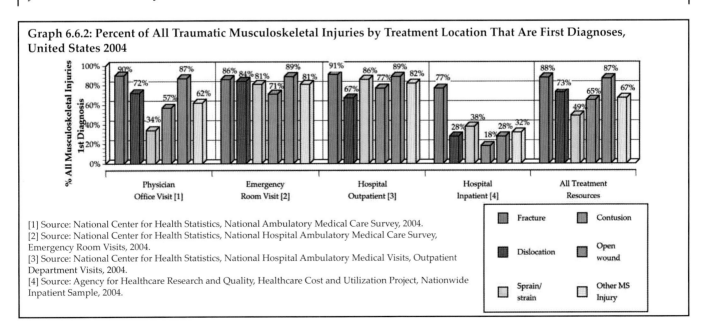

Graph 6.6.2: Percent of All Traumatic Musculoskeletal Injuries by Treatment Location That Are First Diagnoses, United States 2004

[1] Source: National Center for Health Statistics, National Ambulatory Medical Care Survey, 2004.
[2] Source: National Center for Health Statistics, National Hospital Ambulatory Medical Care Survey, Emergency Room Visits, 2004.
[3] Source: National Center for Health Statistics, National Hospital Ambulatory Medical Visits, Outpatient Department Visits, 2004.
[4] Source: Agency for Healthcare Research and Quality, Healthcare Cost and Utilization Project, Nationwide Inpatient Sample, 2004.

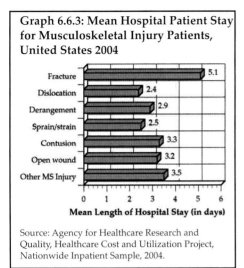

Graph 6.6.3: Mean Hospital Patient Stay for Musculoskeletal Injury Patients, United States 2004

Source: Agency for Healthcare Research and Quality, Healthcare Cost and Utilization Project, Nationwide Inpatient Sample, 2004.

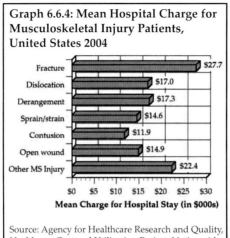

Graph 6.6.4: Mean Hospital Charge for Musculoskeletal Injury Patients, United States 2004

Source: Agency for Healthcare Research and Quality, Healthcare Cost and Utilization Project, Nationwide Inpatient Sample, 2004

for, as well as data on the cost, scope, and breadth of health insurance held by and available to U.S. workers. Currently MEPS collects data from two major components: households and insurance companies. The Household Component (HC) provides data from individual households and their members, which is supplemented by data from their medical providers. The Insurance Component is a separate survey of employers that provides data on employer-based health insurance. MEPS also includes a Medical Provider Component (MPC), which covers hospitals, physicians, home health care providers, and pharmacies identified by MEPS-HC respondents. Its purpose is to supplement and/or replace information received from the MEPS-HC respondents.[6]

hospital, representing 4.9 million hospitalized days and total estimated hospital costs of $26.65 billion. (Table 6.35 and Graph 6.6.3) The mean hospital cost per patient for treatment of a musculoskeletal injury was $25,600. (Graph 6.6.4) Eighty-one percent (81%) of persons hospitalized with a primary (1st) diagnosis of a musculoskeletal injury were treated for a fracture, yet fractures represented 88% of the estimated total cost of treatment. The average hospital length of stay for a fracture was 5.1 days, for a total of 4.3 million hospital days; the average hospital charge per patient was $27,740, for a total cost of $23.44 billion.

Section 6.7: Economic Cost of Musculoskeletal Injuries

Chapter 9 (Health Care Utilization and Economic Costs of Musculsokeletal Diseases) summarizes the cost of musculoskeletal conditions based on analysis of the Medical Expenditures Panel Survey (MEPS) from 1996 to 2004. The MEPS, which began in 1996, is a set of large-scale surveys of families and individuals, their medical providers (doctors, hospitals, pharmacies, etc.), and employers across the United States. MEPS collects data on the specific health services that Americans use, how frequently they use them, the cost of these services, and how they are paid

As with the National Health Interview Survey (NHIS), data in the household component is self-reported. As noted earlier, the NHIS is believed to underreport the incidence of injuries. Comparison of incidence between the two databases indicates injuries in the MEPS may also be underreported. In 2004, the NHIS reported 20.2 million persons sustained a musculoskeletal injury. An annual average of 24.7 million persons reported a musculoskeletal injury between 2002 and 2004 in the MEPS, a relatively stable number since the 1996 to 1998 MEPS data. (Table 6.36) This compares to the 52.7 million injury treatment episodes reported in the four major health care databases for physician offices, emergency rooms, hospital outpatient clinics, and inpatient care.

The estimated annual cost for medical care of musculoskeletal injuries in 2004 utilizing the MEPS data was $127.4 billion or an average of

$5,160 for each of the 24.7 million persons who sustained a musculoskeletal injury. A breakdown of the $127.4 billion cost due to musculoskeletal injuries shows 33% for ambulatory care, 31% for emergency room or inpatient care, 17% for prescription drugs, and 18% for other expenses. The cost of musculoskeletal injuries, in 2004 dollars, rose from $93 billion in 1996 to $127.4 billion in 2004, an increase of 37%. The increasing cost of prescription drugs accounts for the largest percentage of this total cost increase, rising from 11% of total cost to 17% over the 9-year period. (Graph 6.7.1)

1. Centers for Disease Control and Prevention (CDC): *2003 National Health Interview Survey (NHIS) Public Use Data Release*. Available at: http://www.cdc.gov/nchs/about/major /nhis/quest_data_related_1997_forward.htm. Accessed May 10, 2007.

2. Praemer A, Furner S, Rice DP: *Musculoskeletal Conditions in the United States*, ed 2. Rosemont, IL: American Academy of Orthopaedic Surgeons, 1999, p 182.

3. National Safety Council: *Injury Facts, 2005-2006*. Itasca, IL: National Safety Council, 2006.

4. Finkelstein EA, Corso PS, Miller TR: *The Incidence and Economic Burden of Injuries in the United States*. New York, NY: Oxford University Press, Inc., 2006, p 187.

5. National Institute for Occupational Safety and Health (NIOSH): *Workers Health Chartbook*. Cincinnati, OH: Department of Health and Human Services, Centers for Disease Control and Prevention, 2004, p 58.

6. Agency for Health Care Quality and Research: *Medical Expenditure Panel Survey Background*, 2007. Available at: http://www.meps.ahrq.gov/mepsweb/about_meps/surve y_back.jsp. Accessed May 7, 2007.

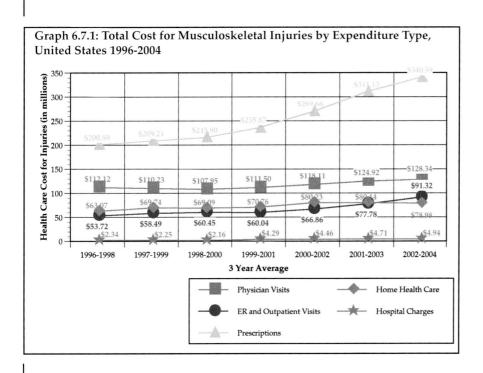

Graph 6.7.1: Total Cost for Musculoskeletal Injuries by Expenditure Type, United States 1996-2004

Section 6.8: Musculoskeletal Injuries Data Tables

Table 6.1: Comparison of Incidence of Unintentional Injuries, United States 1985, 1992-1994, 2000, and 2004

| | Incidence of Injuries (in 000s) | | | | | | | |
| | Rice, 1985 [1] | | MSCUS, 1992-1994 [2] | | Finkelstein, 2000 [3] | | BMUS 2008 | |
	Incidence	% of Total	Incidence	% of Total	Incidence	% of Total	Incidence	% of Total
Total Injuries	56,443		57,885		50,127		95,298	
Fatal Unintentional Injuries	143	0.3%	NA		149	0.3%	111 [4]	0.1%
Hospitalized Injuries	2,300	4.1%	NA		1,870	3.7%	5,167 [5]	5.4%
Non-hospitalized, Medically Treated Injuries	54,000	95.7%	NA		48,108	96.0%	90,131 [6]	94.6%
Musculoskeletal Injuries	NA		36,901		33,460		57,270	
Fatal Uunintentional Injuries	NA		NA		33 [7]	0.1%	20 [8]	0.0%
Hospitalized Injuries	NA		NA		1,273 [7]	3.8%	1,610 [9]	2.8%
Non-hospitalized, Medically Treated Injuries	NA		NA		32,154 [7]	96.1%	55,640 [9]	97.2%
Musculoskeletal as % of All Unintentional Injuries	NA		63.7%		66.8%		60.1%	

[1] Rice DP, MacKenzie EJ: *Cost of Injury in the United States: A Report to Congress*, 1989. San Francisco, CA: Institute for Health & Aging, University of California and Injury Prevention Center, The Johns Hopkins University, 1989.

[2] Praemer A, Furner S, Rice DP: *Musculoskeletal Conditions in the United States*, ed 2. Rosemont, IL: American Academy of Orthopaedic Surgeons, 1999, p 83.

[3] Finkelstein EA, Corso PS, Miller TR: *The Incidence and Economic Burden of Injuries in the United States*. New York, NY: Oxford University Press, 2006, p 8.

[4] National Safety Council: *Injury Facts, 2005-2006*. Itasca, IL: National Safety Council, 2006, p 8.

[5] Agency for Healthcare Research and Quality, Healthcare Cost and Utilization Project, Nationwide Inpatient Sample, 2004.

[6] National Center for Health Statistics: National Ambulatory Medical Care Survey, 2004; National Hospital Ambulatory Medical Care Survey, Emergency Room Visits, 2004; National Hospital Ambulatory Medical Visits, Outpatient Department Visits, 2004.

[7] Defined as spinal cord, vertebral column, torso, upper extremity, lower extremity injuries. Finkelstein EA, Corso PS, Miller TR. *The Incidence and Economic Burden of Injuries in the United States*. New York, NY: Oxford University Press, 2006, p 13.

[8] Defined as falls. National Safety Council: *Injury Facts, 2005-2006*. Itasca, IL: National Safety Council, 2006, p 8.

[9] Defined as fracture, derangement, dislocation, sprain/strain, contusion, crushing injury, open wound, traumatic amputation, and late effects of injury. National Center for Health Statistics: National Ambulatory Medical Care Survey, 2004; National Hospital Ambulatory Medical Care Survey, Emergency Room Visits, 2004; National Hospital Ambulatory Medical Visits, Outpatient Department Visits, 2004.

Table 6.2: Resource Utilization for Traumatic Injuries by Treatment Location and Sex, United States 2004

	Total Visits (in 000s) [1]					
	Physician Office Visits [2]	**Emergency Room Visits** [3]	**Hospital Outpatient Visits** [4]	**Inpatient Stays** [5]	**Total All Treatment Sites**	**% All Diagnoses for All Treatment Locations**
Fractures	9,129	4,065	991	1,103	15,288	25%
Dislocations	4,362	536	196	50	5,144	8%
Sprains and Strains	10,981	4,256	948	98	16,283	26%
Contusions	3,319	4,540	330	182	8,371	14%
Open Wounds	4,887	4,643	579	225	10,334	17%
All Other Musculoskeletal Injuries	4,225	1,403	502	153	6,283	10%
Total All Musculoskeletal Traumatic Injuries	34,372	17,888	3,380	1,610	57,250	
All Injury Treatment Episodes	54,168	30,770	5,192	5,161	95,291	
Proportion of Total Diagnoses that are Musculoskeletal	63%	58%	65%	31%	60%	

[1] All listed diagnoses for inpatients discharged from short-stay hospitals.

[2] Source: National Center for Health Statistics, National Ambulatory Medical Care Survey, 2004.

[3] Source: National Center for Health Statistics, National Hospital Ambulatory Medical Care Survey, Emergency Room Visits, 2004.

[4] Source: National Center for Health Statistics, National Hospital Ambulatory Medical Visits, Outpatient Department Visits, 2004.

[5] Source: Agency for Healthcare Research and Quality, Healthcare Cost and Utilization Project, Nationwide Inpatient Sample, 2004.

Table 6.3 : Distribution of Injury Treatment Episodes and Self-Reported Injuries by Type of Musculoskeletal Injury, United States 2004

	Total Injury Treatment Episodes [1-4]						
	Total	Females	Males	<18 Years	18-44 Years	45-64 Years	65 & Over
Fractures	25%	24%	25%	30%	18%	22%	37%
Dislocations	8%	9%	8%	5%	7%	11%	8%
Sprains and Strains	26%	28%	25%	24%	32%	28%	16%
Contusions	14%	14%	13%	14%	13%	11%	19%
Open Wounds	17%	14%	20%	18%	19%	15%	14%
All Other Musculoskeletal Injuries	10%	11%	9%	9%	11%	13%	6%
	Total Injury Treatment Episodes (in 000s)						
Total All Musculoskeletal Traumatic Injuries	57,250	29,193	28,045	13,502	19,633	14,422	9,615
	Self-Reported Injury Episodes [5]						
Fractures	22%	24%	20%	32%	15%	18%	29%
Dislocations	2%	2%	2%	3%	3%	1%	0%
Sprains and Strains	38%	40%	36%	33%	45%	37%	28%
Contusions	14%	16%	12%	11%	9%	17%	26%
Open Wounds	17%	12%	22%	15%	23%	16%	10%
All Other Musculoskeletal Injuries	7%	6%	8%	6%	5%	11%	7%
	Self-Reported Injury Episodes (in 000s)						
Total All Musculoskeletal Traumatic Injuries	20,227	9,529	10,700	5,139	7,219	5,197	2,672

[1] Source: National Center for Health Statistics, National Ambulatory Medical Care Survey, 2004,

[2] Source: National Center for Health Statistics, National Hospital Ambulatory Medical Care Survey, Emergency Room Visits, 2004,

[3] Source: National Center for Health Statistics, National Hospital Ambulatory Medical Visits, Outpatient Department Visits, 2004,

[4] Source: Agency for Healthcare Research and Quality, Healthcare Cost and Utilization Project, Nationwide Inpatient Sample, 2004,

[5] National Center for Health Statistics, National Health Interview Survey, 2005,

Table 6.4: Injury Treatment Episodes and Rate by Type of Musculoskeletal Injury by Sex and Age, United States 2004

TOTAL POPULATION

Injury Treatment Episodes (in 000s)

	Total		Under 18 Years		18-44 Years		45-64 years		65 Years & Over	
	Injury Treatment Episodes	Rate per 100 Population	Injury Treatment Episodes	Rate per 100 Population	Injury Treatment Episodes	Rate per 100 Population	Injury Treatment Episodes	Rate per 100 Population	Injury Treatment Episodes	Rate per 100 Population
Fractures	15,288	5.2	4,306	5.9	3,825	3.4	3,356	4.8	3,800	10.5
Dislocations	5,144	1.8	652	0.9	1,596	1.4	1,747	2.5	848	2.3
Sprains and Strains	16,283	5.5	3,477	4.7	6,810	6.0	4,393	6.2	1,593	4.4
Contusions	8,371	2.9	1,987	2.7	2,801	2.5	1,685	2.4	1,898	5.2
Open Wounds	10,334	3.5	2,498	3.4	4,026	3.6	2,382	3.4	1,429	3.9
All Other Musculoskeletal Injuries	6,283	2.1	1,340	1.8	2,268	2.0	2,067	2.9	607	1.7
Total All Musculoskeletal Traumatic Injuries	57,250	19.5	13,502	18.4	19,633	17.3	14,422	20.4	9,615	26.5
All Injuries	95,298	32.5	22,609	30.9	32,940	29.1	22,936	32.5	16,806	46.3
Total Population (in 000s)	293,657		73,258		113,373		70,623		36,333	

MALES

Injury Treatment Episodes Males (in 000s)

	Total		Under 18 Years		18-44 Years		45-64 years		65 Years & Over	
Fractures	7,675	5.3	2,859	8.0	2,271	4.1	1,402	3.9	1,143	5.4
Dislocations	2,540	1.8	416	1.2	1,006	1.8	865	2.4	255	1.2
Sprains and Strains	7,532	5.2	1,578	4.4	3,390	6.1	1,898	5.2	666	3.1
Contusions	3,832	2.7	1,062	3.0	1,372	2.5	678	1.9	720	3.4
Open Wounds	5,979	4.1	1,315	3.7	2,432	4.3	1,418	3.9	816	3.9
All Other Musculoskeletal Injuries	2,654	1.8	735	2.1	1,030	1.8	770	2.1	120	0.6
Total All Musculoskeletal Traumatic Injuries	28,045	19.4	7,568	21.2	10,423	18.6	6,614	18.2	3,440	16.3
All Injuries	47,205	32.7	13,490	37.7	16,874	30.2	10,819	29.9	6,890	32.6
Total Population (in 000s)	144,535		35,763		55,952		36,243		21,164	

FEMALES

Injury Treatment Episodes Females (in 000s)

	Total		Under 18 Years		18-44 Years		45-64 years		65 Years & Over	
Fractures	7,604	5.1	1,443	3.8	1,552	2.7	1,954	5.7	2,656	17.5
Dislocations	2,804	1.9	236	0.6	590	1.0	1,183	3.4	595	3.9
Sprains and Strains	8,739	5.9	1,899	5.1	3,418	6.0	2,496	7.2	925	6.1
Contusions	4,540	3.0	924	2.5	1,430	2.5	1,008	2.9	1,178	7.8
Open Wounds	4,354	2.9	1,183	3.2	1,596	2.8	963	2.8	613	4.0
All Other Musculoskeletal Injuries	3,628	2.4	604	1.6	1,238	2.2	1,298	3.8	488	3.2
Total All Musculoskeletal Traumatic Injuries	29,193	19.6	5,930	15.8	9,282	16.2	7,807	22.7	6,174	40.7
All Injuries	48,074	32.2	9,112	24.3	16,061	28.0	14,654	42.5	9,917	65.4
Total Population (in 000s)	149,121		37,496		57,421		34,450		15,169	

Sources: National Center for Health Statistics: National Ambulatory Medical Care Survey, 2004; National Hospital Ambulatory Medical Care Survey, Emergency Room Visits, 2004; National Hospital Ambulatory Medical Visits, Outpatient Department Visits, 2004. Agency for Healthcare Research and Quality, Healthcare Cost and Utilization Project, Nationwide Inpatient Sample, 2004.

Table 6.5: Trends in Fracture Treatment Episodes for Selected Anatomic Sites by Treatment Location, United States 1998-2004

Emergency Room Visits

ICD-9-CM	Description	Total Visits (rounded to nearest 000) [1]						
		1998	1999	2000	2001	2002	2003	2004
Upper Limb								
812	Fracture of Upper Arm (Humerus)	261	346	417	297	329	398	342
813	Fracture of Lower Arm (Radius/Ulna)	647	628	588	745	583	563	763
814-817	Fracture of Wrist/Hand/Fingers	832	1,007	1,033	1,079	970	895	1,093
Lower Limb								
820-821	Fracture of Hip/Upper Leg (Femur)	324	313	297	298	282	302	307
823	Fracture of Lower Leg (Tibia/Fibula)	244	234	209	292	212	197	264
824-826	Fracture of Ankle/Foot/Toes	787	697	836	968	740	816	783
All Anatomic Sites [2]								
812-817	Fracture of Upper Limb	1,726	1,965	2,009	2,097	1,853	1,841	2,163
820-821, 823-826	Fracture of Lower Limb	1,339	1,233	1,331	1,551	1,217	1,311	1,348
812-817, 820-821, 823-826	All Fractures of Upper/Lower Limb	3,041	3,190	3,308	3,624	3,058	3,148	3,495

Source: National Center for Health Statistics, National Hospital Ambulatory Medical Care Survey, Emergency Room Visits, 1998-2004.

Physician Office Visits

ICD-9-CM	Description	Total Visits (rounded to nearest 000) [1]						
		1998	1999	2000	2001	2002	2003	2004
Upper Limb								
812	Fracture of Upper Arm (Humerus)	*	*	*	*	*	*	*
813	Fracture of Lower Arm (Radius/Ulna)	2,429	1,437	1,852	1,685	2,710	1,116	1,485
814-817	Fracture of Wrist/Hand/Fingers	2,691	1,846	2,450	2,675	2,740	2,464	1,988
Lower Limb								
820-821	Fracture of Hip/Upper Leg (Femur)	*	*	*	*	*	*	*
823	Fracture of Lower Leg (Tibia/Fibula)	*	*	*	*	*	*	*
824-826	Fracture of Ankle/Foot/Toes	2,170	1,804	1,883	2,210	2,555	2,228	2,100
All Anatomic Sites [2]								
812-817	Total Upper Limb Fractures	5,718	3,963	5,203	5,005	5,915	4,234	4,203
820-821, 823-826	Total Lower Limb Fractures	4,027	2,750	3,244	3,344	4,008	3,692	3,862
812-817, 820-821, 823-826	All Fractures of Upper/Lower Limb	9,746	6,644	8,349	8,184	9,816	7,731	7,976

Source: National Center for Health Statistics, National Hospital Ambulatory Medical Visits, Physician Visits, 1998-2004.

Inpatient Hospitalization

ICD-9-CM	Description	Total Visits (rounded to nearest 000) [1]						
		1998	1999	2000	2001	2002	2003	2004
Upper Limb								
812	Fracture of Upper Arm (Humerus)	90	98	91	105	890	102	102
813	Fracture of Forearm (Radius/Ulna)	96	98	98	106	92	108	94
814-817	Fracture of Wrist/Hand/Fingers	42	43	41	38	37	35	39
Lower Limb								
820-821	Fracture of Hip/Upper Leg (Femur)	445	443	423	434	431	422	449
823	Fracture of Lower Leg (Tibia/Fibula)	91	99	94	95	86	91	88
824-826	Fracture of Ankle/Foot/Toes	164	172	169	176	166	170	173
All Anatomic Sites [2]								
812-817	Total Upper Limb Fractures	216	225	221	237	209	231	224
820-821, 823-826	Total Lower Limb Fractures	682	694	663	686	665	664	689
812-817, 820-821, 823-826	All Fractures of Upper/Lower Limb	863	887	850	889	843	867	885

Source: National Center for Health Statistics, National Hospital Discharge Survey, 1998-2004.

Table 6.5a: Total Fracture Treatment Episodes for Physician Office Visits, Emergency Room Visits, and Inpatient Hospitalization for Selected Anatomic Sites, United States 1998-2004

Total Visits (rounded to nearest 0000) [1]

ICD-9-CM	Description	1998	1999	2000	2001	2002	2003	2004
Upper Limb								
812	Fracture of Upper Arm (Humerus)	351	444	509	401	418	500	444
813	Fracture of Forearm (Radius/Ulna)	3,172	2,164	2,539	2,536	3,385	1,786	2,342
814-817	Fracture of Wrist/Hand/Fingers	3,564	2,896	3,524	3,793	3,746	3,394	3,120
Lower Limb								
820-821	Fracture of Hip/Upper Leg (Femur)	769	756	720	732	713	724	756
823	Fracture of Lower Leg (Tibia/Fibula)	334	333	303	387	298	288	352
824-826	Fracture of Ankle/Foot/Toes	3,121	2,673	2,888	3,354	3,461	3,213	3,057
All Anatomic Sites [2]								
812-817	Total Upper Limb Fractures	7,661	6,153	7,433	7,339	7,977	6,307	6,591
	Total Lower Limb Fractures	6,049	4,678	5,237	5,582	5,890	5,666	5,898
812-817, 820-821, 823-826	All Fractures of Upper/Lower Limb	13,650	10,722	12,507	12,696	13,718	11,746	12,356

Proportion of Total Visits

ICD-9-CM	Description	1998	1999	2000	2001	2002	2003	2004
Upper Limb		56.1%	57.4%	59.4%	57.8%	58.2%	53.7%	53.3%
812	Fracture of Upper Arm (Humerus)	4.6%	7.2%	6.8%	5.5%	5.2%	7.9%	6.7%
813	Fracture of Forearm (Radius/Ulna)	41.4%	35.2%	34.2%	34.6%	42.4%	28.3%	35.5%
814-817	Fracture of Wrist/Hand/Fingers	46.5%	47.1%	47.4%	51.7%	47.0%	53.8%	47.3%
Lower Limb		44.3%	43.6%	41.9%	44.0%	42.9%	48.2%	47.7%
820-821	Fracture of Hip/Upper Leg (Femur)	12.7%	16.2%	13.8%	13.1%	12.1%	12.8%	12.8%
823	Fracture of Lower Leg (Tibia/Fibula)	5.5%	7.1%	5.8%	6.9%	5.1%	5.1%	6.0%
824-826	Fracture of Ankle/Foot/Toes	51.6%	57.1%	55.1%	60.1%	58.8%	56.7%	51.8%
Location	Emergency Room Visits	22.3%	29.8%	26.5%	28.5%	22.3%	26.8%	28.3%
	Physician Office Visits	71.4%	62.0%	66.8%	64.5%	71.6%	65.8%	64.6%
	Inpatient Hospitalization	6.3%	8.3%	6.8%	7.0%	6.1%	7.4%	7.2%

[1] All diagnoses

[2] Totals may not add due to rounding and inclusion of additional anatomic sites

* Estimate does not meet standards for reliability

Sources: National Center for Health Statistics: National Hospital Discharge Survey, 1998-2004; National Center for Health Statistics, National Hospital Ambulatory Medical Care Survey, Emergency Room Visits, 1998-2004; National Center for Health Statistics, National Hospital Ambulatory Medical Visits, Physician Visits, 1998-2004.

Table 6.6: Location of Musculoskeletal Injury Episode Occurrence, United States 2004

	Total Occurrences (in 000s) [1]	% of Total Occurrences
Inside Home	5,300	24.6%
Outside Home	4,469	20.7%
School	1,624	7.5%
Street or Highway	1,965	9.1%
Sport or Recreation Facility	1,975	9.2%
Shopping Center/Restaurant	638	3.0%
Other	5,288	24.5%
Unknown	295	1.4%
All Musculoskeletal Injuries	21,554	100.0%

[1] All listed diagnoses for persons reporting a musculoskeletal injury in the 3 month period prior to the interview.

* Totals may not add due to rounding.

Source: National Center for Health Statistics, National Health Interview Survey, Injury Database, 2004.

Table 6.7: Nonfatal Unintentional Injuries Treated in Hospital Emergency Departments, United States 2003

Cause of Injury	Total Nonfatal Unintentional Injuries (in 000s)	% of Total Nonfatal Unintentional Injuries	Rate of Nonfatal Unintentional Injuries per 1,000 Persons
Falls	7,895	29%	27.1
Struck By/Against	4,422	16%	15.2
Overexertion	3,325	12%	11.4
Motor Vehicle Ooccupant	3,027	11%	10.4
Cut/Pierce	2,236	8%	7.7
Other Causes	3,641	14%	12.5
Unknown	2,581	10%	
Total All Causes	27,127	100%	93.3

Source: National Safety Council: *Injury Facts, 2005-2006*. Itasca, IL: National Safety Council, 2006, p 13.

Table 6.8: Nonfatal Unintentional Injuries Treated in Emergency Departments by Age, United States 2003

Age	Total Nonfatal Unintentional Injuries	Total Nonfatal Falls	% of Total Nonfatal Injuries that are Falls	Rank as Leading Cause of Nonfatal Injury
0-4 years	2,230,531	987,485	44.3%	1
5-9 years	1,824,466	670,107	36.7%	1
10-14 years	2,373,485	678,897	28.6%	1
15-24 years	5,181,929	973,073	18.8%	3
25-34 years	4,143,055	754,691	18.2%	1
35-44 years	3,953,767	812,270	20.5%	1
45-54 years	2,909,772	739,365	25.4%	1
55-64 years	1,631,619	563,973	34.6%	1
65 years & over	2,878,852	1,822,157	63.3%	1
Total All Ages	27,127,477	7,895,385	29.1%	1

Source: National Safety Council: *Injury Facts, 2005-2006*. Itasca, IL: National Safety Council, 2006, p 13.

Table 6.9: Deaths Due to Falls from Unintentional Injury Episodes by Age, United States 2003

Age	Total Population (in 000s)	Total Unintentional Injury Deaths	Total Deaths Due to Falls	Rate of Unintentional Injury Deaths Due to Falls (per 100,000 persons)	% of Total Unintentional Injury Deaths Due to Falls
0-4 years	19,547	2,587	53	0.3	2.0%
5-9 years	19,962	1,176	18	0.1	1.5%
10-14 years	21,116	1,542	24	0.1	1.6%
15-19 years	20,351	7,137	83	0.4	1.2%
20-34 years	60,046	20,844	471	0.8	2.3%
35-54 years	84,750	31,385	809	1.0	2.6%
55-64 years	26,582	8,345	1,089	4.1	13.0%
65-74 years	18,280	8,086	3,219	17.6	39.8%
75-84 years	12,759	12,904	5,901	46.2	45.7%
85 years & older	4,546	12,651	5,990	131.8	47.3%
Total All Ages	287,939	106,657	17,657	6.1	16.6%

Source: National Safety Council: *Injury Facts, 2005-2006*. Itasca, IL: National Safety Council, 2006, p 32-33.

Table 6.10: Trends in Deaths Due to Falls, United States 1984-2004

Year	Total Unintentional Injury Deaths Occurring All Locations [1]			Total Unintentional Injury Deaths Occurring in the Home [2]			% All Deaths Due to Falls that Occurred in the Home
	Total Unintentional Injury Deaths	Death Due to Falls	% of Deaths Due to Falls	Total Home Injury Deaths	Death Due to Falls	% of Deaths due to Falls	
1984	92,911	11,937	12.8%	21,200	6,400	30.2%	53.6%
1985	93,457	12,001	12.8%	21,600	6,500	30.1%	54.2%
1986	95,277	11,444	12.0%	21,700	6,100	28.1%	53.3%
1987	95,020	11,733	12.3%	21,400	6,300	29.4%	53.7%
1988	97,100	12,096	12.5%	22,700	6,600	29.1%	54.6%
1989	95,028	12,151	12.8%	22,500	6,600	29.3%	54.3%
1990	91,983	12,313	13.4%	21,500	6,700	31.2%	54.4%
1991	89,347	12,662	14.2%	22,100	6,900	31.2%	54.5%
1992	86,777	12,646	14.6%	24,000	7,700	32.1%	60.9%
1993	90,523	13,141	14.5%	26,100	7,900	30.3%	60.1%
1994	91,437	13,450	14.7%	26,300	8,100	30.8%	60.2%
1995	93,320	13,986	15.0%	27,200	8,400	30.9%	60.1%
1996	94,948	14,986	15.8%	27,500	9,000	32.7%	60.1%
1997	95,644	15,447	16.2%	27,700	9,100	32.9%	58.9%
1998	97,835	16,274	16.6%	29,000	9,500	32.8%	58.4%
1999	97,860	13,162	13.4%	30,500	7,600	24.9%	57.7%
2000	97,900	13,322	13.6%	29,200	7,100	24.3%	53.3%
2001	101,537	15,019	14.8%	33,200	8,600	25.9%	57.3%
2002	106,742	16,257	15.2%	36,200	9,700	26.8%	59.7%
2003	108,900	19,800	18.2%	37,600	11,900	31.6%	60.1%
2004	111,000	20,200	18.2%	37,400	12,800	34.2%	63.4%

[1] Source: National Safety Council. *Injury Facts, 2005-2006*. Itasca, IL: National Safety Council, 2006, p 42.

[2] Source: National Safety Council. *Injury Facts, 2005-2006*. Itasca, IL: National Safety Council, 2006, p 127.

Table 6.11: Proportion of Unintentional Injury Episodes by Type and Cause of Injury, United States 2005

	Total Injury Episodes [2]	Proportion of Unintentional Injury Episodes by Injury Type [1]					
		Motor Vehicle	Bike, Scooter, Skateboard, Skis, etc.	Pedestrian (Struck)	Boat, Train, Plane	Fall	Burn
Spain, Strain or Twist	32.2%	49.3%	34.0%	34.2%	39.8%	31.7%	0.0%
Cut or Scrape	22.0%	16.1%	22.0%	8.1%	33.2%	23.1%	4.0%
Fracture	20.4%	13.8%	35.4%	52.7%	9.9%	29.4%	4.1%
Bruise or Contusion	15.8%	27.1%	15.4%	44.0%	0.0%	21.0%	0.0%
Other	13.8%	20.2%	7.3%	12.0%	0.0%	10.1%	0.0%
Bite (Insect or Animal)	3.1%	0.0%	0.0%	0.0%	9.4%	0.0%	0.0%
Burn	1.4%	0.4%	2.4%	0.0%	7.7%	0.3%	92.0%
Total Injury Episodes (in 000s)	7,409	725	273	39	36	2,533	90

[1] Self-reported injury type in the 3 month period prior to the interview.

[2] Multiple injury types per injury episode possible. Totals may not equal 100%.

Source: National Center for Health Statistics. National Health Interview Survey, Injury Database, 2005

Table 6.12: Incidence and Rates of Injuries by Body Region, United States 2000

	Fatal		Hospitalized		Nonhospitalized		Total	
	Incidence (in 000s)	Rate/ 100,000	Incidence (in 000s)	Rate/ 100,000	Incidence (in 000s)	Rate/ 100,000	Incidence (in 000s)	Rate/ 100,000
Traumatic Brain Injury	40	15	156	56	1,147	415	1,343	486
Other Head /Neck Injury	5	2	144	52	6,392	2,312	6,541	2,366
Spinal Cord Injury	1	0	10	4	16	6	27	10
Vertebral Column Injury	1	0	86	31	4,619	1,671	4,706	1,702
Torso	23	8	245	89	3,888	1,406	4,155	1,503
Upper Extremity	1	0	275	100	13,047	4,720	13,324	4,820
Lower Extremity	7	3	656	237	10,584	3,829	11,247	4,069
Other/Unspecified	32	12	18	7	5,789	2,094	5,839	2,113
Systemwide Injuries	39	14	279	101	2,626	950	2,945	1,065
Total	149	54	1,870	676	48,108	17,405	50,127	18,135

Source: Finkelstein EA, Corso PS, Miller TR. *The Incidence and Economic Burden of Injuries in the United States*. New York, NY: Oxford University Press, 2006, p 12.

Table 6.13: Visits to Physicians in Office-Based Practice for Fractures, Sprains and Strains, and Dislocation Injuries at Selected Anatomic Sites by Gender, United States 2004

Visits for Fractures

	Total Visits (in 000s) [1]			% of Total Visits
	Male	Female	Total	
Hand and Fingers	913	616	1,529	15.5%
Radius and Ulna (Arm)	864	621	1,485	15.0%
Ankle	592	641	1,234	12.5%
Ribs and Sternum	*	*	912	9.2%
Tibia and Fibula (Leg)	337	573	910	9.2%
Foot and Toes	346	521	867	8.8%
Humerus (Shoulder)	227	516	743	7.5%
Vertebral Column	*	*	541	5.5%
Neck of Femur (Hip)	*	343	523	5.3%
Wrist	*	357	459	4.6%
Femur	234	*	390	3.9%
Pelvis	*	*	59	0.6%
Clavicle or Scapula	*	*	184	1.9%
Patella (Knee)	*	*	57	0.6%
All Fractures [2]			9,893	100%
Total Fracture Episodes Treated in Physician's Office			9,129	

Visits for Sprains and Strains

	Total Visits (in 000s) [1]			% of Total Visits
	Male	Female	Total	
Back and Sacroiliac	2,370	2,440	4,810	33.6%
Shoulder	1,779	1,316	3,095	21.6%
Elbow and Arm	*	*	253	1.8%
Hand and Wrist	*	*	853	6.0%
Hip	390	886	1,275	8.9%
Knee and Leg	529	572	1,101	7.7%
Ankle and Foot	1,441	1,485	2,926	20.4%
All Sprains and Strains [2]			14,313	100%
Total Sprain and Strain Episodes Treated in Physician's Office			10,981	

Visits for Dislocation Injuries

	Total Visits (in 000s) [1]			% of Total Visits
	Male	Female	Total	
Knee and Leg Joint [3]	1,801	1,860	3,661	62.7%
Shoulder*	91	241	333	5.7%
All Other Sites	706	1,143	1,849	31.7%
All Dislocations [2]			5,842	100%
Total Dislocation Episodes Treated in Physician's Office			4,362	

* Estimate does not meet standards for reliability

[1] All listed diagnoses

[2] Multiple anatomic sites per injury episode possible

[3] The high proportion of dislocation injuries attributed to the knee is due to an ICD-9 coding anomaly. Isolated acute ligamentous injuries of the knee (ACL, MCL, PCL, LCL disruptions) are coded as dislocations using ICD-9 methodology, whereas, equivalent injuries in other joints are coded as sprains/strains. True complete dislocations of the knee joint are actually quite rare, and associated with marked morbidity.

Source: National Center for Health Statistics, National Ambulatory Medical Care Survey, 2004

Table 6.14: Prevalence of Self-Reported Musculoskeletal Injury Episodes by Anatomic Site by Age, United States 2004

	Total Identified Anatomic Site Injuries (in 000s) [1]	% of Total Injuries by Anatomic Site	Prevalence of Self-Reported Injury Sites for All Musculoskeletal Injury Episodes (in 000s) [2]				Proportion of All Injury Sites for All Musculoskeletal Injury Episodes [2]			
			< 18	18 to 44	45 to 64	65 & older	< 18	18 to 44	45 to 64	65 & older
Ankle	3,103	11.6%	774	1,333	682	315	12.9%	13.5%	9.4%	8.4%
Knee	3,050	11.4%	559	1,169	977	345	9.3%	11.9%	13.4%	9.3%
Finger/Thumb	2,399	9.0%	519	1,128	580	172	8.6%	11.4%	8.0%	4.6%
Shoulder	2,230	8.3%	428	887	575	340	7.1%	9.0%	7.9%	9.1%
Foot or toe	2,370	8.8%	691	880	616	242	11.5%	8.9%	8.5%	6.5%
Lower leg	1,568	5.9%	423	389	457	300	7.0%	3.9%	6.3%	8.0%
Hand	1,623	6.1%	259	795	393	175	4.3%	8.1%	5.4%	4.7%
Back	1,485	5.5%	190	675	376	244	3.2%	6.9%	5.2%	6.5%
Wrist	1,319	4.9%	504	310	325	180	8.4%	3.1%	4.5%	4.8%
Forearm	1,167	4.4%	482	236	329	120	8.0%	2.4%	4.5%	3.2%
Elbow	894	3.3%	287	309	197	102	4.8%	3.1%	2.7%	2.7%
Hip	839	3.1%	94	187	244	314	1.6%	1.9%	3.4%	8.4%
Thigh	597	2.2%	127	149	215	106	2.1%	1.5%	3.0%	2.8%
Upper Arm	636	2.4%	190	100	190	156	3.2%	1.0%	2.6%	4.2%
Other	3,521	13.1%	490	1,305	1,108	618	8.1%	13.2%	15.3%	16.6%
All Musculoskeletal Injury Episode Anatomic Sites*	26,801	100.0%	6,017	9,852	7,264	3,729	100.0%	100.0%	100.0%	100.0%

* Totals may not add due to rounding

[1] All listed diagnoses for persons reporting a musculoskeletal injury in the 3 month period prior to the interview.

[2] Multiple anatomic sites per injury episode possible.

Source: National Center for Health Statistics. National Health Interview Survey, Injury Database, 2004

Table 6.15: Activity Limitations due to Fracture or Bone/Joint Injury by Gender and Aged for Persons Age 18 and Over, United States 2003-2004

	Rate of Reported Limitations due to Fracture or Bone/Joint Injury [1] (per 100 persons)		
	Male	Female	Total
18-44 years	3.5	2.2	2.8
45-64 years	7.5	6.2	6.9
65 & over	10.4	11	10.8
All ages	4.2	3.8	4.0

[1] "What condition or health problem causes you to have difficulty with or need help with the following activities?"

Source: National Center for Health Statistics. National Health and Nutrition Examination Survey, 2003-2004

Table 6.16: Activity Limitations Due to Fracture of Bone/Joint Injury for Persons Aged 18 and Over, United States 2003-2004

Activity Limitation Reported [1]	Degree of Limitation for Persons Reporting a Limitation [2]			Total % With Difficulty
	Some Difficulty	Much Difficulty	Unable to Do	
Stooping, crouching, or kneeling	46.5%	20.6%	16.7%	83.8%
Standing on feet for 2 hours	27.5%	16.3%	18.8%	62.6%
Push or pull large objects like a chair	32.3%	11.3%	15.9%	59.5%
Sitting for 2 hours	34.7%	9.8%	4.9%	49.4%
Doing chores around the houe	27.1%	8.1%	5.0%	40.2%
Standing up from armless straight chair	26.7%	7.1%	5.8%	39.6%
Lifting/carrying 10 pound item	23.4%	5.8%	8.1%	37.3%
Getting in and out of bed	29.3%	6.0%	0.7%	36.0%
Reaching over head	23.7%	5.9%	4.3%	33.9%
Walking quarter mile (2-3 blocks)	24.6%	4.8%	3.0%	32.4%
Going shopping, to movies or events	20.6%	7.6%	4.0%	32.2%
Dressing self (tying shoes, zippers, buttons)	23.3%	2.7%	0.1%	26.1%
Waking up 10 steps without resting	19.0%	5.1%	0.8%	24.9%
Participating in social activities	17.1%	2.1%	4.2%	23.4%
Using fingers to grasp small objects	19.3%	3.2%	0.3%	22.8%
Moving around rooms on same level	12.1%	1.7%	2.2%	16.0%
Managing money or paying bills	12.2%	1.5%	2.1%	15.8%
Relaxing at home, watching TV, sewing	12.8%	0.7%	0.2%	13.7%
Preparing own meals	10.0%	2.2%	1.3%	13.5%
Eating with utensils or drinking from a glass	7.0%	1.0%	0.0%	8.0%

[1] "What condition or health problem causes you to have difficulty with or need help with the following activities . . . ?"

[2] "By yourself and without using any special equipment, how much difficulty do you have . . .?"

Source: National Center for Health Statistics. National Health and Nutrition Examination Survey, 2003-2004

Table 6.17: Bed Days Due to Major Health Conditions by Gender for Persons Aged 18 and Over, United States 2005

	Bed Days [1]				Bed Days [1]		
	Persons Reporting Bed Days (in 000s)	Mean Bed Days	Total Bed Days (in 000s)		Persons Reporting Bed Days (in 000s)	Mean Bed Days	Total Bed Days (in 000s)
All Causes [2]				**Other Major Health Conditions**			
				Heart Problem [7]			
Total Population	76,170	13.2	1,005,444	Total Population	2,821	40.8	115,097
Male	32,113	11.8	378,933	Male	1,349	36.8	49,643
Female	44,056	14.1	621,190	Female	1,472	44.5	65,504
18 to 44 Years	41,186	9.0	370,674	18 to 44 Years	288	42.0	12,096
45 to 64 Years	25,117	16.5	414,431	45 to 64 Years	1,108	39.8	44,098
65 Years & Over	9,867	22.2	219,047	65 Years & Over	1,425	41.4	58,995
Musculoskeletal Conditions							
All Musculoskeletal Injuries or Conditions [3]				**Stroke** [8]			
Total Population	25,910	28.0	725,697	Total Population	784	55.5	43,512
Male	9,687	27.1	262,475	Male	335	49.6	16,616
Female	16,224	28.5	462,601	Female	449	60.0	26,940
18 to 44 Years	8,152	28.5	232,438	18 to 44 Years	56	118.0	6,608
45 to 64 Years	11,898	30.2	359,800	45 to 64 Years	235	43.6	10,246
65 Years & Over	5,859	24.8	145,418	65 Years & Over	492	54.2	26,666
Fracture/Bone/Joint Injury [4]				**Hypertension** [9]			
Total Population	4,444	28.6	126,921	Total Population	1,951	49.1	95,794
Male	2,090	29.6	61,822	Male	664	46.0	30,544
Female	2,355	27.7	65,139	Female	1,287	50.7	65,251
18 to 44 Years	1,961	24.7	48,442	18 to 44 Years	313	72.2	22,599
45 to 64 Years	1,879	29.5	55,425	45 to 64 Years	1,043	45.2	47,144
65 Years & Over	604	38.0	22,963	65 Years & Over	595	43.8	26,061
Back/Neck Problem [5]				**Other Injury** [10]			
Total Population	10,632	29.4	312,581	Total Population	1,021	27.7	28,251
Male	4,118	29.2	120,246	Male	493	30.4	14,972
Female	6,514	29.5	192,163	Female	527	25.2	13,254
18 to 44 Years	4,205	29.4	123,627	18 to 44 Years	162	8.7	1,403
45 to 64 Years	4,729	33.6	158,894	45 to 64 Years	285	25.1	7,148
65 Years & Over	1,698	25.2	42,790	65 Years & Over	483	31.8	15,369
Arthritis/Rheumatism [6]							
Total Population	10,834	26.4	286,018				
Male	3,479	23.1	80,365				
Female	7,355	27.9	205,205				
18 to 44 Years	1,986	30.4	60,374				
45 to 64 Years	5,290	27.5	145,475				
65 Years & Over	3,557	22.4	79,677				

[1] A bed day is defined as 1/2 or more days in bed due to injury or illness in past 12 months, excluding hospitalization.

[2] Respondents reported "Yes" when asked "Are you limited in any way in any activities because of physical, mental or emotional problems." AND Respondents reporting a limitation reported "Yes" when asked if limitation was caused by "arthritis/rheumatism back/neck problem fracture/bone/joint injury other injury heart problem stroke hypertension."

[3] Respondents reporting a limitation reported "Yes" when asked if limitation was caused by "Fracture/bone/joint injury Back/neck problem Arthritis/Rheumatism"

[4] Respondents reporting a limitation reported "Yes" when asked if limitation was caused by "Fracture/bone/joint injury."

[5] Respondents reporting a limitation reported "Yes" when asked if limitation was caused by "Back/neck problem."

[6] Respondents reporting a limitation reported "Yes" when asked if limitation was caused by "Arthritis/rheumatism."

[7] Respondents reporting a limitation reported "Yes" when asked if limitation was caused by "Heart problem."

[8] Respondents reporting a limitation reported "Yes" when asked if limitation was caused by "Stroke."

[9] Respondents reporting a limitation reported "Yes" when asked if limitation was caused by "Hypertension."

[10] Respondents reporting a limitation reported "Yes" when asked if limitation was caused by "Other injury."

Source: National Center for Health Statistics. National Health Interview Survey, 2005

The Burden of Musculoskeletal Diseases in the United States - Copyright © 2008

Table 6.18: Lost Work Days Due to Major Health Conditions by Gender for Persons Aged 18 and Over, United States 2005

	Work Days Lost [1]				Work Days Lost [1]		
	Persons Reporting Lost Work Days (in 000s)	Mean Work Days Lost	Total Work Days Lost (in 000s)		Persons Reporting Lost Work Days (in 000s)	Mean Work Days Lost	Total Work Days Lost (in 000s)
All Causes [2]				**Other Major Health Conditions**			
				Heart Problem [7]			
Total Population	68,222	9.6	654,931	Total Population	501	46.4	23,246
Male	32,599	9.7	316,210	Male	240	52.6	12,624
Female	35,622	9.4	334,847	Female	260	40.6	10,556
18 to 44 Years	42,703	7.4	316,002	18 to 44 Years	109	33.0	3,597
45 to 64 Years	23,910	13.0	310,830	45 to 64 Years	302	61.4	18,543
65 Years & Over	1,609	15.4	24,779	65 Years & Over	90	12.3	1,107
Musculoskeletal Conditions							
All Musculoskeletal Injuries or Conditions [3]				**Stroke** [8]			
Total Population	14,346	21.1	302,294	Total Population	91	42.1	3,831
Male	6,156	21.7	133,415	Male	42	63.4	2,663
Female	8,190	20.6	168,810	Female	48	23.3	1,118
18 to 44 Years	6,103	18.0	109,946	18 to 44 Years	17	6.0	102
45 to 64 Years	7,625	24.0	183,118	45 to 64 Years	63	46.1	2,904
65 Years & Over	616	15.1	9,330	65 Years & Over	10	80.8	808
Fracture/Bone/Joint Injury [4]				**Hypertension** [9]			
Total Population	2,908	24.8	72,118	Total Population	510	37.1	18,921
Male	1,458	24.8	36,158	Male	254	47.7	12,116
Female	1,450	24.9	36,105	Female	256	26.5	6,784
18 to 44 Years	1,512	19.8	29,938	18 to 44 Years	111	21.9	2,431
45 to 64 Years	1,315	30.6	40,239	45 to 64 Years	380	42.5	16,150
65 Years & Over	81	25.7	2,082	65 Years & Over	19	17.1	325
Back/Neck Problem [5]				**Other Injury** [10]			
Total Population	6,360	21.5	136,740	Total Population	830	48.7	40,421
Male	2,823	21.5	60,695	Male	452	56.1	25,357
Female	3,537	21.4	75,692	Female	378	39.8	15,044
18 to 44 Years	3,172	18.2	57,730	18 to 44 Years	409	39.8	16,278
45 to 64 Years	2,949	25.2	74,315	45 to 64 Years	417	57.8	24,103
65 Years & Over	238	18.1	4,308	65 Years & Over	4	4.0	16
Arthritis/Rheumatism [6]							
Total Population	5,078	18.4	93,435				
Male	1,875	19.5	36,563				
Female	3,203	17.8	57,013				
18 to 44 Years	1,419	15.7	22,278				
45 to 64 Years	3,361	20.4	68,564				
65 Years & Over	297	9.9	2,940				

[1] A missed work day is defined as absence from work due to illness or injury in the past 12 months, excluding maternity or family leave.

[2] Respondents reported 'Yes' when asked "Are you limited in any way in any activities because of physical, mental or emotional problems." AND Respondents reporting a limitation reported 'Yes' when asked if limitation was caused by "arthritis/rheumatis back/neck problem fracture/bone/joint injury other injury heart problem stroke hypertension."

[3] Respondents reporting a limitation reported 'Yes' when asked if limitation was caused by "Fracture/bone/joint injury Back/neck problem Arthritis/Rheumatism"
[4] Respondents reporting a limitation reported 'Yes' when asked if limitation was caused by "Fracture/bone/joint injury."
[5] Respondents reporting a limitation reported 'Yes' when asked if limitation was caused by "Back/neck problem."
[6] Respondents reporting a limitation reported 'Yes' when asked if limitation was caused by "Arthritis/rheumatism."
[7] Respondents reporting a limitation reported 'Yes' when asked if limitation was caused by "Heart problem."
[8] Respondents reporting a limitation reported 'Yes' when asked if limitation was caused by "Stroke."
[9] Respondents reporting a limitation reported 'Yes' when asked if limitation was caused by "Hypertension."
[10] Respondents reporting a limitation reported 'Yes' when asked if limitation was caused by "Other injury."
Source: National Center for Health Statistics. National Health Interview Survey, 2005

Table 6.19: Summary of Bed and Lost Work Days Due to Health Problems for Persons Age 18 and Over, United States 2005

Cause of Bed/ Lost Work Days [1]	Bed Days [2] Total (in 000s)	% of Total	Lost Work Days [3] Total (in 000s)	% of Total
Musculoskeletal Injury or Condition	725,697	72%	302,294	46%
Heart Problem	115,097	11%	23,246	4%
Hypertension	95,794	10%	18,921	3%
Stroke	43,512	4%	3,831	1%
Other Injury	28,282	3%	40,421	6%
Other Health Conditions		0%	266,218	41%
Musculoskeletal Injury or Condition				
Back/Neck Pain	312,581	31%	136,740	21%
Arthritis/Rheumatism	286,018	28%	93,435	14%
Fracture/Bone/Joint Pain	126,921	13%	72,118	11%
All Causes	1,005,444		654,931	

[1] Respondents reported "Yes" when asked "Are you limited in any way in any activities because of physical, mental or emotional problems."

[2] A bed day is defined as 1/2 or more days in bed due to injury or illness in past 12 months, excluding hospitalization.

[3] A missed work day is defined as absence from work due to illness or injury in the past 12 months, excluding maternity or family leave.

Source: National Center for Health Statistics. National Health Interview Survey, 2005

Table 6.20: Musculoskeletal Disorders (MSDs) for Work-Related Injuries and Illnesses Involving Days Away from Work, United States 2000-2005

	All Cases of Work-related Injuries and	MSDs	% of Full-time Workers Away From Work
1992	2,331,098	784,145	33.6%
1993	2,252,591	762,727	33.9%
1994	2,236,639	755,594	33.8%
1995	2,040,929	695,789	34.1%
1996	1,880,525	647,355	34.4%
1997	1,833,380	626,352	34.2%
1998	1,730,534	592,544	34.2%
1999	1,702,420	582,340	34.2%
2000	1,664,018	577,814	34.7%
2001	1,537,567	522,528	34.0%
2002	1,436,194	487,915	34.0%
2003	1,315,920	435,180	33.1%
2004	1,259,320	402,700	32.0%
2005	1,234,860	375,540	30.4%

Source 1998 to 2005: U.S. Department of Labor, Bureau of Labor Statistics: Case and Demographic Characteristics for Work-related Injuries and Illnesses Involving Days Away from Work. Supplemental Table 11: Number of nonfatal occupational injuries and illnesses involving days away from work by selected worker and case characteristics and musculoskeletal disorders, All United States, private industry, 2000-2005. Available at: http://www.bls.gov/iif/oshcdnew.htm#Resource%20Table%20categories%20-%202005. Accessed July 27, 2007.
Source 1992 to 1997: U.S. Department of Labor, Bureau of Labor Statistics: Worker Health Chartbook 2004. Available at: http://www2a.cdc.gov/niosh-Chartbook/imagedetail.asp?imgid=77. Accessed August 24, 2007.

Table 6.21: Musculoskeletal Disorders for Work-Related Injuries and Illnesses Involving Days Away from Work by Nature of Injury, United States 2000-2005

Nature of Injury [1]	2000 Number	Percent	2001 Number	Percent	2002 Number	Percent	2003 Number	Percent	2004 Number	Percent	2005 Number	Percent
Sprains, Strains	442,839	71.2%	399,722	76.5%	369,785	70.2%	331,020	72.1%	306,210	76.0%	287,970	72.4%
Carpal Tunnel Syndrome	27,571	4.4%	26,522	5.1%	22,583	4.3%	22,110	4.8%	18,760	4.7%	16,440	4.1%
Tendonitis	12,577	2.0%	12,131	2.3%	8,105	1.5%	6,740	1.5%	5,940	1.5%	5,040	1.3%
Soreness, Pain	57,139	9.2%	22,346	4.3%	56,887	10.8%	45,580	9.9%	46,230	11.5%	41,930	10.5%
Back Pain	31,685	5.1%	27,894	5.3%	30,953	5.9%	23,650	5.2%	23,770	5.9%	22,050	5.5%
All Other (including MS system and connective diseases and disorders and hernia)	50,265	8.1%	33,913	6.5%	38,660	7.3%	29,740	6.5%	1,790	0.4%	24,170	6.1%
Total Cases	577,814	100.0%	522,528	100.0%	487,915	100.0%	435,180	100.0%	402,700	100.0%	375,540	100.0%

[1] Multiple injuries per case possible percentages based on total injuries, which may be > total cases.

Source: U.S. Department of Labor, Bureau of Labor Statistics: Case and Demographic Characteristics for Work-related Injuries and Illnesses Involving Days Away from Work. Supplemental Tables, Table 11: Number of nonfatal occupational injuries and illnesses involving days away from work by selected worker and case characteristics and musculoskeletal disorders, All United States, private industry, 2000-2005. Available at: http://www.bls.gov/iif/oshcdnew.htm#Resource%20Table%20categories%20-%202005. Accessed July 27, 2007.

Table 6.22: Trends in MSD Injuries Involving Days Away from Work in Private Industry by Sex, United States 2000 to 2005

All MSD Injuries

		Male	Female	Total
2000	Number	358,949	216,014	574,963
	Percent	62.4%	37.6%	
2001	Number	324,935	194,910	519,845
	Percent	62.5%	37.5%	
2002	Number	300,128	186,966	487,915
	Percent	61.6%	38.4%	
2003	Number	267,530	166,780	435,180
	Percent	61.6%	38.4%	
2004	Number	254,220	147,750	402,700
	Percent	63.2%	36.8%	
2005	Number	238,630	136,340	375,540
	Percent	63.5%	36.3%	

Source: U.S. Department of Labor, Bureau of Labor Statistics: Case and Demographic Characteristics for Work-related Injuries and Illnesses Involving Days Away from Work. Supplemental Tables 2005, Table 11: Number of nonfatal occupational injuries and illnesses involving days away from work by selected worker and case characteristics and musculoskeletal disorders, all United States, private industry, 2000-2005. Available at: http://www.bls.gov/iif/oshcdnew.htm#Resource%20Table%20categories%20-%202005. Accessed July 27, 2007.

Table 6.23: Distribution of Nonfatal Injury and Illness Cases Involving Days Away from Work in Private Industry for Musculoskeletal Disorders by Sex, United States 2005

Nonfatal Injuries by Injury Type, 2005

		Male	Female	Total
All Nonfatal Injuries and Illnesses	Number	814,250	415,880	1,234,680
	Percent	65.9%	33.7%	
All MSD Injuries	Number	238,630	136,340	375,540
	Percent	63.5%	36.3%	
All Sprains, Strains & Tears [1]	Number	320,350	181,100	503,350
	Percent	63.6%	36.0%	
Carpal Tunnel Syndrome	Number	5,890	10,560	16,460
	Percent	35.8%	64.2%	
Tendonitis	Number	2,570	3,160	5,720
	Percent	44.9%	55.2%	

[1] Totals are greater than shown in Table 11 for MDS sprains & strains due to inclusion of all sprains and strains.

Source: U.S. Department of Labor, Bureau of Labor Statistics: Case and Demographic Characteristics for Work-related Injuries and Illnesses Involving Days Away from Work. Supplemental Tables 2005, Table 9: Number of nonfatal occupational injuries and illnesses involving days away from work by selected worker case characteristics and nature of injury or illness, All United States, private industry, 2000-2005. Available at: http://www.bls.gov/iif/oshcdnew.htm#Resource%20Table%20categories%20-%202005. Accessed July 27, 2007.

Table 6.24: Musculoskeletal Disorders (MSDs) for Work-Related Injuries and Illnesses Involving Days Away from Work by Race, United States 2005

Race or Ethnicity [2]	Nonfatal Injuries and Illnesses [1] Number	Percent	MSDs Number	Percent	Sprains, Strains & Tears Number	Percent	Carpal Tunnel Syndrome Number	Percent	Tendonitis Number	Percent
White	567,790	66.2%	175,600	70.0%	229,560	68.5%	9650	79.0%	2660	66.0%
Black/African American	163,440	19.0%	37,630	15.0%	41,810	12.5%	1000	8.2%	370	9.2%
Hispanic or Latino	101,170	11.8%	29,950	11.9%	53,870	16.1%	1190	9.7%	750	18.6%
Other	25,870	3.0%	7,680	3.1%	9,840	2.9%	370	3.0%	250	6.2%
Total	858,270		250,860		335,080		12,210		4,030	
Not Reported	376,550		124,660		168,450		4260		1670	

[1] Nonfatal injuries and illnesses include the total of all nonfatal injuries and illnesses involving days away from work

[2] Percentages based on number of cases for which race is reported.

Source: U.S. Department of Labor, Bureau of Labor Statistics: Case and Demographic Characteristics for Work-related Injuries and Illnesses Involving Days Away from Work. Supplemental Tables 2005, Table 9: Number of nonfatal occupational injuries and illnesses involving days away from work by selected worker case characteristics and nature of injury or illness, All United States, private industry, 2005 and Table 11: Number of nonfatal occupational injuries and illnesses involving days away from work by selected worker and case characteristics and musculoskeletal disorders, All United States, private industry, 2005. Available at: http://www.bls.gov/iif/oshcdnew.htm#Resource%20Table%20categories%20-%202005. July 27, 2007.

Table 6.25: Musculoskeletal Disorders (MSDs) for Work-Related Injuries and Illnesses Involving Days Away from Work by Age, United States 2005

	Nonfatal Injuries and Illnesses		MSDs		Sprains, Strains and Tears		Carpal Tunnel Syndrome		Tendonitis	
	Number	Percent	Number	Percent	Number	Percent	Number	Percent	Number	Percent
Under 14 Years	*	*	*	*	*	*	*	*	*	*
14-15	90	0.0%	*	*	*	*	*	*	*	*
16-19	41,530	3.4%	7,940	2.1%	12,510	2.5%	40	0.2%	40	0.7%
20-24	133,760	10.9%	33,560	9.0%	47,900	9.6%	340	2.1%	500	8.8%
25-34	290,880	23.8%	89,070	23.9%	121,430	24.3%	2,710	16.5%	1,350	23.8%
35-44	311,880	25.5%	106,480	28.6%	138,500	27.7%	4,580	27.9%	1,860	32.7%
45-54	282,310	23.1%	92,830	24.9%	118,470	23.7%	6,200	37.8%	1,410	24.8%
55-64	135,290	11.1%	37,330	10.0%	52,070	10.4%	2,410	14.7%	490	8.6%
65 Years & Older	27,050	2.2%	5,380	1.4%	8,350	1.7%	120	0.7%	30	0.5%
Total	1,234,680		375,540		503,530		16,460		5,720	

* Data does not meet publication guidelines

Source: U.S. Department of Labor, Bureau of Labor Statistics: Case and Demographic Characteristics for Work-related Injuries and Illnesses Involving Days Away from Work. Supplemental Tables 2005, Table 9: Number of nonfatal occupatonal injuries and illnesses involving days away from work by selected worker case characteristics and nature of injury or illness, all United States, private industry, 2005, and Table 11: Number of nonfatal occupational injuries and illnesses involving days away from work by selected worker and case characteristics and musculoskeletal disorders, all United States, private industry, 2005. Available at: http://www.bls.gov/iif/oshcdnew.htm#Resource%20Table%20categories%20-%202005. Accessed July 27, 2007.

Table 6.26: Musculoskeletal Disorders (MSDs) for Work-Related Injuries and Illnesses Involving Days Away from Work by Body Part Affected, United States 2005

Body Part Affected	All Natures		MSDs		Sprains, Strains and Tears		Carpal Tunnel Syndrome		Tendonitis	
	Number	Percent	Number	Percent	Number	Percent	Number	Percent	Number	Percent
Head (total)	81,090	6.6%	50	0.0%	160	0.0%	0	0.0%	0	0.0%
Head (except eye) [1]	46,350	3.8%	30	0.0%	70	0.0%	0	0.0%	0	0.0%
Eye	34,740	2.8%	20	0.0%	90	0.0%	0	0.0%	0	0.0%
Neck	18,470	1.5%	6,440	1.7%	13,730	2.7%	0	0.0%	0	0.0%
Trunk (total)	428,500	34.7%	269,020	71.6%	290,330	57.7%	0	0.0%	980	17.2%
Trunk (except shoulder and back) [1]	79,810	6.5%	38,670	10.3%	23,530	4.7%	0	0.0%	30	0.5%
Shoulder	77,800	6.3%	45,910	12.2%	54,260	10.8%	0	0.0%	950	16.6%
Back	270,890	21.9%	184,440	49.1%	212,540	42.2%	0	0.0%	0	0.0%
Upper Extremities (total)	284,750	23.1%	55,450	14.8%	43,410	8.6%	16,460	100.0%	4,250	74.4%
Upper Extremities (except wrist, hand and finger) [1]	70,390	5.7%	19,650	5.2%	18,480	3.7%	0	0.0%	1,860	32.6%
Wrist	56,250	4.6%	29,350	7.8%	15,880	3.2%	16,460	100.0%	1,820	31.9%
Hand (except finger)	47,020	3.8%	3,020	0.8%	3,470	0.7%	0	0.0%	280	4.9%
Finger	111,090	9.0%	3,430	0.9%	5,580	1.1%	0	0.0%	290	5.1%
Lower Extremities (total)	271,740	22.0%	29,390	7.8%	119,810	23.8%	0	0.0%	310	5.4%
Lower Extremities (except knee, foot and toe) [1]	127,340	10.3%	8,870	2.4%	55,020	10.9%	0	0.0%	90	1.6%
Knee	100,560	8.1%	19,170	5.1%	58,310	11.6%	0	0.0%	130	2.3%
Foot, Toe	43,840	3.6%	1,350	0.4%	6,480	1.3%	0	0.0%	90	1.6%
Body Systems	17,950	1.5%	0	0.0%	0	0.0%	0	0.0%	0	0.0%
Multiple Parts	120,960	9.8%	14,710	3.9%	35,090	7.0%	0	0.0%	150	2.6%
All Other [1]	11,220	0.9%	480	0.1%	1,000	0.2%	0	0.0%	20	0.4%
Total Cases	1,234,680		375,540		503,530		16,460		5,720	

[1] Computed value

Source: U.S. Department of Labor, Bureau of Labor Statistics: Case and Demographic Characteristics for Work-related Injuries and Illnesses Involving Days Away from Work. Supplemental Tables 2005, Table 9: Number of nonfatal occupatonal injuries and illnesses involving days away from work by selected worker case characteristics and nature of injury or illness, all United States, private industry, 2005, and Table 11: Number of nonfatal occupational injuries and illnesses involving days away from work by selected worker and case characteristics and musculoskeletal disorders, all United States, private industry, 2005. Available at: http://www.bls.gov/iif/oshcdnew.htm#Resource%20Table%20categories%20-%20200. Accessed July 27, 2007.

Table 6.27: Incidence Rates per 10,000 Full Time Workers for Injuries and Illnesses by Nature of Injury or Illness for Nonfatal Occupational Injuries Involving Days Away from Work, United States 1996-2005

	Rate per 10,000 Full-time Workers										**Incidence Rate Change 1996-2005**
	1996	**1997**	**1998**	**1999**	**2000**	**2001**	**2002**	**2003**	**2004**	**2005**	
Sprains, Strains	97.6	92.5	85.6	81.8	79.2	73.7	69.9	64.3	59.0	55.3	-43.3%
Bruises, Contusions	20.8	19.2	17.3	17.3	16.5	15.0	14.4	13.5	12.9	11.8	-43.3%
Cuts, Lacerations, Punctures	15.8	15.5	15.5	14.6	13.2	12.6	12.5	11.0	11.1	11.2	-29.1%
Fractures	14.3	13.8	13.0	12.6	12.7	11.9	11.2	10.8	10.6	10.5	-26.6%
Heat Burns	3.5	3.5	3.2	3.0	2.6	2.8	2.4	2.2	2.1	1.9	-45.7%
Carpal Tunnel Syndrome	3.6	3.4	3.0	3.1	3.0	3.0	2.6	2.5	2.1	1.8	-50.0%
Tendonitis	2.1	2.1	1.9	1.8	1.6	1.6	1.1	0.9	0.8	0.6	-71.4%
Chemical Burns	1.4	1.4	1.3	1.3	1.0	1.0	<1.0	0.9	0.8	0.7	-50.0%
Amputations	1.2	1.3	1.2	1.1	1.1	1.0	1.0	0.9	0.9	0.9	-25.0%
Multiple Traumatic Injuries	7.2	6.9	6.5	6.6	6.5	5.9	5.9	5.5	5.7	5.5	-23.6%
MSD Injuries All Cases	223.8	212.3	195.0	188.3	181.1	169.1	162.6	150.0	141.3	135.7	-39.4%

Source: U.S. Department of Labor, Bureau of Labor Statistics: Survey of Occupational Injuries and Illnesses. Table 6 (1996-2002) or 7 (2003-2005): Incidence rates for nonfatal occupational injuries and illnesses involving days away from work per 10,000 full-time workers for selected characteristics and major industry sector: Nature of injury or illness. Lost work time:1995-2005. Available at: www.bls.gov/iif/oshcdnew.htm. Accessed July 7, 2007.

Table 6.28: Incidence Rates for Injuries and Illnesses by Industry for Nonfatal Occupational Injuries Involving Days Away from Work by Body Part Affected, United States 2005

	Total Private Industry	**Goods Producing**				**Service Providing**						
		Total Goods	**Natural Resources and Mining**	**Con-struction**	**Manu-facturing**	**Total Service**	**Trade, Transport and Utilities**	**Infor-mation**	**Financial Activities**	**Education and Health Services**	**Leisure and Hospi-tality**	**Other Services**
Head (total)	8.9	14.0	16.1	19.6	11.3	7.2	11.0	3.6	4.1	6.8	5.6	8.1
Eye	3.8	7.7	7.7	9.7	6.8	2.6	3.9	1.2	1.6	2.0	1.0	4.4
Neck	2.0	2.2	2.0	3.6	1.6	2.0	2.8	1.4	1.0	2.8	0.8	1.1
Trunk (total)	47.1	56.3	57.4	73.8	48.1	44.1	64.5	23.5	15.2	61.2	32.2	28.3
Shoulder	8.6	11.1	10.8	12.2	10.7	7.7	12.3	4.1	2.1	9.4	5.8	4.3
Back	29.8	33.0	30.9	46.0	27.2	28.7	39.9	15.4	10.1	43.7	20.6	18.2
Upper Extremities (total)	31.3	50.3	42.0	57.3	47.9	25.1	33.7	15.4	10.5	22.7	35.3	27.0
Wrist	6.2	8.4	5.4	7.8	8.9	5.5	7.1	4.6	3.6	6.2	4.7	6.1
Hand (except finger)	5.2	8.5	5.6	10.9	7.7	4.1	5.2	1.9	1.3	3.2	7.3	5.2
Finger	12.2	22.3	21.3	24.0	21.6	8.9	12.2	3.7	3.1	6.1	15.6	10.3
Lower Extremities (total)	29.9	37.6	45.4	59.8	26.6	27.4	41.2	18.1	11.9	27.9	23.1	21.4
Knee	11.1	12.7	15.7	19.3	9.4	10.5	15.5	6.5	4.7	12.0	9.1	7.7
Foot (except toe)	4.8	7.0	6.2	10.7	5.3	4.1	6.9	3.4	1.7	3.4	3.0	3.2
Toe	1.4	1.8	1.7	2.4	1.5	1.3	2.2	0.8	0.4	1.0	0.8	1.5
Body Systems	2.0	2.1	3.5	2.5	1.8	1.9	1.7	2.1	2.4	2.5	1.8	1.6
Multiple Parts	13.3	13.0	16.4	20.9	9.1	13.4	16.4	10.1	7.2	20.6	9.7	9.1
Rate All Cases	135.7	176.9	184.5	239.5	147.1	121.1	171.3	74.2	52.3	144.5	108.5	96.6

Source: U.S. Department of Labor, Bureau of Labor Statistics: Survey of Occupational Injuries and Illnesses. Table 7: Incidence rates for nonfatal occupational injuries and illnesses involving days away from work per 10,000 full-time workers for selected characteristics and major industry sector: Part of body affected by the injury or illness. Lost work time:1995-2005. Available at: www.bls.gov/iif/oshcdnew.htm. Accessed July 7, 2007.

Table 6.29: Musculoskeletal Disorders (MSDs) for Work-Related Injuries and Illnesses Involving Days Away from Work by Occupation, United States 2005

Industry	All Natures		MSDs		Sprains, Strains and Tears		Carpal Tunnel Syndrome		Tendonitis	
	Number	Percent	Number	Percent	Number	Percent	Number	Percent	Number	Percent
Management, Business, Financial	28,110	2.3%	6,360	1.7%	8,780	1.7%	1,250	7.6%	70	1.2%
Professional and Related	83,060	6.7%	28,210	7.5%	40,310	8.0%	1,150	7.0%	540	9.4%
Service	247,270	20.0%	77,390	20.6%	107,470	21.4%	1,440	8.7%	680	11.9%
Sales and Related	80,020	6.5%	24,770	6.6%	36,030	7.2%	940	5.7%	420	7.3%
Office and Administrative Support	91,400	7.4%	31,010	8.3%	37,800	7.5%	3,430	20.8%	750	13.1%
Farming, Fishing, and Forestry	15,540	1.3%	2,380	0.6%	4,790	1.0%	50	0.3%	40	0.7%
Construction and Extractive	152,490	12.4%	36,330	9.7%	53,170	10.6%	840	5.1%	630	11.0%
Installation, Maintenance and Repair	107,770	8.7%	31,120	8.3%	40,840	8.1%	1,120	6.8%	410	7.2%
Production	173,440	14.1%	57,390	15.3%	60,100	11.9%	4,790	29.1%	1,580	27.6%
Transportation and Material Moving	253,570	20.6%	80,480	21.4%	113,910	22.6%	1,450	8.8%	600	10.5%
Total	1,234,680	100.0%	315,540	100.0%	503,530	100.0%	16,460	100.0%	5,720	100.0%

Source: U.S. Department of Labor, Bureau of Labor Statistics: Case and Demographic Characteristics for Work-related Injuries and Illnesses Involving Days Away from Work. Supplemental Tables 2005, Table 9: Number of nonfatal occupatonal injuries and illnesses involving days away from work by selected worker case characteristics and nature of injury or illness, All United States, private industry, 2005 and Table 11: Number of nonfatal occupational injuries and illnesses involving days away from work by selected worker and case characteristics and musculoskeletal disorders, all United States, private industry, 2005. Available at: http://www.bls.gov/iif/oshcdnew.htm#Resource%20Table%20categories%20-%202005. Accessed July 27, 2007.

Table 6.30: Median Days Away from Work for Nonfatal Injuries and Illnesses by Nature of Injury or Illnesses, United States 1996-2005

	Median Days Away From Work									
	1996	1997	1998	1999	2000	2001	2002	2003	2004	2005
Sprains, Strains (MSD & Other)	6	6	6	6	6	6	7	8	8	8
Bruises, Contusions	3	3	3	3	3	3	4	4	4	4
Cuts, Lacerations, Punctures	3	3	3	3	3	3	3	4	4	4
Fractures	17	21	19	20	20	21	29	30	28	27
Heat Burns	25	4	4	4	4	5	4	5	5	5
Carpal Tunnel Syndrome (MSD & other)	4	25	24	27	27	25	30	32	28	27
Tendonitis (MSD & other)	9	11	10	9	10	10	15	11	13	12
Chemical Burns	2	2	2	3	2	2	2	2	3	3
Amputations	20	18	18	18	18	18	26	30	25	22
Multiple Traumatic Injuries	8	7	7	7	8	8	9	9	9	8
Musculoskeletal Disorders	*	*	7	7	7	8	9	10	10	9
Total All Cases	8	5	5	6	6	6	7	8	7	7

	Total Cases (in 000s)									
Musculoskeletal disorder cases	*	*	592.5	582.3	577.8	522.5	487.9	435.2	402.7	375.5
All cases	1,880.5	1,833.3	1,730.5	1,702.5	1,664.0	1,537.6	1,36.2	1,315.9	1,259.3	1,234.7

* Data not available

Source: U.S. Department of Labor, Bureau of Labor Statistics: Survey of Occupational Injuries and Illnesses. Table 9 (1996-2002) and Table 11 (2003-2005): Percent distribution of nonfatal occupational injuries and illnesses involving days away from work by selected injury or illness characteristics and and number of days away from work: Nature of injury or illness. Lost work time: 1996-2005. Available at: www.bls.gov/iif/oshcdnew.htm. Accessed July 7, 2007.

Table 6.31: Median Days Away from Work for Nonfatal Injuries and Illnesses by Part of Body Affected, United States 1996-2005

	1996	1997	1998	1999	2000	2001	2002	2003	2004	2005
Head (total)	2	2	2	2	2	2	2	2	2	2
Eye	2	2	2	2	2	2	2	2	2	2
Neck	5	5	4	6	5	5	7	8	6	7
Trunk (total)	6	7	6	7	7	7	8	9	9	8
Shoulder	8	9	9	10	10	12	15	18	17	15
Back	6	6	6	6	6	6	7	7	7	7
Upper Extremities (total)	6	6	5	6	5	6	7	7	7	7
Wrist	12	12	11	12	12	13	15	17	14	14
Hand (except finger)	4	5	4	5	4	4	5	5	5	5
Finger	4	5	4	4	4	5	5	5	5	5
Lower Extremities (total)	6	6	6	7	7	7	9	9	9	9
Knee	9	9	10	10	10	11	14	14	15	12
Foot (except toe)	5	5	5	5	5	6	7	7	6	7
Toe	4	5	4	5	5	5	6	6	6	5
Body Systems	3	4	3	3	3	4	4	4	5	7
Multiple Parts	7	8	8	8	8	8	10	10	10	8
Total All Cases	5	5	5	6	6	6	7	8	7	7
Total Cases (in 000s)	1,880.5	1,833.4	1,730.5	1,702.5	1,664.0	1,537.6	1,436.2	1,315.9	1,259.3	1,234.7

Source: U.S. Department of Labor, Bureau of Labor Statistics: Survey of Occupational Injuries and Illnesses. Table 11: Percent distribution of nonfatal occupational injuries and illnesses involving days away from work by selected injury or illness characteristics and and number of days away from work: Part of body affected by the injury or illnesss. Lost work time:1996-2005. Available at: : www.bls.gov/iif/oshcdnew.htm. Accessed July 7, 2007

Table 6.32: Resource Utilization for Traumatic Musculoskeletal (MS) Injuries by Treatment Location and Sex, United States 2004

	Total Visits (in 000s) [1]					% All Diagnoses for All Treatment Locations	% Total Diagnoses by Treatment Location			
	Physician Office Visits [2]	Emergency Room Visits [3]	Hospital Out-patient Visits [4]	Inpatient Stays [5]	Total All Treatment Sites		Physician Office Visits [2]	Emergency Room Visits [3]	Hospital Out-patient Visits [4]	Inpatient Stays [5]
Fractures										
All Fractures	9,129	4,065	991	1,103	15,288	24.8%	60%	27%	6%	7%
Males	4,554	2,079	565	477	7,675	25.4%	59%	27%	7%	6%
Females	4,575	1,986	426	617	7,604	24.0%	60%	26%	6%	8%
Dislocations										
All Dislocations	4,362	536	196	50	5,144	8.3%	85%	10%	4%	1%
Males	2,112	299	100	29	2,540	8.4%	83%	12%	4%	1%
Females	2,450	237	96	21	2,804	8.9%	87%	8%	3%	1%
Sprains and Strains										
All Sprains and Strains	10,981	4,256	948	98	16,283	26.4%	67%	26%	6%	1%
Males	5,072	2,024	387	49	7,532	24.9%	67%	27%	5%	1%
Females	5,909	2,222	560	48	8,739	27.6%	68%	25%	6%	1%
Contusions										
All Contusions	3,319	4,540	330	182	8,371	13.6%	40%	54%	4%	2%
Males	1,498	2,122	135	77	3,832	12.7%	39%	55%	4%	2%
Females	1,821	2,418	196	105	4,540	14.3%	40%	53%	4%	2%
Open Wounds										
All Open Wounds	4,887	4,643	579	225	10,334	16.7%	47%	45%	6%	2%
Males	2,502	2,956	377	144	5,979	19.8%	42%	49%	6%	2%
Females	2,385	1,687	202	80	4,354	13.7%	55%	39%	5%	2%
Other Musculoskeletal Injuries										
All Other MS Injuries	4,225	1,403	502	153	6,283	10.2%	67%	22%	8%	2%
Males	1,620	698	252	84	2,654	8.85	61%	26%	9%	3%
Females	2,605	705	250	68	3,628	11.5%	72%	19%	7%	2%
Total Musculoskeletal Traumtatic Injuries										
All MS Traumatic Injuries	34,372	17,888	3,380	1,610	57,250		60%	31%	6%	3%
Males	16,177	9,382	1,747	739	28,045	49.0%	58%	33%	6%	3%
Females	18,195	8,506	1,632	860	29,193	51.0%	62%	29%	6%	3%
All Injury Treatment Episodes	54,168	30,770	5,192	5,161	95,291		57%	32%	5%	5%

[1] All listed diagnoses for inpatients discharged from short-stay hospitals. Multiple diagnoses per case possible; percentages based on total diagnoses.

[2] Source: National Center for Health Statistics, National Ambulatory Medical Care Survey, 2004.

[3] Source: National Center for Health Statistics, National Hospital Ambulatory Medical Care Survey, Emergency Room Visits, 2004.

[4] Source: National Center for Health Statistics, National Hospital Ambulatory Medical Visits, Outpatient Department Visits, 2004.

[5] Source: Agency for Healthcare Research and Quality, Healthcare Cost and Utilization Project, Nationwide Inpatient Sample, 2004.

Table 6.33: Resource Utilization for Traumatic Musculoskeletal (MS) Injuries by Treatment Location and Age, United States 2004

	Total Visits (in 000s) [1]						% Total Visits at Treatment Location			
	Physician Office Visits [2]	Emer-gency Room Visits [3]	Hospital Out-patient Visits [4]	In-patient Stays [5]	Total All Treatment Sites	% All Diagnoses for All Treatment	Physician Office Visits [2]	Emer-gency Room Visits [3]	Hospital Out-patient Visits [4]	In-patient Stays [5]
Fractures										
All Fractures	9,129	4,065	991	1,103	15,288					
Under 18 Years	2,507	1,286	429	84	4,306	28%	27%	32%	43%	8%
18-44 Years	2,048	1,269	279	229	3,825	25%	22%	31%	28%	21%
45-64 Years	2,233	716	188	219	3,356	22%	24%	18%	19%	20%
65 Years & Over	2,342	794	96	568	3,800	25%	26%	20%	10%	51%
Dislocations										
All Dislocations	4,362	536	196	50	5,144					
Under 18 Years	382	177	89	4	652	13%	9%	33%	45%	8%
18-44 Years	1,285	223	69	19	1,596	31%	29%	42%	35%	38%
45-64 Years	1,626	85	23	13	1,747	34%	37%	16%	12%	26%
65 Years & Over	769	51	15	13	848	16%	18%	10%	8%	26%
Sprains and Strains										
All Sprains and Strains	10,981	4,256	948	98	16,283					
Under 18 Years	2,186	1,013	274	4	3,477	21%	20%	24%	29%	4%
18-44 Years	4,204	2,174	403	29	6,810	42%	38%	51%	43%	30%
45-64 Years	3,335	807	223	28	4,393	27%	30%	19%	24%	29%
65 Years & Over	1,256	252	48	37	1,593	10%	11%	6%	5%	38%
Contusions										
All Contusions	3,319	4,540	330	182	8,371					
Under 18 Years	666	1,151	159	11	1,987	24%	20%	25%	48%	6%
18-44 Years	568	2,096	97	40	2,801	33%	17%	46%	29%	22%
45-64 Years	826	773	49	37	1,685	20%	25%	17%	15%	20%
65 Years & Over	1,259	520	25	94	1,898	23%	38%	11%	8%	52%
Open Wounds										
All Open Wounds	4,887	4,643	579	225	10,334					
Under 18 Years	1,022	1,314	138	24	2,498	24%	21%	28%	24%	11%
18-44 Years	1,593	2,056	266	111	4,026	39%	33%	44%	46%	49%
45-64 Years	1,356	848	132	46	2,382	23%	28%	18%	23%	20%
65 Years & Over	916	425	44	44	1,429	14%	19%	9%	8%	20%
Other Musculoskeletal Injuries										
All Other MS Injuries	4,225	1,403	502	153	6,283					
Under 18 Years	817	404	106	13	1,340	21%	19%	29%	21%	8%
18-44 Years	1,365	661	189	53	2,268	36%	32%	47%	38%	35%
45-64 Years	1,667	239	122	39	2,067	33%	39%	17%	24%	25%
65 Years & Over	376	98	85	48	607	10%	9%	7%	17%	31%
Total Musculoskeletal Traumatic Injuries										
All MS Traumatic Injuries	34,372	17,888	3,380	1,610	57,250					
Under 18 Years	7,241	4,994	1,143	124	13,502	24%	21%	28%	34%	8%
18-44 Years	10,327	7,769	1,143	394	19,633	34%	30%	43%	34%	24%
45-64 Years	10,246	3,133	706	337	14,422	25%	30%	18%	21%	21%
65 Years & Over	6,558	1,993	312	752	9,615	17%	19%	11%	9%	47%
All Injury Treatment Episodes	54,168	30,770	5,192	5,161	95,291					
Under 18 Years	11,415	9,131	1,702	361	22,609	24%	21%	30%	33%	7%
18-44 Years	16,855	13,013	1,892	1,180	32,940	35%	31%	42%	36%	23%
45-64 Years	15,184	5,307	1,061	1,384	22,936	24%	28%	17%	20%	27%
65 Years & Over	10,714	3,319	537	2,236	16,806	18%	20%	11%	10%	43%

[1] All listed diagnoses for inpatients discharged from short-stay hospitals. Multiple diagnoses per case possible; percentages based on total diagnoses.

[2] Source: National Center for Health Statistics, National Ambulatory Medical Care Survey, 2004.

[3] Source: National Center for Health Statistics, National Hospital Ambulatory Medical Care Survey, Emergency Room Visits, 2004.

[4] Source: National Center for Health Statistics, National Hospital Ambulatory Medical Visits, Outpatient Department Visits, 2004.

[5] Source: Agency for Healthcare Research and Quality, Healthcare Cost and Utilization Project, Nationwide Inpatient Sample, 2004.

Table 6.34: Percent Resource Utilization for Traumatic Musculoskeletal (MS) Injuries by Treatment Location for All Injury Diagnoses versus Primary (1st) Diagnosis, United States 2004

	Percent of All Injury Diagnoses that are Primary (1st) Diagnosis				
	Physician Office Visits [1]	Emergency Room Visits [2]	Hospital Outpatient Visits [3]	Inpatient Stays [4]	Total All Treatment Sites
Fractures	90%	86%	91%	77%	88%
Dislocations	72%	84%	67%	28%	73%
Sprains and Strains	34%	81%	86%	38%	49%
Contusions	57%	71%	77%	18%	65%
Open Wounds	87%	89%	90%	28%	87%
All Other MS Iinjuries	62%	81%	82%	32%	67%
Total All MS Traumatic Injuries	84%	89%	90%	65%	85%

[1] Source: National Center for Health Statistics, National Ambulatory Medical Care Survey, 2004.

[2] Source: National Center for Health Statistics, National Hospital Ambulatory Medical Care Survey, Emergency Room Visits, 2004.

[3] Source: National Center for Health Statistics, National Hospital Ambulatory Medical Visits, Outpatient Department Visits, 2004.

[4] Source: Agency for Healthcare Research and Quality, Healthcare Cost and Utilization Project, Nationwide Inpatient Sample, 2004.

Table 6.35 : Patient Days and Estimated Total Cost for Hospital Care for Traumatic Musculoskeletal (MS) Injury Patients, United States 2004

	Total Patients (in 000s) [1]	Hospital Stay			Hospital Cost		
		Mean Length of Stay (in days)	Total Patient Days (in 000s)	% of Total Patient Days [2]	Mean Charge per Patient [3]	Estimated Total Cost (in billion $) [3]	% of Total Cost [2]
Fractures							
Fracture of Upper Limb	160	3.1	496	10.1%	$20,080	$3.21	12.1%
Fracture of Lower Limb	584	5.6	3270	66.4%	$30,260	$17.67	66.3%
Fracture of Trunk/Multiple Sites	101	5.6	566	11.5%	$25,330	$2.56	9.6%
All fractures	845	5.1	4310	87.5%	$27,740	$23.44	88.0%
Derangement Injuries							
Derangement of Knee	8	1.8	14	0.3%	$16,110	$0.13	0.5%
Other Joint Derangement	16	2.6	42	0.8%	$17,470	$0.28	1.0%
All Derangement Injuries	24	2.4	58	1.2%	$17,010	$0.41	1.5%
Dislocation Injuries							
Dislocations of Upper Limb	4	2.2	9	0.2%	$14,420	$0.06	0.2%
Dislocations of Lower Limb	9	3.2	29	0.6%	$18,880	$0.17	0.6%
All Dislocation Injuries	14	2.9	41	0.8%	$17,310	$0.24	0.9%
Sprain and Strain Injuries							
Sprains of Upper Limb	16	1.9	30	0.6%	$16,140	$0.26	1.0%
Sprains of Lower Limb	19	3.0	57	1.2%	$14,010	$0.27	1.0%
All Sprains and Strain Injuries	37	2.5	93	1.9%	$14,560	$0.54	2.0%
Other Musculoskeletal Injuries							
Contusions	32	3.3	106	2.1%	$11,870	$0.38	1.4%
Crushing Injuries	6	6.9	41	0.8%	$44,230	$0.27	1.0%
Open Wounds	64	3.2	205	4.2%	$14,930	$0.96	3.6%
Traumatic Amputation	10	4.7	47	1.0%	$28,600	$0.29	1.1%
Late Effects/Consequences of Traumatic Injuries	9	2.9	26	0.5%	$15,060	$0.14	0.5%
All Other MS Injuries	121	3.5	424	8.6%	$16,690	$2.02	7.6%
Total All MS Traumatic Injuries	1,041	4.7	4,893	100.0%	$25,600	$26.65	100.0%

[1] First listed diagnosis for inpatients discharged from short-stay hospitals.

[2] Due to rounding, totals may not equal sum of the individual components.

[3] Rounded to nearest ten.

Source: Agency for Healthcare Research and Quality, Healthcare Cost and Utilization Project, Nationwide Inpatient Sample, 2004.

Table 6.36: Number and Percent of Population with Musculoskeletal Injuries and Distribution of Persons with Injuries by Age, United States 1996-2004

Year	Total Population (in millions)	Persons with MS Injury		Age Distribution of Persons with MS Injuries			
		# individuals (in millions)	% Total Population	≤18	18-44	45-64	65 & Over
1996-1998	271.2	23.4	8.6%	24.2%	43.4%	19.4%	13.0%
1997-1999	273.7	22.5	8.2%	24.8%	41.8%	20.0%	13.3%
1998-2000	276.1	21.6	7.8%	24.5%	41.8%	21.0%	12.7%
1999-2001	279.7	21.4	7.7%	23.0%	41.8%	22.4%	12.8%
2000-2002	283.6	22.3	7.9%	21.4%	41.8%	23.4%	13.4%
2001-2003	287.7	23.6	8.2%	21.0%	41.1%	24.1%	13.8%
2002-2004	290.8	24.7	8.5%	21.2%	40.2%	24.6%	14.0%

Source: Medical Expenditures Panel Survey (MEPS) 1996 to 2004. Agency for Healthcare Research and Quality, Rockville, MD.

Chapter 7

Congenital and Infantile Developmental Conditions of the Musculoskeletal System

Congenital and infantile developmental conditions of the musculoskeletal system include a variety of defects and range from clinically minor anomalies, such as extra fingers or toes, to more serious and disabling conditions, such as spina bifida. This chapter focuses on musculoskeletal conditions among infants for which population-based surveillance data are available. Although the overall birth prevalence of these conditions is relatively low in comparison to other types of musculoskeletal conditions, due to the seriousness of some of these conditions (e.g., spina bifida, limb deficiencies, skeletal dysplasias, and cerebral palsy), they place a lifetime burden on patients, their families, and the medical community. Further surveillance and research efforts are needed: (1) to gain a better understanding of the magnitude of the public health impact of these conditions, including morbidity, mortality, and health services needs, and of possible disparities in prevalence and outcomes by race/ethnicity, socioeconomic status, and geography; (2) to identify possible causes and factors that may influence health status, development, and level of functioning; and (3) to develop and evaluate potential interventions for prevention.

The primary data sources available on congenital and developmental conditions are the National Birth Defects Prevention Network (NBDPN), from which estimates of prevalence for selected defects are drawn based on state birth defects surveillance programs; the Centers for Disease Control and Prevention (CDC) Metropolitan Atlanta Congenital Defects Program (MACDP), which collects data on birth defects; and the CDC Metropolitan Atlanta Developmental Disabilities Surveillance Program (MADDSP), which monitors the occurrence of selected developmental disabilities in school-age children. Data were analyzed and prepared by the Division of Birth Defects and Developmental Disabilities, Centers for Disease Control and Prevention, Atlanta, Georgia.

Section 7.1: Prevalence of Congenital and Infantile Developmental Conditions of the Musculoskeletal System

Estimated prevalence of selected musculoskeletal conditions at birth using a 95% confidence interval ranges from a low of 1.2 cases per 10,000 births for skeletal dysplasias to 15.5 cases per 10,000 births for polydactyly. (Table 7.1 and Graph 7.1.1) For the few conditions reported by both the national NBDPN and Atlanta based MACDP studies, prevalence is slightly higher in the NBDPN study than found in the MACDP.

Utilizing data from the NBDPN or MACDP and the average number of births in the United States of 4.05 million for the years 1999 to 2003, the estimated number of infants born each year with a congenital musculoskeletal or developmental condition is greater than 17,000 identified for the conditions presented. (Table 7.2) During this time period, there were between 1,030 and 1,500 births with spina bifida without anencephalus, 2,300 and 2,500 with development dysplasia of the hip (DDH), 4,100 with clubfoot without neural tube

Graph 7.1.1: 95% Confidence Intervals around the Estimated Prevalence of Selected Musculoskeletal Congenital and Development Conditions at Birth, United States 1999-2003

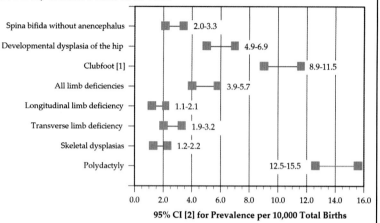

95% CI [2] for Prevalence per 10,000 Total Births

[1] Talipes equinovarus and clubfoot of unspecified type without a neural tube defect
[2] 95% confidence interval (CI) based on Metropolitan Atlanta Congenital Defects Program data, 1999-2003
Correa A, Cragan JD, Kucik JE, et al: Reporting birth defects surveillance data 1968-2003. *Birth Defects Research A Clin Mol Teratol* 2007;79(2):65–186.

defect (NTD), 1,900 with limb deficiencies, 600 with skeletal dysplasias, and 5,600 with polydactyly each year. (Graph 7.1.2)

Congenital musculoskeletal defects show some variation by race and ethnicity. (Table 7.3) Based

Graph 7.1.2: Estimated Number of Infants Born per Year in the United States with Selected Congenital Musculoskeletal Defects, 1999-2003

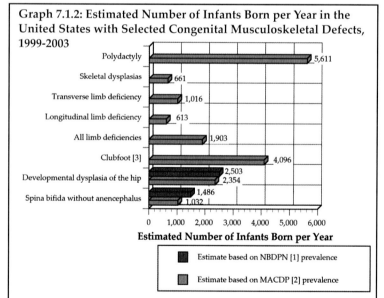

Estimated Number of Infants Born per Year

■ Estimate based on NBDPN [1] prevalence
▨ Estimate based on MACDP [2] prevalence

[1] National Birth Defects Prevention Network
[2] Metropolitan Atlanta Congenital Defects Program
[3] Talipes equinovarus and clubfoot of unspecified type without a neural tube defect
Sources:
(1) National Birth Defects Prevention Network: Birth defects surveillance data from selected states, 1999-2003. *Birth Defects Research A ClinMol Teratol* 2006;76(12):894-960.
(2) Correa A, Cragan JD, Kucik JE, et al: Reporting birth defects surveillance data 1968-2003. *Birth Defects Research A Clin Mol Teratol* 2007;79(2).65–186.

on NBDPN data, the prevalence of spina bifida without anencephalus was highest among Hispanics/Latinos (4.3 per 10,000 total births) and lowest among births of "Other" race or ethnicity (3.2 per 10,000). The prevalence of developmental dysplasia of the hip, or developmental hip dislocation, was highest among whites (7.5 per 10,000) and lowest among blacks/ African Americans (3.0 per 10,000).

Based on MACDP data, the prevalence of spina bifida without anencephalus was also highest among Hispanics/Latinos (5.2 per 10,000 total births) and lowest among Others (0.7 per 10,000). (Table 7.4 and Graph 7.1.3). For developmental dysplasia of the hip, the prevalence was again highest among whites (8.8 per 10,000) and lowest among blacks/African Americans (1.5 per 10,000).

Among those conditions presented only in the MACDP data, the prevalence of clubfoot without NTD and skeletal dysplasia was highest among Whites (12.2 per 10,000 and 2.1 per 10,000, respectively), while both were lowest among Others (8.5 per 10,000 total births and 1.3 per 10,000, respectively.) Polydactyly shows the highest prevalence among Blacks/ African Americans (18.7 per 10,000) and lowest among Whites (10.4 per 10,000). The prevalence of all limb deficiencies varied little by race and ethnicity.

Cerebral palsy (CP), which is reported only in the MADDSP, had a prevalence of 3.1 per 1000 among children aged 8 years in 2000. (Table 7.4) The prevalence of cerebral palsy is slightly higher among blacks/African Americans than among whites (3.6/1000

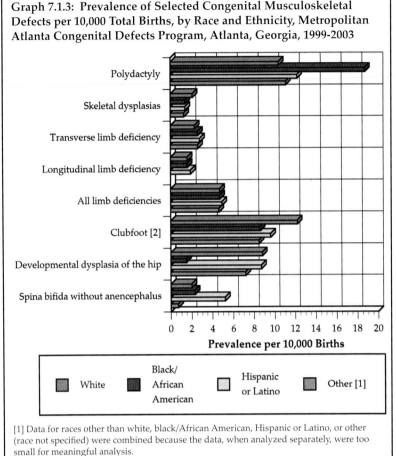

Graph 7.1.3: Prevalence of Selected Congenital Musculoskeletal Defects per 10,000 Total Births, by Race and Ethnicity, Metropolitan Atlanta Congenital Defects Program, Atlanta, Georgia, 1999-2003

Polydactyly
Skeletal dysplasias
Transverse limb deficiency
Longitudinal limb deficiency
All limb deficiencies
Clubfoot [2]
Developmental dysplasia of the hip
Spina bifida without anencephalus

0 2 4 6 8 10 12 14 16 18 20
Prevalence per 10,000 Births

White
Black/African American
Hispanic or Latino
Other [1]

[1] Data for races other than white, black/African American, Hispanic or Latino, or other (race not specified) were combined because the data, when analyzed separately, were too small for meaningful analysis.
[2] Talipes equinovarus and clubfoot of unspecified type without a neural tube defect.
Source: Correa A, Cragan JD, Kucik JE et al: Reporting birth defects surveillance data 1968–2003. *Birth Defects Research A Clin Mol Teratol* 2007;79(2):65–186.

versus 2.9/1000), and among males than females (3.6 per 1000 versus 2.6 per 1000). The majority of children in the study had spastic cerebral palsy (61%) compared with nonspastic CP (5%) and CP not otherwise specified (33%).[1]

Section 7.2: Selected Congenital and Infantile Development Conditions of the Musculoskeletal System

Section 7.2.1: Spina Bifida

Spina bifida consists of a bony defect in the spine through which the cerebrospinal fluid, meninges, nerves, spinal cord, or a combination thereof can herniate. It results from failure of the neural tube to close during the first 28 days after conception

and is classified embryologically as a congenital anomaly of the central nervous system. The most common types of spina bifida are meningocele and myelomeningocele. In meningocele, only the meninges and cerebrospinal fluid herniate through the spinal defect. In myelomeningocele, the nerves, the spinal cord, or both also herniate. The spinal defect in spina bifida can be either covered by normal skin (closed) or in communication with the environment (open). Additional defects of other organs are present in about 20% of infants with spina bifida.[2]

Spina bifida can be diagnosed prenatally through screening for elevated alpha-fetoprotein in maternal serum and prenatal ultrasonography. While many spina bifida defects can be repaired surgically, affected children have lifelong complications such as hydrocephalus, neurologic deficit, bowel and bladder incontinence, and decreased long-term survival.[2,3] A decline in the prevalence of spina bifida since the mid-1970s has been reported in the United States, Europe, Australia, and New Zealand.[4,5] Spina bifida is seen more frequently at birth among females than males, and most frequently among infants of Hispanic or Latino ethnicity, particularly those born in Mexico.[6-10]

In the early 1990s, randomized clinical trials in Great Britain and Hungary demonstrated that consumption of the vitamin folic acid during the periconceptional period (before and during the early weeks of pregnancy) could prevent the recurrence[11] and occurrence[12] of anencephaly and spina bifida. As a result, in 1992, the U.S. Public Health Service recommended that all women of childbearing age who are capable of becoming pregnant consume 4.0 mg of folic acid daily to reduce their risk of having a baby with anencephaly or spina bifida.[13] Subsequently, in 1996, the U.S. Food and Drug Administration established regulations requiring that flour and other enriched grain products be fortified with 140 micrograms of folic acid per 100 grams of grain by January 1, 1998.[14] Since these regulations were implemented, serum and red blood cell folate levels have increased among women of reproductive age in the United States, and declines in the prevalence of anencephaly and spina bifida have been observed.[9,15-18]

Section 7.2.2: Developmental Dysplasia of the Hip

Developmental dysplasia of the hip (DDH) refers to a spectrum of abnormalities that includes an unstable, subluxed, or dislocated hip, or malformed acetabulum. DDH can originate early in gestation as the lower limbs develop, during the second trimester as the hip muscles develop, or late in the third trimester as a result of mechanical forces associated with oligohydramnios or breech presentation. It also can develop in the weeks following delivery or during infancy and childhood. The clinical symptoms of DDH can change and evolve over time. If untreated, persistent subluxation or dislocation can lead to permanent changes in the hip, including a shallow acetabulum, muscle contractures, and constriction of the hip capsule. Newborns and young infants can be treated effectively with a Pavlik harness, while older infants and children can require closed or open surgical reduction.

Diagnosing DDH can be difficult, particularly among newborns. It is usually detected by physical examination, radiography, or ultrasound, although false positives and false negatives occur with all of these methods. Among older infants, limited abduction of the hip is usually the most consistent finding. The

Committee on Quality Improvement, Subcommittee on Developmental Dysplasia of the Hip, American Academy of Pediatrics has developed clinical practice guidelines for pediatric health care providers on the early detection of DDH.[19]

DDH can occur unilaterally or bilaterally. When unilateral, the left side is involved approximately three times more often than the right. DDH is more common among girls, first-born children, and those with a positive family history in a parent or sibling. It can occur as part of a more general neuromuscular disorder or clinical syndrome. However, "typical" hip dislocation occurs among otherwise healthy infants.[19] The prevalence of DDH can differ depending on the age of the child at diagnosis, the type of examination used for screening, the experience of the examiner, and the diagnostic criteria and terminology used.

Section 7.2.3: Clubfoot

Congenital talipes equinovarus (TEV), more commonly referred to as clubfoot, is a common congenital disorder of the lower limb. A clubfoot is fixed in adduction, supination, and varus, that is, the forefoot turned in, the ankle turned inward, and the foot pointed down.[20] True TEV requires active treatment, including casting, manipulation, and sometimes surgery to place the foot in the correct anatomical position.[21] Clubfoot can occur as an isolated finding, as a result of another abnormality such as spina bifida, or as part of a clinical syndrome. The treatment of clubfoot can be particularly challenging if an infant has associated abnormalities.[22]

Isolated TEV occurs almost twice as often among males as in females, regardless of ethnicity.[23] It is bilateral in 50% or more of cases. When unilateral, the right side is involved more frequently than the left.[24] In metropolitan Atlanta, the prevalence of clubfoot not associated with an NTD declined remarkably from 1968 through 2003.[25] Studies have suggested that maternal smoking might be a risk factor for clubfoot, particularly among those with a family history of clubfoot.[26] However, the corresponding decline in smoking over this period probably was not sufficient to fully explain the decline in clubfoot.

Section 7.2.4: Limb Deficiencies

Limb deficiencies, also known as limb reduction defects, are defined by the absence (or severe hypoplasia) of part or all of bony structures of the extremities. The most common type of this defect is a transverse terminal limb deficiency, characterized by the absence of the distal segments of any limb while the proximal segments remain intact. People with transverse digital deficiencies are missing part or all of any phalanx with intact metacarpal or metatarsal bones and proximal segments. The functional consequences of these defects can be considerable when the thumb and multiple fingers are involved. Other categories include preaxial and postaxial deficiencies, often grouped together as longitudinal limb deficiencies, as well as split hand or split foot malformations. The least common category of deficiency is the intercalary type (classic phocomelia), defined by the absence of proximal parts of limbs with distal structures totally or partially present.

Although specific genetic loci for several limb defect syndromes have been identified in recent years, the causes of limb deficiencies currently cannot be easily identified for many affected infants.[27] Certain phenotypes, particularly those involving split hand or split foot, intercalary, radial ray, or postaxial deficiencies, have been associated with single-gene mutations (e.g., the Holt-Oram "heart/hand" syndrome or familial split hand or split foot malformation). Other rare

causes include chromosome abnormalities such as aneuploidies or exposure to known teratogens such as thalidomide and valproic acid. Because chromosomal abnormalities account for a small proportion of limb deficiencies overall, advancing maternal age has not been shown to be a risk factor for these defects.[28] The hypothesis of a vascular pathogenesis for transverse terminal limb deficiencies is supported by animal, epidemiologic, autopsy, and family studies, but often specific vasoactive exposures cannot be identified for individual infants. However, even for the distinctive amniotic band phenotype, there is controversy regarding the intrinsic versus extrinsic nature of limb disruption.[29]

Prenatal ultrasonography has resulted in early identification of a significant proportion of limb deficiencies among countries where this procedure has become routine, but primary prevention of most of these defects has remained elusive.[30] There is some suggestion from limb deficiency case-control studies that periconceptional multivitamin use might be protective for longitudinal or transverse terminal deficiencies,[31,32] and this hypothesis is being further investigated along with studies of gene-environment interactions that might shed light on mechanisms of nutritional protective factors or vasoactive risk factors.

Section 7.2.5: Skeletal Dysplasias

Skeletal dysplasias belong to a heterogeneous group of birth defects. They include over 200 disorders (e.g., chondrodystrophies, osteodystrophies, dwarfisms, and generalized skeletal dysplasias) characterized by abnormalities of cartilage and bone growth resulting in an abnormal shape and size of the skeleton and a disproportion of the long bones, spine, and head.[33] Most of them are genetic conditions. Most fetuses with skeletal dysplasia now can be diagnosed prenatally.[34] However, some skeletal dysplasias do not manifest until short stature and other complications arise during childhood. Skeletal dysplasias differ in inheritance patterns, severity, natural histories, and prognoses. Modes of inheritance include both autosomal and X-linked dominant and recessive forms. Several genetic mutations have been described and associated with skeletal dysplasias.[35,36] Males are primarily affected in X-linked recessive disorders; X-linked dominant disorders can be lethal in males. Severity of skeletal dysplasias ranges from mild forms (nonlethal) to severe (lethal) forms.[37] The most common lethal skeletal dysplasias include thanatophoric dysplasia, achondrogenesis, and osteogenesis imperfecta.[38] Achondroplasia is the most common nonlethal skeletal dysplasia. Prognosis and life expectancy of children with nonlethal skeletal dysplasias depend on the degree of skeletal abnormalities and other associated anomalies.

Treatment is usually supportive. With early intervention from specialists, patients with nonlethal skeletal dysplasias can avoid or minimize the many complications associated with these disorders.[39] Orthopaedic surgery is one of the pillars of treatment to prevent neurologic and orthopaedic complications due to spinal cord compression, joint instability, and long bone deformity. The International Skeletal Dysplasia Registry is a referral center for the diagnosis, management, and the etiology of skeletal dysplasia.[40]

Section 7.2.6: Polydactyly

Polydactyly is a heterogeneous group of anomalies described by excessive partition of the digital rays of the hands and feet that can appear in isolation or in association with other birth defects. Clinically, it generally manifests as an extra digit. It is the most common congenital digital anomaly of the hand and foot. Isolated polydactyly is often autosomal dominant or occasionally sporadic, while polydactyly associated with other major defects can be autosomal recessive.[41] Polydactyly is classified into postaxial and preaxial types. Postaxial polydactyly, the most common type in the United States, typically involves an extra digit on the ulnar or fibular side of the limb. Preaxial polydactyly refers to duplication on the radial or tibial side. Central polydactyly is a term used primarily in clinical settings, usually in the rare situation when syndactyly is associated with duplication of the second, third, or fourth digit.

In general, there is a significant racial predilection for polydactyly. Postaxial polydactyly is more frequent among blacks/African Americans than among whites, and is more frequent among male children.[42] This higher prevalence among African Americans is largely due to a higher prevalence of postaxial skin tags, which generally are not considered to be a major abnormality. Postaxial skin tags in African Americans are not included in the data from MACDP on polydactyly presented in the tables and graphs. Other factors associated with postaxial hand polydactyly in one study included twinning, low maternal education, parental consanguinity, and recurrence in first-degree relatives.[43]

All types of polydactylies are rarely associated with other congenital anomalies. In a recent study, trisomy 13, Meckel syndrome, and Down syndrome accounted for most cases of syndromic polydactyly.[44] Treatment of polydactyly depends greatly on the complexity of the malformation and varies from tying the base of the finger with a suture to complex surgical correction.

Section 7.2.7: Cerebral Palsy

Cerebral palsy (CP) describes a group of permanent disorders of movement and posture that are attributed to nonprogressive disturbances in the developing brain of the fetus or infant. The motor disorders of CP are often accompanied by: (1) disturbances of sensation, perception, cognition, communication, and behavior; (2) epilepsy; and (3) secondary musculoskeletal problems.[45] This definition of CP covers a wide array of clinical presentations and degrees of activity limitation. Traditional classification schemes have focused principally on the distributional patterns of affected limbs (e.g., hemiplegia or diplegia), with an added modifier describing the predominant type of tone or movement abnormality (e.g., spastic or dyskinetic.)[45] The etiology of CP is not fully understood. Factors associated with an increased risk for CP include low birth weight, intrauterine infections, and multiple gestation.[46,47] However, anywhere from 17% to 60% of cases of CP have no known perinatal or neonatal complications.[46]

The prevalence of CP, estimated to occur in slightly over 3 persons in 1,000, has been generally stable for several decades except for a modest increase in recent years. This recent increase in prevalence has been attributed to an increase among very low birth weight infants, which, in turn, has been attributed to their

increased survival resulting from newborn intensive care.[48] CP occurs more frequently in males than in females, and is higher among blacks/African Americans than found in other race or ethnic groups. (Table 7.5 and Graph 7.2.1)

Section 7.3: Birth Defects Surveillance Programs

The National Birth Defects Prevention Network (NBDPN) is composed of state-based birth defects surveillance programs and individuals working in birth defects surveillance, research, and prevention at the local, state, and national levels. NBDPN publishes an annual report of surveillance data from participating programs. In 2006, prevalence data for selected birth defects from 11 states with active case-finding for births in 1999-2003 were published, from which data were pooled to calculate prevalence estimates for spina bifida without anencephaly and developmental dysplasia of the hip (developmental hip dislocation) used in this chapter.[49]

The CDC's Metropolitan Atlanta Congenital Defects Program (MACDP) is a population-based surveillance system for birth defects that was established in 1967. Since that time, the program has conducted ongoing surveillance for birth defects among infants, fetuses, and children born to residents of the five central counties of metropolitan Atlanta through the use of active case-finding methods and multi-source ascertainment.[36] Prevalence data from MACDP are presented for the period 1999-2003 for comparison with prevalence estimates from the NBDPN for the same period. In 2003, there were 51,676 live births to residents of the five counties.

The CDC's Metropolitan Atlanta Developmental Disabilities Program (MADDSP) is a population-based surveillance system that has been monitoring the occurrence of selected developmental disabilities, including cerebral

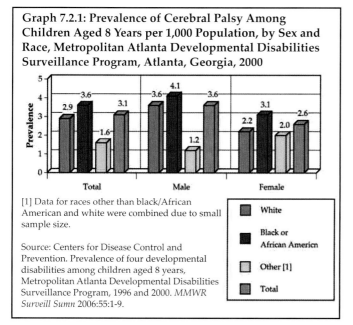

Graph 7.2.1: Prevalence of Cerebral Palsy Among Children Aged 8 Years per 1,000 Population, by Sex and Race, Metropolitan Atlanta Developmental Disabilities Surveillance Program, Atlanta, Georgia, 2000

[1] Data for races other than black/African American and white were combined due to small sample size.

Source: Centers for Disease Control and Prevention. Prevalence of four developmental disabilities among children aged 8 years, Metropolitan Atlanta Developmental Disabilities Surveillance Program, 1996 and 2000. *MMWR Surveill Summ* 2006;55:1-9.

palsy, among school-aged children since 1991 in the same population as MACDP. Prevalence data on CP are presented for children aged 8 years during 2000.[1] In 2000, the population in Metropolitan Atlanta included 43,593 children aged 8 years.

1. Centers for Disease Control and Prevention (CDC): Prevalence of four developmental disabilities among children aged 8 years Metropolitan Atlanta Developmental Disabilities Surveillance Program, 1996 and 2000. *MMWR Surveill Summ*;2006;55:1-9.

2. Botto LD, Moore CA, Khoury MJ, et al: Neural-tube defects. *N Engl J Med* 1999;341:1509-1519.

3. Wong LC, Paulozzi LJ: Survival of infants with spina bifida: A population study, 1979-1994. *Paediatr Perinat Epidemiol* 2001;15:374-378.

4. Elwood JM, Little J, Elwood JH: *Epidemiology and Control of Neural Tube Defects*. New York, NY: Oxford University Press, 1992.

5. Yen IH, Khoury MJ, Erickson JD, et al: The changing epidemiology of neural tube defects, United States, 1968-1989. *Am J Dis Child* 1992;146:857-861.

6. Canfield MA, Annegers JF, Brender JD, et al: Hispanic origin and neural tube defects in Houston/Harris County, Texas: II. Risk factors. *Am J Epidemiol* 1996;143:12-24.

7. Khoury M, Erickson JD, James LM: Etiologic heterogeneity of neural tube defects: Clues from epidemiology. *Am J Epidemiol* 1982;115:538-548.

8. Shaw GM, Velie EM, Wasserman CR: Risk for neural tube defect-affected pregnancies among women of Mexican descent and white women in California. *Am J Public Health* 1997;87:1467-1471.

9. Williams LJ, Rasmussen SA, Flores A, et al: Decline in the prevalence of spina bifida and anencephaly by race/ethnicity: 1995-2002. *Pediatrics* 2005;116:580-586.

10. Canfield MA, Honein MA, Yuskiv N, et al: National estimates and race/ethnic-specific variations of selected birth defects in the United States, 1991-2001. *Birth Defects Research A Clin Mol Teratol* 2006;76:747-756.

11. MRC Vitamin Study Research Group: Prevention of neural tube defects: results of the Medical Research Council Vitamin Study. *Lancet* 1991;338:131-137.

12. Czeizel AE, Dudas I: Prevention of the first occurrence of neural-tube defects by periconceptional vitamin supplementation. *N Engl J Med* 1992;327:1832-1835.

13. Centers for Disease Control and Prevention (CDC): Recommendations for the use of folic acid to reduce the number of cases of spina bifida and other neural tube defects. *MMWR Recomm Rep* 1992;41:1-7.

14. U.S. Food and Drug Administration: Food standards: amendment of standards of identity for enriched grain products to require addition of folic acid. *Fed Regist* 1996;61:8781-8797.

15. Centers for Disease Control and Prevention (CDC): Foliate status in women of childbearing age, by race/ethnicity, United States, 1999-2000. *MMWR Morb Mortal Wkly Rep* 2002;51:808-810.

16. Honein MA, Paulozzi LJ, Mathews TJ, et al: Impact of folic acid fortification of the US food supply on the occurrence of neural tube defects. *JAMA* 2001;285:2981-2986.

17. Honein MA, Paulozzi LJ, Mathews TJ, et al: Erratum on: impact of folic acid fortification of the US food supply on the occurrence of neural tube defects. *JAMA* 2001;286:2236.

18. Williams LJ, Mai CT, Edmonds LD, et al: Prevalence of spina bifida and anencephaly during the transition to mandatory folic acid fortification in the United States. *Teratology* 2002;66:33-39.

19. Committee on Quality Improvement, Subcommittee on Developmental Dysplasia of the Hip, American Academy of Pediatrics: Clinical practice guidelines: early detection of developmental dysplasia of the hip. *Pediatrics* 2000;105:896-905.

20. Miedzybrodzka Z: Congenital talipes equinovarus (clubfoot): a disorder of the foot but not hand. *J Anat* 2003;202:37-42.

21. Dietz F: The genetics of idiopathic clubfoot. *Clin Orthop Relat Res* 2002;401:39-48.

22. Cummings RJ, Davidson RS, Armstrong PF, et al: Congenital clubfoot. *J Bone Joint Surg Am* 2002;84:290-308.

23. Lochmiller C, Johnston D, Scott A, et al: Genetic epidemiology of idiopathic talipes equinovarus. *Am J Med Genet* 1998;79:90-96.

24. Paulozzi LJ, Lary JM: Laterality patterns in infants with external birth defects. *Teratology* 1999;60:265-271.

25. Correa A, Cragan JD, Kucik JE, et al: Reporting birth defects surveillance data 1968-2003. *Birth Defects Research A Clin Mol Teratol* 2007;79:65-186.

26. Honein MA, Paulozzi LJ, Moore CA: Family history, maternal smoking, and clubfoot: An indication of a gene-environment interaction. *Am J Epidemiol* 2000;152:658-665.

27. McGuirk CK, Westgate MN, Holmes LB: Limb deficiencies in newborn infants. *Pediatrics* 2001;108:E64.

28. Reefhuis J, Honein MA: Maternal age and non-chromosomal birth defects, Atlanta, 1968-2000. *Birth Defects Research A Clin Mol Teratol* 2004;70:572-579.

29. Orioli IM, Ribeiro MG, Castilla EE: Clinical and epidemiological studies of amniotic deformity, adhesion, and mutilation (ADAM) sequence in a South American (ECLAMC) population. *Am J Med Genet* 2003;118:135-145.

30. Stoll C, Wiesel A, Queisser-Luft A, et al: Evaluation of the prenatal diagnosis of limb reduction deficiencies: EUROSCAN Study Group. *Prenat Diagn* 2000;20:811-818.

31. Shaw GM, O'Malley CD, Wasserman CR, et al: Maternal periconceptional use of multivitamins and reduced risk for conotruncal heart defects and limb deficiencies among offspring. *Am J Med Genet* 1995;59:536-545.

32. Yang Q, Khoury MJ, Olney RS, et al: Does periconceptional multivitamin use reduce the risk for limb deficiency in offspring? *Epidemiology* 1997;8:157-161.

33. Romero R, Athanassiadis AP, Jeanty P: Fetal skeletal anomalies. *Radiol Clin North Am* 1990;28:75-99.

34. Mortier G: The diagnosis of skeletal dysplasias: A multidisciplinary approach. *Eur J Radiol* 2001;40:161-167.

35. Baitner AC, Maurer SG, Gruen MB, et al: The genetic basis of the osteochondrodysplasias. *Journal of Pediatric Orthopaedics* 2000;20:594-605.

36. Superti-Furga A, Bonafe L, Rimoin DL: Molecular-pathogenetic classification of genetic disorders of the skeleton. *Am J Med Genet* 2001;106:282-293.

37. Azouz EM, Teebi AS, Eydoux P, et al: Bone dysplasias: an introduction. *Can Assoc Radiol J* 1998;49:105-109.

38. Lemyre E, Azouz EM, Teebi AS, et al: Bone dysplasia series. Achondroplasia, hypochondroplasia and thanatophoric dysplasia: review and update. *Can Assoc Radiol J* 1999;50:185-197.

39. Hurst JA, Firth HV, Smithson S: Skeletal dysplasias. *Semin Fetal Neonatal Med* 2005;10:233-241.

40. International Skeletal Dysplasia Registry, Cedars-Sinai Medical Center. Available at: http://www.csmc.edu/9934.html. Accessed October 12, 2007.

41. Hosalkar HS, Shah H, Gujar P, et al: Crossed polydactyly. *J Postgrad Med* 1999;45:90-92.

42. Finley WH, Gustavson KH, Hall TM, et al: Birth defects surveillance: Jefferson County, Alabama, and Uppsala County, Sweden. *South Med J* 1994;87:440-445.

43. Castilla EE, da Graca Dutra M, Lugarinho da Fonseca R, et al: Hand and foot postaxial polydactyly: Two different traits. *Am J Med Genet* 1997;73:48-54.

44. Castilla EE, Lugarinho R, da Graca Dutra M, et al: Associated anomalies in individuals with polydactyly. *Am J Med Genet* 1998;80:459-465.

45. Rosenbaum P, Panet N, Leviton A, et al: A report: the definition and classification of cerebral palsy. *Dev Med Child Neurol Suppl* 2007;49:8-14.

46. Davis D: Review of cerebral palsy, part I: description, incidence, and etiology. *Neonatal Netw* 1997;16:7-12.

47. Odding E, Roebroeck ME, Stam HJ: The epidemiology of cerebral palsy: incidence, impairments, and risk factors. *Disabil Rehabil* 2006;28:183-191.

48. Paneth N, Hong T, Korzeniewski S: The descriptive epidemiology of cerebral palsy. *Clinical Perinatology* 2006;33:251-267.

49. National Birth Defects Prevention Network: Birth defects surveillance data from selected states, 1999-2003. *Birth Defects Research A Clin Mol Teratol* 2006;76:894-960

Section 7.4: Congenital and Infantile Developmental Conditions of the Musculoskeletal System Data Tables

Table 7.1: Estimated Prevalence of Selected Congenital Musculoskeletal Defects, National Birth Defects Prevention Network and Metropolitan Atlanta Congenital Defects Program, 1999-2003

Musculoskeletal Defect	NBDPN [1] 1999-2003		MACDP [2] 1999-2003	
	Prevalence per 10,000 Total Births	95% CI [3]	Prevalence per 10,000 Total Births	95% CI [3]
Spina Bifida without Anencephalus	3.7	3.5 – 3.9	2.6	2.0 - 3.3
Developmental Dysplasia of the Hip	6.2	5.9 – 6.4	5.8	4.9 - 6.9
Clubfoot [4]			10.2	8.9 - 11.5
All Limb Deficiencies			4.7	3.9 - 5.7
Longitudinal Limb Deficiency			1.5	1.1 -2.1
Transverse Limb Deficiency			2.5	1.9 -3.2
Skeletal Dysplasias			1.6	1.2 -2.2
Polydactyly			13.9	12.5 -15.5

[1] National Birth Defects Prevention Network

[2] Metropolitan Atlanta Congenital Defects Program

[3] Confidence interval

[4] Talipes equinovarus and clubfoot of unspecified type without a neural tube defect

Source 1: National Birth Defects Prevention Network: Birth defects surveillance data from selected states, 1999-2003. *Birth Defects Research A Clin Mol Teratol* 2006;76(12):894-960.

Source 2: Correa A, Cragan JD, Kucik JE, et al: Reporting birth defects surveillance data 1968-2003. *Birth Defects Research A Clin Mol Teratol* 2007;79(2):65-186.

Table 7.2: Estimated Number of Infants Born per Year in the United States with Selected Congenital Musculoskeletal Defects, 1999 -2003

Musculoskeletal Defect	Estimate Based on NBDPN [1] Prevalence	95% CI [2]	Estimate Based on MACDP [3] Prevalence	95% CI [2]
Spina Bifida without Anencephalus	1,486	1,411 – 1,564	1,032	970 – 1,097
Developmental Dysplasia of the Hip	2,503	2,406 – 2,603	2,354	2,260 – 2,451
Clubfoot [4]			4,096	3,971 – 4,223
All limb Deficiencies			1,903	1,818 – 1,990
Longitudinal Limb Deficiency			613	565 – 663
Transverse Limb Deficiency			1,016	954 – 1,080
Skeletal Dysplasias			661	612 – 713
Polydactyly			5,611	5,466 – 5,760

[1] National Birth Defects Prevention Network

[2] Confidence interval

[3] Metropolitan Atlanta Congenital Defects Program

[4] Talipes equinovarus and clubfoot of unspecified type without a neural tube defect

Source 1: National Birth Defects Prevention Network:Birth defects surveillance data from selected states, 1999-2003. *Birth Defects Research A Clin Mol Teratol* 2006;76(12):894-960.

Source 2: Correa A, Cragan JD, Kucik JE, et al: Reporting birth defects surveillance data 1968-2003. *Birth Defects Research A Clin Mol Teratol* 2007;79(2):65–186.

Table 7.3: Prevalence of Selected Congenital and Infantile Developmental Musculoskeletal Defects per 10,000 Total Births, by Race and Ethnicity, National Birth Defects Prevention Network, 11 States With Active Surveillance Systems, 1999-2003

Musculoskeletal Defect	White Prevalence	White 95% CI [2]	Black/African American Prevalence	Black/African American 95% CI [2]	Hispanic or Latino Prevalence	Hispanic or Latino 95% CI [2]	Other [1] Prevalence	Other [1] 95% CI [2]
Spina Bifida without Anencephalus [3]	3.4	3.2 - 3.7	3.4	2.9 - 3.9	4.3	4.0 - 4.7	3.2	2.6 -4.0
Developmental Dysplasia of the Hip (developmental hip dislocation) [4]	7.5	7.1 - 7.9	3.0	2.6 - 3.5	5.9	5.4 - 6.4	5.5	4.5 -6.6

[1] Data for races other than white, black/African American, Hispanic or Latino were combined due to small sample size.

[2] Confidence interval

[3] Prevalence estimates based on pooled data from 11 states with active case finding during this time period: Alabama, Arkansas, California, Georgia, Hawaii, Iowa, Massachusetts, North Carolina, Oklahoma, Texas, and Utah.

[4] Prevalence estimates based on pooled data from 8 states with active case finding during this time period: Alabama, Arkansas, Georgia, Hawaii, Iowa, North Carolina, Oklahoma, and Texas.

Source: National Birth Defects Prevention Network: Birth defects surveillance data from selected states, 1999-2003. *Birth Defects Research A Clin Mol Teratol* 2006;76(12):894-960.

Table 7.4: Prevalence of Selected Congenital Musculoskeletal Defects per 10,000 Total Births, by Race and Ethnicity Metropolitan Atlanta Congenital Defects Program, Atlanta, Georgia, 1999-2003

Musculoskeletal Defect	White Prevalence	95% CI [2]	Black/African American Prevalence	95% CI [2]	Hispanic or Latino Prevalence	95% CI [2]	Other [1] Prevalence	95% CI [2]
Spina Bifida without Anencephalus	2.0	1.2 – 3.1	2.3	1.4 – 3.5	5.2	3.2 – 7.8	0.7	0.0 – 3.6
Developmental Dysplasia of the Hip	8.8	7.0 – 10.9	1.5	0.8 – 2.4	8.7	6.1 – 12.0	7.2	3.6 – 12.9
Clubfoot [3]	12.2	10.1 – 14.7	8.6	6.9 – 10.7	9.6	6.9 – 13.1	8.5	4.5 – 14.6
All Limb Defiencies	4.7	3.4 – 6.3	4.7	3.4 – 6.3	4.9	3.1 – 7.6	4.6	1.8 – 9.4
Longitudinal Limb Deficiency	1.6	0.9 – 2.6	1.6	0.9 – 2.6	1.9	0.8 – 3.7	-	-
Transverse Limb Deficiency	2.3	1.4 – 3.5	2.6	1.7 – 3.8	2.8	1.5 – 4.9	2.6	0.7 – 6.7
Skeletal Dysplasias	2.1	1.3 – 3.2	1.4	0.7 – 2.3	1.4	0.5 – 3.1	1.3	0.2 – 4.7
Polydactyly	10.4	8.4 – 12.6	18.7	16.1 – 21.6	12.2	9.1 – 16.0	11.1	6.5 – 17.8

[1] Data for races other than white, black /African American, Hispanic or Latino were combined due to small sample size.

[2] Confidence interval

[3] Talipes equinovarus and clubfoot of unspecified type without a neural tube defect.

Source: Correa A, Cragan JD, Kucik JE et al: Reporting birth defects surveillance data 1968–2003. *Birth Defects Research A Clin Mol Teratol* 2007;79(2):65–186.

Table 7.5: Prevalence of Cerebral Palsy Among Children Aged 8 Years per 1,000 Population, by Sex and Race, Metropolitan Atlanta Developmental Disabilities Surveillance Program, Atlanta, Georgia, 2000

	Number	Prevalence	95% CI [1]
MALE			
White	33	3.6	2.6 – 5.1
Black/African American	40	4.1	3.0 – 5.6
Other [2]	4	1.2	0.5 – 3.3
Total	79	3.6	2.9 – 4.5
FEMALE			
White	20	2.2	1.4 – 3.5
Black/African American	30	3.1	2.2 – 4.5
Other [2]	6	2.0	0.9 – 4.4
Total	56	2.6	2.0 – 3.4
TOTAL			
White	53	2.9	2.2 – 3.8
Black or African American	70	3.6	2.9 – 4.6
Other [2]	10	1.6	0.9 – 3.0
TOTAL [3]	135	3.1	2.6 – 3.7

[1] Confidence interval.

[2] Data for races other than white black/African American were combined due to small sample size.

[3] Total includes two children whose race was not indicated.

Source: Centers for Disease Control and Prevention. Prevalence of four developmental disabilities among children aged 8 years, Metropolitan Atlanta Developmental Disabilities Surveillance Program, 1996 and 2000. *MMWR Surveill Summ*;2006:55:1-9.

Chapter 8

Neoplasms of Bone and Connective Tissue

Bone and connective tissue neoplasms are rare when compared with other cancers and with other musculoskeletal conditions, accounting for about 1.5% of annual cancer cases between 2000 and 2004. However, it is estimated that in 2007, 2,370 persons will be diagnosed with cancer of the bones and joints, with more than one in four diagnoses for children and youth under the age of 20. Myeloma, a malignant tumor of the bone marrow, will be diagnosed in 19,900 persons.[1] In addition, 1,330 persons will die of cancer of the bone and joints, while 10,790 will die of myeloma in 2007.

Data from the Surveillance Epidemiology and End Results (SEER) program of the National Cancer Institute, used to present the burden of bone and connective tissue neoplasms, is the most comprehensive source of information on cancer incidence, prevalence, mortality, survival, and lifetime risks. Data is currently available from 1974 to 2004. The SEER program is one of the most comprehensive sources of neoplasm data; it is based on data representing approximately 10% of the U.S. population. In addition, data from the American College of Surgeons' Commission on Cancer National Cancer Data Base (NCDB) was utilized in the analysis of the three main bone sarcomas: osteosarcoma, chondrosarcoma and Ewing's sarcoma. This database is maintained by the American College of Surgeons and contains the same standardized data as that collected by the SEER database. Data are collected from all institutions wishing to be accredited by the American College of Surgeons Commission on Cancer. Each accredited institution is required to report all patients with cancer treated at their institution, including annual follow-up data. Site visits and interaction between American College of Surgeons cancer database personnel and the local reporting institutions verifies a minimum of 90% case capture and reporting for each institution. Multiple internal checks verify the data accuracy. It is estimated the approximately 1,700 reporting institutions each year treat approximately 75% of all patients with malignancies in the United States.

Section 8.1: Incidence of Neoplasms of Bone and Connective Tissue

Musculoskeletal cancers are classified into bone and joint cancers and myeloma. The three most common classifications of cancers of bones and joints are osteosarcoma, Ewing's sarcoma, and chondrosarcoma. The ages at which these cancers are most prevalent vary. *Osteosarcoma*, a malignant bone tissue tumor, is the most common, occurring most frequently in teens and young adults. *Ewing's sarcoma*, a tumor often located in the shaft of long bones and in the pelvic bones, occurs most frequently in children and youth. *Chondrosarcoma*, a sarcoma of malignant cartilage cells, most likely occurs as a secondary cancer by malignant degeneration of pre-existing cartilage cells within bone, including chondromas (a benign tumor), and is primarily found among older adults. However, the vast majority of chondromas never undergo malignant change and, therefore, the routine resection of benign chondromas is unwarranted. Of these three, Ewing's sarcoma is generally considered to have the worst prognosis. By definition, all cases of Ewing's sarcoma are high grade, the most aggressive category of cancer, with full potential to metastasize and bring about death.

Approximately 6% to 20% of osteosarcomas are of lower grade; chondrosarcoma has a higher proportion of low grade cases than the other two bone and joint cancers.

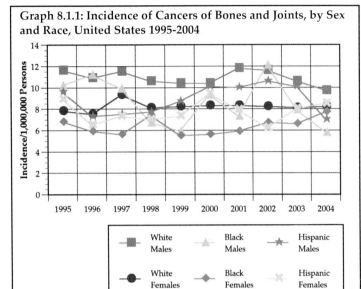

Graph 8.1.1: Incidence of Cancers of Bones and Joints, by Sex and Race, United States 1995-2004

Source: Ries LAG, Harkins D, Krapcho M, et al (eds): *SEER Cancer Statistics Review, 1975-2003, Overview.* Bethesda, MD: National Cancer Institute, 2006. Available at http://seer.cancer.gov/csr/1975_2003/. Accessed June 19, 2007.

Bone cancers are found more frequently in males than females, and more frequently among whites than those of any other race. (Table 8.1 and Graph 8.1.1) The average annual incidence of bone cancers between 2000 and 2004 was 9 in one million persons; the rate among all males was 10 in one million, while among all females it was 8 in one million. Among white males, the overall incidence jumped to 11 in one million persons. The incidence of cancer of the bones and joints in the United States is comparable to several site-specific oral cancers (i.e., lip, salivary gland, floor of the mouth), cancers of the bile duct, cancers of the eye, and Kaposi's sarcoma, which affects the skin and mucous membranes and is often associated with immunodeficient individuals with AIDS.

Myeloma, a malignant primary tumor of the bone marrow that can form in any of the

bone-marrow cells and usually involves multiple bones at the same time, occurs five to six times as frequently as bone cancers. It occurs most frequently in adults between the ages of 50 and 70. The average annual incidence of myeloma between 2000 and 2004 was 56 cases in one million persons. (Table 8.2 and Graph 8.1.2) Again, males have a higher incidence of myeloma than do females, with an average of 70 cases in one million males to 45 cases in one million females. The incidence of myeloma in the United States is comparable to esophageal, liver, cervical, ovarian, brain, and lymphocytic leukemia cancers.

The isolated single bone version of myeloma is called plasmacytoma, but virtually all cases of isolated plasmacytoma develop into full-fledged multiple myeloma over the subsequent 5 to 10 years after diagnosis.

Although annual rates of cancers of the bones and joints and myeloma vary somewhat, the overall incidence has remained relatively constant since the mid-1970s.[2]

With a median age of 39 years at time of diagnosis, cancers of the bones and joints attack

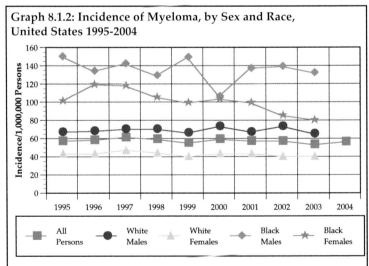

Graph 8.1.2: Incidence of Myeloma, by Sex and Race, United States 1995-2004

Source: Ries LAG, Harkins D, Krapcho M, et al (eds): *SEER Cancer Statistics Review, 1975-2003, Overview.* Bethesda, MD: National Cancer Institute, 2006. Available at http://seer.cancer.gov/csr/1975_2003/. Accessed June 19, 2007.

younger patients than most other broad categories of cancer. (Table 8.3) Males are typically diagnosed with bone cancers 5 years earlier than females. Myeloma, on the other hand, is primarily a cancer found among elderly persons, with a median age of 70 at the time of diagnosis. Again, males are typically diagnosed with myeloma at ages several years younger than females.

Section 8.2: Mortality and Survival Rates for Neoplasms of Bones and Connective Tissue

Annual population-based mortality rates due to cancers of bones and joints are low, averaging four deaths per one million persons per year between 2000 and 2004. Over the past 35 years, the mortality rate from bone and joint cancer dropped by approximately 50% from that of the late 1970s.[1] However, there has been no significant improvement over the past 20 years.[3] Males have a higher mortality rate than females for all races. The overall 5-year survival rate is 54% for osteosarcoma, 75% for chondrosarcoma, and 51% for Ewing's sarcoma. The osteosarcoma survival rate varies with age: 5-year survival was 60% for persons under 30 years of age, 50% for those aged 30 to 49, and 30% for those 50 years old and older.[3]

The overall 5-year relative survival rate for bone and joint cancers is 68%, and is comparable to a number of more common cancers such as lymphoma, urinary, cervical/ovarian, and soft tissue cancers. (Table 8.4 and Graph 8.2.1) The annual population-based mortality rate of myeloma was an average of 37 persons per one million population between 2000 and 2004.[1] The mortality rate from myeloma has remained relatively constant since the mid-1970s.[1] The 5-year survival rate for myeloma, 34%, is one of the lowest for all cancers.

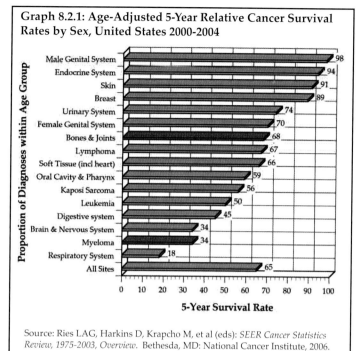

Graph 8.2.1: Age-Adjusted 5-Year Relative Cancer Survival Rates by Sex, United States 2000-2004

Source: Ries LAG, Harkins D, Krapcho M, et al (eds): *SEER Cancer Statistics Review, 1975-2003, Overview.* Bethesda, MD: National Cancer Institute, 2006. Available at http://seer.cancer.gov/csr/1975_2003/. Accessed June 19, 2007.

Section 8.3: Bone and Joint Cancer Among Children and Young Adults

While myeloma is primarily a cancer of middle aged to older adults, cancers of bones and joints are found among persons under the age of 30 in higher proportion than expected for the overall incidence. In 2000-2003, 45% of bone and joint cancers were diagnosed in persons under the age of 35, with 28% occurring among children and adolescents under the age of 20. This compares to less than 4% of all cancer sites in persons aged 35 and younger, and only 1% in those younger than 20 years. (Table 8.5 and Graph 8.3.1)

Deaths from bone and joint cancer follow a similar pattern. (Table 8.6 and Graph 8.3.2) Between 2000 and 2003, 15% of deaths from bone and joint cancer occurred in children and youth under the age of 20, and an additional 14% among young adults aged 20 to 34. The mortality rate among younger persons from bone and joint cancer comprises 1.3% of deaths from all types of cancer. The relative proportion of deaths from

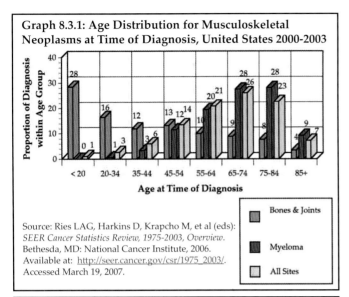

Graph 8.3.1: Age Distribution for Musculoskeletal Neoplasms at Time of Diagnosis, United States 2000-2003

Source: Ries LAG, Harkins D, Krapcho M, et al (eds): *SEER Cancer Statistics Review, 1975-2003, Overview.* Bethesda, MD: National Cancer Institute, 2006. Available at: http://seer.cancer.gov/csr/1975_2003/. Accessed March 19, 2007.

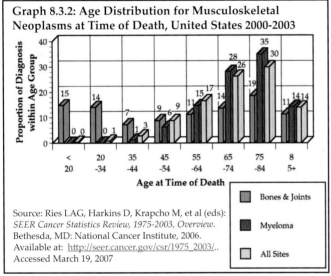

Graph 8.3.2: Age Distribution for Musculoskeletal Neoplasms at Time of Death, United States 2000-2003

Source: Ries LAG, Harkins D, Krapcho M, et al (eds): *SEER Cancer Statistics Review, 1975-2003, Overview.* Bethesda, MD: National Cancer Institute, 2006. Available at: http://seer.cancer.gov/csr/1975_2003/.. Accessed March 19, 2007

bone and joint cancer was higher in children, youth, and young adults than all other cancer types that disproportionately affect younger people, including brain and nervous system, leukemia and soft tissue cancers.

During the same time period, 2000-2003, osteosarcoma accounted for 59% of the malignant bone tumors diagnosed in persons under the age of 20, with 46% of osteosarcoma diagnoses occurring in persons younger than 20 years of age. The majority of the remaining tumors in the age 20 and under group were Ewing's sarcoma (31%), accounting for 66% of Ewing's sarcoma diagnoses. In the young adult population (age 20

to 34 years) diagnosed with malignant bone tumors, chondrosarcoma accounted for 37% and osteosarcoma for 36%, Ewing's sarcoma was diagnosed 17% of the time; this represented 16%, 17%, and 21% of all diagnoses for these tumors, respectively. (Table 8.7 and Graph 8.3.3)

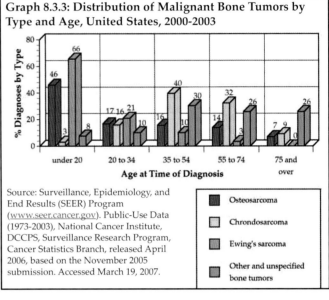

Graph 8.3.3: Distribution of Malignant Bone Tumors by Type and Age, United States, 2000-2003

Source: Surveillance, Epidemiology, and End Results (SEER) Program (www.seer.cancer.gov). Public-Use Data (1973-2003), National Cancer Institute, DCCPS, Surveillance Research Program, Cancer Statistics Branch, released April 2006, based on the November 2005 submission. Accessed March 19, 2007.

The overall incidence of malignant bone tumors from 1975 to 2000 in persons under the age of 30 peaked between the ages of 15-19 years and 10-14 years at 14.8 and 13.1 per million persons, respectively. The incidence of osteosarcoma peaks in these ages at 8.2 and 7.6 per million, respectively, while Ewing's sarcoma peaks at 4.6 and 4.3, respectively. (Graph 8.3.4)

The high incidence and mortality rate of bone cancers among children, youth and young adults creates a significant burden on the productivity and life of future generations. Apart from the financial costs, emotional toil, and lost lives from the initial treatments, survivors carry significant functional burdens and continuing care costs. At least 75% of surviving bone and joint cancer patients are treated with limb salvaging surgery. These surgeries most often require implantation of massive bone-replacing endoprostheses that have limited life span and compromised function, requiring periodic surveillance and revision

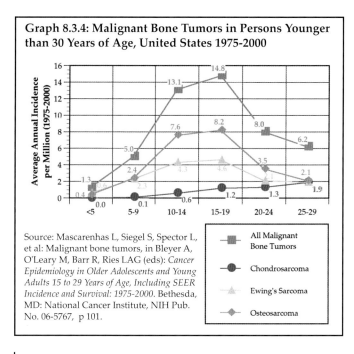

Graph 8.3.4: Malignant Bone Tumors in Persons Younger than 30 Years of Age, United States 1975-2000

Source: Mascarenhas L, Siegel S, Spector L, et al: Malignant bone tumors, in Bleyer A, O'Leary M, Barr R, Ries LAG (eds): *Cancer Epidemiology in Older Adolescents and Young Adults 15 to 29 Years of Age, Including SEER Incidence and Survival: 1975-2000.* Bethesda, MD: National Cancer Institute, NIH Pub. No. 06-5767, p 101.

surgery to repair or replace worn parts. The amputated survivors will require prosthetic limbs, the function of which is clearly limiting in comparison to normal activity. Both procedures are expensive, with cost estimates of $25,000 per year for replacement of an amputated limb in an active 20- to 30-year-old man in 1997 dollars, and estimates of $23,500 for implant, rehabilitation, monitoring, and replacement with limb salvaging endoprothesis.[4] Due to chronic pain and overall dysfunction, a large number of such survivors will end up on disability, requiring public support for the majority of their adult lifetime.

Section 8.4: Economic Cost of Malignant Bone Tumors

Information on insurance coverage at time of treatment was only available for roughly one-third of patients (8,342) and the patterns of coverage were similar between osteosarcoma and Ewing's sarcoma. For chondrosarcoma, due to the older mean age of the patients, relatively more patients were covered by Medicare (8.6%) or Medicare with supplement (16.7%). At the time of diagnosis, insurance coverage was most

commonly through managed care (38.5%) for all groups. Private insurance was the next most common recorded insurance coverage (27.4%), followed by Medicare with supplement (10%), although the majority of those patients had chondrosarcoma. Only 0.3% of patients overall were covered by Medicaid.

Section 8.5: Soft Tissue Sarcomas

Soft tissue sarcomas are malignant (cancerous) tumors that develop in any part of the body, including fat, muscle, nerve, fibrous tissues surrounding joints, blood vessel, or deep skin tissues. Approximately 55% to 60% of sarcomas develop in the arms or legs; the rest begin in the trunk (15% to 20%), head and neck area (8% to 10%), internal organs, or the retroperitoneum or back of the abdominal cavity (15%).[5]

In terms of case numbers, the musculoskeletal health burden in the United States from soft tissue sarcomas is two to three times greater than that of bone and joint sarcomas. Soft tissue sarcomas come in a wide variety of forms which affect different age groups, but the most frequently encountered soft tissue sarcomas affect older adults.

As previously noted, the National Cancer Data Base (NCDB), a joint program of the Commission on Cancer and the American College of Surgeons, maintains the most thorough database on the prevalence of soft tissue sarcomas. Although the NCDB was not created to serve as an incidence-based registry currently gathers data on approximately 75% of the cancers treated in the United States. It should be noted this percentage varies from year to year based on the participation and reporting by hospitals to this voluntary database.

Over the past 20 years, 86,355 soft tissue sarcomas of the extremities, shoulders and pelvic girdles and trunk have been treated. This number excludes approximately 32,250 soft tissue sarcomas of the head and neck, thoracic, and abdominal areas; these patients are generally cared for by non-musculoskeletal specialists. Using a 20-year average and assuming 75% of annual cases are included in NCDB, over 5,700 cases of soft tissue sarcoma have been reported annually.

In the 5 years between 2000-2004, soft tissue sarcomas, including those of the head, neck, thoracic, and abdominal areas, averaged 8,700 cases per year, and represented approximately 0.7% of all cancer cases.[6] This compares to an average of 2,700 cases of bone and joint sarcomas, (0.2% of all cancer cases.) (Table 8.8)

In 2007, it is expected about 9,220 new soft tissue sarcomas will have been diagnosed in the United States. Of these, 5,050 cases will be diagnosed in males, and 4,710 cases will be diagnosed in females. During 2007, it is expected 3,560 Americans (1,840 males and 1,720 females) will die of soft tissue sarcomas. These statistics include both adults and children.[7]

Section 8.5.1: Soft Tissue Sarcoma Survival Rates

For high-grade soft tissue sarcomas, the most important prognostic factor is the stage at which the tumor is identified. Staging criteria for soft tissue sarcomas are primarily determined by whether the tumor has metastasized or spread elsewhere in the body. Size is highly correlated with risk of metastasis and survival. In general, the prognosis for a soft tissue sarcoma is poorer if the sarcoma is large. As a general rule, high-grade soft tissue sarcomas over 10 centimeters in diameter have an approximate 50% mortality rate and those over 15 centimeters in diameter have an approximate 75% mortality rate.

The National Cancer Institute (NCI) has reported the overall 5-year relative survival of people with sarcomas is approximately 66%. The NCI statistics staging classification of sarcomas is (1) confined to the primary site (localized—54% of sarcomas are diagnosed at this stage), (2) spread to regional lymph nodes or directly beyond the primary site (regional—22%), or (3) metastasized (distant—15%). For the remaining cases, the staging information was unknown. The corresponding 5-year relative survival rates reported are 84% for localized sarcomas; 62% for regional stage sarcomas; 16% for sarcomas with distant spread; and 54% for unstaged sarcomas. The 10-year relative survival rate is only slightly worse for these stages, meaning that most people who survive 5 years are cured.[8]

Using the staging criteria of soft tissue sarcomas of the American Joint Committee on Cancer (AJCC) produces similar results for sarcomas found in the limbs (arms or legs): 90% 5-year survival rate for stage 1 sarcomas; 81% for stage 2; and 56% for stage 3. Sarcomas identified as stage 4 have a very low 5-year survival rate. Sarcomas located in other than a limb also have lower survival rates.[8]

Comparing soft tissue sarcomas by stage to the most common types of cancer shows a relatively high proportion of cases that are not identified until stage 3 or stage 4. (Table 8.8 and Graph 8.5.1)

Section 8.5.2: Types of Soft Tissue Sarcoma

There are multiple soft tissue sarcomas with varying degrees of aggressive behavior (Table 8.9), but virtually all have the capacity to metastasize and cause death. Treatment for high-grade soft tissue sarcomas is typically resection (removal) and radiation. Chemotherapy is playing an ever-increasing role, especially in high-grade and metastatic cases.

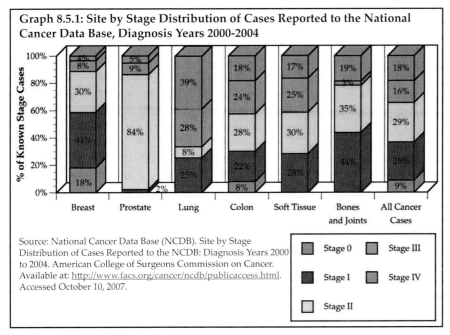

Graph 8.5.1: Site by Stage Distribution of Cases Reported to the National Cancer Data Base, Diagnosis Years 2000-2004

Source: National Cancer Data Base (NCDB). Site by Stage Distribution of Cases Reported to the NCDB: Diagnosis Years 2000 to 2004. American College of Surgeons Commission on Cancer. Available at: http://www.facs.org/cancer/ncdb/publicaccess.html. Accessed October 10, 2007.

The most commonly encountered soft tissue sarcoma is malignant fibrous histiocytoma, a tumor of the fibrous tissue most often occurring in the arms or legs. The least differentiated of the sarcomas, in many cases it represents a poorly defined, high-grade soft tissue sarcoma that cannot be further defined pathologically (histologically). A recent trend is to classify these poorly differentiated sarcomas as pleomorphic or spindle cell sarcomas "not otherwise specified, (NOS)." Poorly differentiated sarcomas typically affect older individuals.

The next most commonly reported soft tissue sarcoma is liposarcoma, malignant tumors of the fat tissues. This sarcoma also is more common in older persons. There are several subtypes ranging from the low-grade lipoma, such as liposarcoma that rarely metastasizes, to the high-grade pleomorphic liposarcoma and round cell liposarcoma, which have a prognosis similar to malignant fibrous histiocytoma.

The third most commonly encountered soft tissue sarcoma is synovial sarcoma, which is more likely to affect younger adults than previously mentioned sarcomas. Many of these cases

respond very favorably to chemotherapy with significant shrinkage of the tumor, although resection and radiation remain the cornerstones of current therapy. The prognosis is similar to malignant fibrous histiocytoma and the other high-grade soft tissue sarcomas mentioned above.

Rhabdomyosarcomas are primarily tumors of children. Clinically and behaviorally they are in a class by themselves. These are treated with aggressive chemotherapy, as well as surgery and/or radiation in many cases. The aggressive treatments often cause permanent life-altering disability, even in survivors.

Section 8.6: Benign Bone Tumors

In addition to the burden of malignant bone and soft tissue tumors, a plethora of benign tumors and tumor-like conditions disable thousands of Americans annually. (Table 8.10) No national databases on which to base estimates of the prevalence or incidence of such tumors exist. The relative frequency of more common benign bone tumors can be discerned from prior publications and extrapolation from the primary contributor's ongoing case registry of consecutive surgical cases treated between 1991 through 2004. Table 8.11 reflects the collected experience reported in the Mayo Clinic publication of 1986, the University of Florida publication from 1983, the J. Mirra experience reported in 1989, and the most recent updated case series reflecting the practice of William G. Ward, a full-time orthopaedic oncologist in practice from 1991 to 2004 at Wake Forest University Health Sciences in Winston-Salem, NC.

It is believed that the experience of Dr. Ward, one of few orthopaedic oncologists in the state of North Carolina, is reflective of the current general prevalence of bone and soft tissue tumors as he treats a wide variety of benign and malignant bone tumors in a broad referral practice. All cases in his case registry reflect recently treated patients, i.e., none were "consult cases" in which only radiographs or pathology slides were reviewed for outside consulting physicians, such as the Mayo and Mirra series included. The earlier data sets were accumulated during time periods prior to the full development of the subspecialty of orthopaedic oncology; thus, only the more unusual cases of bone tumors were referred to major medical centers, making estimates of their incidence less reliable. It is believed that, except for bone cysts, few bone tumors have been treated by general orthopaedic surgeons or other musculoskeletal specialists in North Carolina over the past 15 years, as most are referred to orthopaedic oncologists. Practical experience has confirmed that osteosarcoma is the least likely sarcoma to be treated by anyone other than an orthopaedic oncologist. Dr. Ward and a few other orthopaedic oncologists have treated nearly all patients with an osteosarcoma in North Carolina for the past 15 years. Very few benign bone tumors have been treated by general orthopaedic surgeons. Thus, comparing the cases of benign bone tumors relative to the cases of osteosarcoma treated by Dr. Ward provides a relative index useful in generating a broad estimate of the prevalence of these tumors. By comparing this estimate with the national estimate for the annual occurrence of osteosarcoma, the most commonly encountered primary sarcoma of bone, a rough estimate of the prevalence of these benign bone tumor diseases can be calculated.

The most commonly encountered benign tumor of bone is osteochondroma, estimated to have an annual prevalence of >1,500 cases. Osteochondroma typically arises near the long ends of bones. Osteochondromas are often painful due to formation of bursa overlying the lesion, interference with neurovascular function due to tenting of such structures over the osteochondroma surface, and the potential for deformity in the involved and/or adjacent bones. Long-term complications are uncommon except for rare cases of dedifferentiation into a chondrosarcoma. There is no estimate of the number of patients seen with non-operatively managed osteochondroma, as records are kept only for surgically treated cases managed by Dr. Ward. The prevalence of osteochondroma, thus, is an estimate of only those cases requiring surgery. The estimate is further underestimated due to the fact that some general orthopaedic surgeons provide surgical treatment of osteochondromas.

The second most commonly encountered benign bone lesions are unicameral bone cysts, with an estimated annual prevalence of >1,250 cases. The etiology of these fluid-filled bone cysts, usually found in the growing ends of children's long bones such as the proximal humerus or femur, is unclear. Because they never metastasize and are usually quite characteristic on radiographs, many of these are treated by other orthopaedic surgeons. The true incidence, therefore, is probably significantly higher than that estimated by extrapolation from Dr. Ward's practice experience. These cystic lesions cause weakening of the bone and often require multiple surgeries to rebuild the bone with bone grafts, injections, and other techniques. They occur in children and typically recur multiple times until skeletal maturity is achieved.

Giant cell tumor of bone, with an estimated annual prevalence of >750 cases, is the third most commonly encountered benign bone neoplasm, and accounts for significant disability and dysfunction. This bone-destroying tumor typically occurs near the end of the long bones, most commonly the lower femur or upper tibia, and causes destruction of the bone. The tumor may extend through the cortex of the bone into the soft tissues and, if large enough, prior to treatment can be associated with pathologic fracture of the involved bone. Smaller tumors can be treated with resection and reconstruction of the bone with bone graft or cement filler. More complicated cases require sophisticated reconstruction with massive joint replacements and/or massive allografts and can cause severe long-term disability. On rare occasions, giant cell tumors can metastasize to the lungs. In such cases, they typically respond poorly to chemotherapy and may cause death. These tumors are infrequently treated by general orthopaedic surgeons.

A fourth commonly encountered tumor that requires surgery is enchondroma, estimated at more than 725 annual cases. Bones typically form as cartilage models in embryos that ultimately convert into bone structure. The cartilage-based growth plates add length to the bones from bone growth. Enchondromas are basically tumors derived from these cartilaginous tissues that abnormally remain in the skeleton as remnants from the normal pattern of maturation and development. If these achieve sufficient size, they can cause pain or bony erosion and may present diagnostic challenges requiring biopsy. They often require treatment by curettage and bone grafting. These lesions can dedifferentiate into malignant cartilage tumors, called chondrosarcomas. Many small enchondromas are seen incidentally, cause no symptoms, and are treated with simple observation. Only the surgically treated cases were recorded in Dr. Ward's series, so the total incidence of enchondromas is much higher than that shown. The burden of enchondromas requiring surgical treatment is fairly accurately and conservatively estimated.

There are multiple other benign tumors that are even less commonly encountered. Aneurysmal bone cysts (ABCs) are more aggressive forms of cystic lesions similar to unicameral bone cysts. However, ABCs are more destructive, expanding the weakened bone and causing greater bone destruction. They tend to be filled with blood and tissue, not simple fluid. They usually respond favorably to curettage and bone grafting, but recur in at least 20% of cases. Metaphyseal fibrous defects are deficiencies in normal bone formation within the various bones that occur in 2% to 3% of of children. Most resolve without ever causing symptoms and may never even be detected, but many require surgery, such as bone grafting, to prevent fracture and/or surgery to treat completed fractures that have occurred. Osteoid osteoma is a small tumor typically occurring in children that is associated with severe unrelenting night pain. It usually requires resection and may require bone grafting. When located in the spine it can cause a painful scoliosis. More recently, successful treatment with radio-frequency ablation procedures under radiographic guidance has become the treatment of choice for accessible lesions. Chondroblastoma is an unusual neoplasm that occurs in the ends of growing bones in teenagers and young adults. This requires resection of the lesion and bone grafting. If untreated, it can cause collapse and degenerative arthritis in the associated joint and on rare occasion can metastasize to the lung. These usually are referred to orthopaedic oncologists. Numerous other less common benign bone tumors often are treated similar to giant cell tumors, ABCs, or chondroblastomas with curettage, resection and bone grafting. Most cause some degree of disability and dysfunction of the involved extremity.

Section 8.7: Benign Soft Tissue Tumors

As with the benign bone tumors, there is no national registry of benign soft tissue tumors. By comparing Dr. Ward's 13 years of practice history from 1991 to 2004, and computing an incidence index relative to that of osteosarcoma, some estimate of the prevalence of surgically treated lesions may be obtained. (Table 8.12) From this index estimate, a baseline estimate of the national incidence can be calculated. However, benign soft tissue tumors are the most likely category of tumors to be treated by other surgeons, such as general orthopaedic surgeons and general surgeons; therefore, this national estimate is extremely conservative. The prevalence and burden in the United States from benign soft tissue tumors is significantly higher than estimated herein.

The majority of benign soft tissue tumors cause local growth and may require resection. Benign lesions rarely cause death, and it is quite infrequent that an amputation is required. However, depending on the site of involvement and size of the lesion, significant disability of the involved extremity and/or joint can occur. The true cost of these otherwise benign neoplasms can be quite high in terms of healthcare costs, lost work time, morbidity, emotional cost, and disability expenses.

A summary of "Neoplasms of the Bones & Joints and Soft Tissues, 20-Year Cumulative Case Counts, 1985-2004, National Cancer Data Base of the American College of Surgeons Commission on Cancer" is shown in Table 8.13.

1. Ries LAG, Melbert D, Krapcho M, et al, (eds): *SEER Cancer Statistics Review, 1975-2004*. Bethesda, MD: National Cancer Institute: 2006. Available at: http://seer.cancer.gov/csr/1975_2003/. Accessed June 19, 2007.

2. Praemer A Furner S, Rice DP: *Musculoskeletal Conditions in the United States*. ed 2. Rosemont, IL: American Academy of Orthopaedic Surgeons, 1999, p 182.

3. Damron TA, Ward WG, Stewart A: Osteosarcoma, chondrosarcoma and Ewing's sarcoma: National Cancer Center Data Base Report. *Clin Orthop Relat Res* 2007;459:40-47.

4. Grimer RJ, Carter SR, Pynsent PB: The cost-effectiveness of limb salvage bone tumours. *J Bone Joint Surg Br* 1997;79:558-561.

5. National Cancer Society (NCS): *What Is a Soft Tissue Sarcoma?* Available at: http://www.cancer.org/docroot/ cri/content/cri_2_4_1x_what_is_sarcoma_38.asp?sitearea =cri. Accessed October 10, 2007.

6. National Cancer Data Base (NCDB): *Site by Stage Distribution of Cases Reported to the NCDB: Diagnosis Year 2000 to 2004*. Chicago, IL: American College of Surgeons Commission on Cancer. Available at: http://www.facs.org/cancer/ncdb/publicaccess.html. Accessed October 10, 2007.

7. National Cancer Society (NCS): *What Are the Key Statistics About Soft Tissue Sarcoma?* Available at: http://www.cancer.org/docroot/CRI/content/CRI_2_4_1X _What_are_the_key_statistics_for_sarcoma_38.asp?rnav =cri. Accessed October 10, 2007.

8. National Cancer Society (NCS): *How Are Soft Tissue Sarcomas Staged?* Available at: http://www.cancer.org/ docroot/CRI/content/CRI_2_4_3X_How_is_sarcoma_ staged_38.asp?rnav=cri. Accessed October 10, 2007.

Section 8.8: Neoplasm of Bones and Connective Tissue Data Tables

Table 8.1: Incidence of Cancer of Bones and Joints, by Sex and Race, United States 1995-2004

		Incidence per 1,000,000 Persons										
Year	All Persons	White		Black		Hispanic		American Indian/ Alaska Native		Asian or Pacific Islander	
		Males	Females	Males	Females	Males	Females	Males	Females	Males	Females
1995		11.6	7.8	10.2	6.8	9.6	8.9			9.5	4.1
1996		10.9	7.5	11.2	5.9	7.3	6.5	5.0	30.7	6.3	4.1
1997		11.5	9.3	9.9	5.6	7.5	7.3		20.0	8.4	4.2
1998		10.6	8.1	6.7	7.4	7.7	7.0	4.8	3.6	5.9	5.8
1999		10.4	8.2	5.9	5.5	8.7	7.3			6.8	2.8
2000		10.4	8.3	9.3	5.6	10.1	9.4	27.1	6.7	8.5	7.7
2001		11.8	8.3	7.3	5.9	10.0	7.9	4.1	13.4	6.8	2.5
2002		11.6	8.2	12.1	6.7	10.6	6.2	15.6	6.6	6.4	7.5
2003	9.0	10.6	8.1	7.9	6.6	10.1	8.0	15.7	2.6	6.9	7.1
2004	9.0	9.7	8.2	5.8	7.7	7.0	8.5	2.3	2.3	6.4	2.7

Source: Ries LAG, Harkins D, Krapcho M, et al (eds): *SEER Cancer Statistics Review, 1975-2003, Overview.* Bethesda, MD: National Cancer Institute, 2006. Available at: http://seer.cancer.gov/csr/1975_2003/. Accessed June 19 2007.

Table 8.2: Incidence of Myeloma, by Sex and Race, United States 1995-2004

		Incidence per 1,000,000 Persons			
Year		White		Black	
	All Persons	Males	Females	Males	Females
1995	57	67	43	150	101
1996	58	68	43	134	119
1997	61	70	47	142	118
1998	59	70	44	129	105
1999	55	66	40	149	99
2000	59	73	43	106	103
2001	57	67	43	137	99
2002	57	73	40	139	85
2003	53	65	40	132	80
2004	56				

Source: Ries LAG, Harkins D, Krapcho M, et al (eds): *SEER Cancer Statistics Review, 1975-2003, Overview.* Bethesda, MD: National Cancer Institute, 2006. Available at: http://seer.cancer.gov/csr/1975_2003/. Accessed June 19 2007.

Table 8.3: Median Age of Patients at Diagnosis by Primary Cancer Site by Sex and Race, United States 2000-2003

Type	Median Age at Diagnosis, All Races			Median Age at Diagnosis, Whites			Median Age at Diagnosis, Blacks		
	Total	Males	Females	Total	Males	Females	Total	Males	Females
Bones & Joints	39.0	37.0	42.0	39.0	37.0	43.0	34.0	34.0	34.5
Kaposi's Sarcoma	42.0	41.0	79.0	44.0	42.0	80.0	38.0	37.0	41.0
Endocrine System	47.0	52.0	46.0	47.0	52.0	46.0	49.0	51.0	48.0
Brain & Nervous System	55.0	54.0	56.0	56.0	55.0	57.0	48.0	48.0	50.0
Soft Tissue (incl heart)	56.0	56.0	56.0	57.0	58.0	57.0	48.0	45.0	50.0
Skin	59.0	62.0	55.0	60.0	63.0	55.0	53.0	53.0	53.5
Breast (incl breast in situ)	61.0	67.0	61.0	62.0	67.0	62.0	57.0	62.0	57.0
Female Genital System	61.0	NA	61.0	62.0	NA	62.0	60.0	NA	60.0
Oral Cavity & Pharynx	62.0	61.0	66.0	63.0	62.0	68.0	57.5	58.0	57.0
Lymphoma (Hodgkin and Non-Hodgkin)	64.0	62.0	67.0	65.0	63.0	68.0	52.0	51.0	54.0
Leukemia	67.0	66.0	68.0	68.0	67.0	69.0	61.0	59.0	63.0
Male Genital System	68.0	68.0	NA	68.0	68.0	NA	65.0	65.0	NA
Myeloma	70.0	69.0	72.0	71.0	70.0	73.0	67.0	66.0	68.0
Respiratory System	70.0	70.0	70.0	70.0	70.0	71.0	66.0	65.0	66.0
Urinary System	70.0	70.0	71.0	71.0	70.0	71.0	65.0	64.0	67.0
Digestive system	71.0	69.0	73.0	72.0	70.0	74.0	66.0	65.0	69.0
All Sites	67.0	68.0	66.0	68.0	68.0	67.0	63.0	64.0	62.0

Age-adjusted to the U.S. Standard Population (19 age groups - Census P25-1130)

Source: Ries LAG, Harkins D, Krapcho M, et al (eds): *SEER Cancer Statistics Review, 1975-2003, Overview.* Bethesda, MD: National Cancer Institute, 2006. Available at: http://seer.cancer.gov/csr/1975_2003/. Accessed March 19, 2007.

Table 8.4: Age-Adjusted [1] 5-Year Relative Cancer Survival Rates by Sex, United States 2000-2004

Site	Total	Males	Females
Male Genital System	98.1	98.1	NA
Endocrine System	93.9	88.3	95.8
Skin	90.8	88.8	93.3
Breast (incl breast in situ)	88.6	85.0	88.6
Urinary System	73.5	75.0	70.2
Female Genital System	69.7	NA	69.7
Bones & Joints	67.9	64.4	72.4
Lymphoma (Hodgkin and Non-Hodgkin)	66.8	64.4	69.7
Soft Tissue (incl heart)	66.3	66.6	66.0
Oral Cavity & Pharynx	59.1	57.6	62.6
Kaposi's Sarcoma	56.3	55.8	63.7
Leukemia	49.6	49.7	49.4
Digestive system	44.6	42.6	46.8
Brain & Nervous System	33.9	32.2	36.0
Myeloma	33.7	35.5	31.7
Respiratory System	18.5	18.0	19.1
All Sites	64.9	64.6	65.2

[1] Age-adjusted to the US Standard Population (19 age groups - Census P25-1130)

Source: Ries LAG, Harkins D, Krapcho M, et al (eds): *SEER Cancer Statistics Review, 1975-2003, Overview,* Bethesda, MD: National Cancer Institute, 2006. Available at: http://seer.cancer.gov/csr/1975_2003/. Accessed June 19 2007.

Table 8.5: Age Distribution [1] of Primary Cancer Site at Time of Diagnosis, United States 2000-2003

Type	Age Distribution (%) of Incidence Cases by Site, 2000-2003								Total Cases All Ages
	≤ 20	20-34	35-44	45-54	55-64	65-74	75-84	85+	
Bones & Joints	28.4	16.4	11.9	13.2	10.0	8.9	7.7	3.5	2,691
Brain & Nervous System	13.8	9.5	10.8	15.1	16.1	16.7	14.1	3.8	18,542
Leukemia	10.9	4.8	5.8	9.9	14.5	20.4	23.8	10.0	34,625
Soft Tissue (incl heart)	10.7	10.7	11.8	14.9	14.9	15.4	15.8	5.8	8,755
Endocrine System	3.8	17.5	22.4	22.3	15.2	11.1	6.3	1.4	26,171
Lymphoma (Hodgkin and Non-Hodgkin)	3.1	8.0	9.1	13.8	16.7	20.9	21.0	7.3	62,126
Skin	1.0	8.3	13.3	18.4	18.0	18.4	16.7	5.9	57,447
Urinary System	0.6	0.9	3.7	11.0	19.4	27.4	27.6	9.3	96,064
Oral Cavity & Pharynx	0.5	2.4	7.3	20.5	24.3	22.2	17.0	5.7	29,790
Female Genital System	0.4	4.6	10.6	19.1	22.7	20.2	16.6	5.7	76,273
Digestive System	0.2	1.0	3.7	11.6	18.2	26.2	27.8	11.4	251,329
Male Genital System	0.2	1.7	1.7	8.5	25.9	35.6	21.8	4.6	216,884
Kaposi's Sarcoma	0.1	19.8	36.7	16.7	6.0	6.5	8.4	5.8	2,029
Respiratory System	0.1	0.4	2.3	9.3	21.5	32.3	27.5	6.7	192,800
Breast (incl breast in situ)	0.0	1.9	10.6	22.1	22.8	20.4	16.8	5.4	199,479
Myeloma	0.0	0.6	3.4	11.5	19.5	27.5	28.1	9.3	15,356
All Sites	1.1	2.7	6.0	13.5	20.8	26.0	22.6	7.3	1,327,804

[1] Age-adjusted to the U.S. Standard Population (19 age groups - Census P25-1130)

Source: Ries LAG, Harkins D, Krapcho M, et al (eds): *SEER Cancer Statistics Review, 1975-2003, Overview.* Bethesda, MD: National Cancer Institute, 2006. Available at: http://seer.cancer.gov/csr/1975_2003/, based on November 2005 SEER data submission, posted to the SEER web site, 2006. Accessed March 19, 2007.

Table 8.6: Age Distribution [1] of Primary Cancer Site at Time of Death, United States 2000-2003

Site	Age Distribution (%) of Deaths by Cancer Site, 2000-2003								Total Cases All Ages
	≤ 20	20-34	35-44	45-54	55-64	65-74	75-84	85+	
Bones & Joints	14.8	14.1	7.3	8.9	11.2	13.7	18.6	11.3	4,966
Endocrine System	8.3	2.6	4.9	10.7	15.9	21.7	24.5	11.4	8,895
Brain & Nervous System	4.3	4.1	8.3	15.5	19.7	22.8	19.6	5.7	50,995
Soft Tissue (incl heart)	4.1	6.8	7.9	13.5	16.7	19.8	21.6	9.7	14,556
Leukemia	3.3	3.3	3.7	6.7	11.9	22.6	31.6	17.0	86,118
Lymphoma (Hodgkin and Non-Hodgkin)	0.6	2.5	3.7	7.8	13.9	23.5	32.5	15.6	93,728
Urinary System	0.2	0.3	1.8	7.1	14.8	24.6	32.6	18.5	100,119
Oral Cavity & Pharynx	0.2	0.9	3.6	14.3	22.9	24.9	22.2	11.0	30,707
Skin	0.1	2.4	6.6	13.8	17.4	21.5	24.1	14.0	39,993
Digestive System	0.1	0.5	2.5	9.0	16.0	25.3	30.3	16.3	529,051
Female Genital System	0.0	1.4	5.0	12.0	17.8	23.7	26.9	13.2	107,351
Male Genital System	0.0	0.4	0.4	1.6	6.6	20.9	41.4	28.6	124,235
Respiratory System	0.0	0.1	1.7	7.8	19.4	32.3	30.0	8.6	646,226
Breast (incl breast in situ)	0.0	1.1	6.6	15.4	18.6	20.5	23.1	14.7	166,399
Myeloma	0.0	0.1	1.3	6.3	14.7	28.2	35.0	14.4	43,075
All Sites	0.4	0.9	2.9	8.9	16.6	26.3	30.0	14.1	2,220,994

[1] Age-adjusted to the US Standard Population (19 age groups - Census P25-1130)

Source: Ries LAG, Harkins D, Krapcho M, et al (eds): *SEER Cancer Statistics Review, 1975-2003, Overview.* Bethesda, MD: National Cancer Institute, 2006. Available at: http://seer.cancer.gov/csr/1975_2003/, based on November 2005 SEER data submission, posted to the SEER web site, 2006. Accessed March 19, 2007.

Table 8.7: Annual Distribution of Malignant Bone Tumors and Myeloma by Type and Age, United States 2000-2003

	Annual Prevalence Bone Tumor Cases, 2000-2003					Total Malignant Cases
	≤ 20	20-34	35-44	55-64	75+	All Ages
Malignant Bone Tumors						
Osteosarcoma	421	153	145	130	65	916
Chrondosarcoma	31	156	389	318	91	987
Ewing's sarcoma	221	71	34	11	0	339
Other and unspecified bone tumors	34	45	136	116	116	449
Total Malignant Bone Tumors	708	426	705	577	273	2,691
Myeloma	0	92	2,288	7,217	5,743	15,341

	Proportion (%) of Total Bone Tumor Cases by Type, 2000-2003					Total Malignant Cases
	≤ 20	20-34	35-44	55-64	75+	All Ages
Malignant Bone Tumors						
Osteosarcoma	46.0%	16.8%	15.8%	14.3%	7.1%	100%
Chrondosarcoma	3.2%	15.9%	39.5%	32.3%	9.2%	100%
Ewing's sarcoma	65.5%	21.0%	10.1%	3.4%	0.0%	100%
Other and unspecified bone tumors	7.6%	10.1%	30.4%	25.9%	25.9%	100%
Total Malignant Bone Tumors	26.3%	15.9%	26.2%	21.5%	10.1%	100%
Myeloma	0.0%	0.6%	14.9%	47.0%	37.4%	100%

	Distribution (%) of Total Bone Tumor Cases by Age, 2000-2003					Total Malignant Cases
	≤ 20	20-34	35-44	55-64	75+	All Ages
Malignant Bone Tumors						
Osteosarcoma	59.4%	36.0%	20.6%	22.7%	24.0%	916
Chrondosarcoma	4.4%	36.7%	55.2%	55.2%	33.0%	987
Ewing's sarcoma	31.3%	16.7%	4.8%	2.0%	0.0%	339
Other and unspecified bone tumors	4.8%	10.7%	19.4%	20.2%	43.0%	449
Total Malignant Bone Tumors	100%	100%	100%	100%	100%	2,691

Source: Surveillance, Epidemiology, and End Results (SEER) Program (www.seer.cancer.gov): Public-Use Data (1973-2003). National Cancer Institute, DCCPS, Surveillance Research Program, Cancer Statistics Branch, released April 2006, based on the November 2005 submission. Accessed March 19, 2007.

Table 8.8: Site by Stage Distribution of Cases Reported to the National Cancer Data Base, Diagnosis Years 2000-2004

Primary Site	Proportion of Total Cases with Known Stage, 2000-2004					Stage Unknown	Total Cases	% of Total Cases
	Stage 0	Stage I	Stage II	Stage III	Stage IV			
Breast	18.0%	40.7%	29.9%	7.9%	3.5%	35,762	839,265	17.8%
Prostate	0.0%	2.1%	84.1%	8.5%	5.3%	38,727	612,414	13.0%
Lung, Bronchus-NSCC	0.3%	25.2%	8.1%	27.7%	38.7%	38,309	490,609	10.4%
Colon	7.9%	22.1%	27.5%	24.2%	18.3%	25,862	353,444	7.5%
Bladder	50.6%	23.7%	12.7%	6.0%	7.0%	15,466	190,144	4.0%
Non-Hodgkins Lymphoma	0.0%	32.0%	17.5%	15.9%	34.6%	35,954	172,269	3.7%
Melanoma-Skin	25.8%	43.2%	15.9%	11.0%	4.1%	20,605	158,558	3.4%
Uterus	1.4%	70.3%	8.9%	12.5%	6.9%	17,235	139,009	3.0%
Kidney and Renal Pelvis	0.0%	52.9%	11.3%	15.0%	20.8%	15,380	132,380	2.8%
Rectum	9.1%	31.0%	22.3%	23.3%	14.3%	17,304	109,971	2.3%
Pancreas	0.5%	9.0%	15.1%	14.3%	61.1%	17,105	102,399	2.2%
Lung, Bronchus-SCC	0.3%	6.7%	4.0%	30.3%	58.7%	9,779	96,167	2.0%
Soft Tissue	0.0%	28.3%	30.4%	24.8%	16.6%	12,310	32,622	0.7%
Bones and Joints	0.0%	43.7%	34.6%	2.9%	18.8%	4,339	10,002	0.2%
All Cancer Cases	8.8%	27.9%	28.9%	16.0%	18.7%	858,270	4,708,118	

Source: National Cancer Data Base (NCDB): Site by Stage Distribution of Cases Reported to the NCDB: Diagnosis Years 2000 to 2004. American College of Surgeons Commission on Cancer. Available at: http://www.facs.org/cancer/ncdb/publicaccess.html. Accessed October 10, 2007.

Table 8.9: Malignant Soft Tissue Tumors (Sarcomas)

Tumors of Fat Tissue

Liposarcomas	Malignant tumors of fat tissue. They can develop anywhere in the body, but they most often develop in the thigh, behind the knee, and inside the back of the abdomen. They occur mostly in adults between 50 and 65 years old. Some liposarcomas grow very slowly, others can grow quickly.

Tumors of Muscle Tissue

Smooth muscle sarcomas (Found in internal organs such as stomach, intestines, blood vessels, or uterus (womb) and causes them to contract. These muscles are involuntary.)

Leiomyosarcomas	Malignant tumors of involuntary muscle tissue. They can grow almost anywhere in the body but are most often found in the retroperitoneum and the internal organs and blood vessels where leiomyomas also arise. Less often, they develop in the deep soft tissues of the legs or arms. They tend to occur in adults, particularly the elderly.

Skeletal muscle sarcomas (Muscle that allows movement of arms and legs and other body parts; voluntary movement.)

Rhabdomyosarcomas	Malignant tumors of skeletal muscle. These tumors commonly grow in the arms or legs, but they can also begin in the head and neck area and in reproductive and urinary organs such as the vagina or bladder. Children are affected much more often than adults.

Tumors of Peripheral Nerve Tissue

Malignant schwannomas, neurofibrosarcomas, or neurogenic sarcomas	Malignant tumors of the cells that surround a nerve. A new name for these is malignant peripheral nerve sheath tumors,

Tumors of Joint Tissue

Joints are surrounded by tough tissue called synovium, which produces the fluid that lubricates the joint surfaces so that they move smoothly. Tumors of joints start in the synovium.

Synovial sarcoma	Malignant tumor of the tissue around joints. The most common location is the thigh. Despite the name synovial sarcoma, most do not occur in joints. This sarcoma tends to occur mostly in young adults, but can also occur in childrenand in older people.

Table 8.9 continued next page.

Table 8.9: Malignant Soft Tissue Tumors (Sarcomas) (continued)

Tumors of Blood Vessels and Lymph Vessels

Hemangiopericytoma	A tumor of perivascular tissue. It most often develops in the legs, pelvis, and retroperitoneum (the back of the abdominal cavity). It is most common in adults. These can be either benign or malignant. They don't often spread to distant sites, but tend to come back where they started, even after surgery, unless widely excised.
Hemangioendo-thelioma	A blood vessel tumor that is less aggressive than hemangiosarcoma but still considered a low-grade cancer. It usually invades nearby tissues and sometimes can metastasize. It may develop in soft tissues or in internal organs, such as the liver or lungs.
Angiosarcomas	Malignant tumors that can develop either from blood vessels (hemangiosarcomas) or from lymph vessels (lymphangiosarcomas). These tumors can sometimes develop in a part of the body that has been exposed to radiation. Angiosarcomas are sometimes seen in the breast after radiation therapy for breast cancer or in the arm on the same side as a breast that has been irradiated or removed by mastectomy. They are difficult to cure.
Kaposi's sarcoma	A cancer formed by cells similar to those lining blood or lymph vessels. In the past, Kaposi's sarcoma was an uncommon cancer mostly seen in older people with no apparent immune system problems. It is most common in people with human immunodeficiency virus (HIV) infection and acquired immunodeficiency syndrome (AIDS), but it can also develop in organ transplant patients who are taking medication to suppress their immune system. It is probably related to infection with a virus called human herpesvirus-8 (HHV-8).

Tumors of Fibrous Tissue

Fibrous tissue forms tendons and ligaments and covers bones as well as other organs in the body.

Fibrosarcoma	Cancer of fibrous tissue. It usually affects the legs, arms, or trunk. It is most common between the ages of 20 and 60, but can occur at any age, even in infancy.
Fibromatosis	The name given to fibrous tissue tumor with features in between fibrosarcoma and benign tumors such as fibromas and superficial fibromatosis. They tend to grow slowly but, often, steadily. At one time they were called desmoid tumors, when they were closely attached to skeletal muscles. Now they are called musculoaponeurotic fibromatosis. They do not metastasize, but they can invade nearby tissues and are sometimes fatal. Some doctors consider these to be a type of low-grade fibrosarcoma; others believe they are a unique type of fibrous tissue tumors. Certain hormones, particularly estrogen, increase the growth of some desmoid tumors. Antiestrogen drugs are sometimes useful in treating desmoids that cannot be completely removed by surgery.
Dermatofibrosarcoma protuberans (DFSP)	A slow-growing cancer of the fibrous tissue beneath the skin, usually in the trunk or limbs. It invades nearby tissues but rarely metastasizes.
Malignant fibrous histiocytoma (MFH)	Most often found in the arms or legs. Less often, it can develop inside the back of the abdomen. This sarcoma is most common in older adults. Although it mostly tends to grow locally, it can spread to distant sites. It is the most commonly diagnosed soft tissue sarcoma.

Tumors of Uncertain Tissue Type

Through microscopic examination and other laboratory tests, doctors can usually find similarities between most sarcomas and certain types of normal soft tissues. However, some sarcomas have not been linked to a specific type of normal soft tissue.

Malignant mesenchymoma	A rare type of sarcoma that contains some areas showing features of fibrosarcoma and other areas with features of at least two other types of sarcoma.
Alveolar soft-part sarcoma	A rare cancer that mostly affects young adults. The legs are the most common location of these tumors.
Epithelioid sarcoma	Most often develops in tissues under the skin of the hands, forearms, feet, or lower legs. Adolescents and young adults are often affected.
Clear cell sarcoma	A rare cancer that often develops in tendons of the arms or legs. Under the microscope, it shares some features with malignant melanoma, a type of cancer that develops from pigment-producing skin cells. How cancers with these features develop in parts of the body other than the skin is not known.
Desmoplastic small cell tumor	A rare sarcoma of adolescents and young adults, found most often in the abdomen. Its name means that it is formed by small, round cancer cells surrounded by scar-like tissue.

Other Types of Sarcoma

There are other types of soft tissue sarcomas, however, they are less commonly encountered.

Source: American Cancer Society: What is a soft tissue sarcoma? 2006. Available at: http://www.cancer.org/docroot/cri/content/cri_2_4_1x_what_is_sarcoma_38.asp?sitearea=cri. Accessed October 10, 2007. Editorial revisions provided by William G. Ward, MD.

Table 8.10: Benign Soft Tissue Tumors

Tumors of Fat Tissue

Lipomas	Benign tumors of fat tissue. They are the most common benign soft tissue tumor. Most are found under the skin, but they can develop anywhere in the body.
Lipoblastomas	Benign fat tumors that occur in infants and young children.
Hibernomas	Like lipomas, are also benign fat tissue tumors. They are much less common than lipomas.

Tumors of Muscle Tissue

Smooth muscle sarcomas (Found in internal organs such as stomach, intestines, blood vessels, or uterus (womb) and causes them to contract. These muscles are involuntary.)

Leiomyomas	Benign tumors of smooth muscle (or involuntary muscle). Leiomyomas can arise almost anywhere in the body in either men or women because they can start in tissues as widespread, for example, as blood vessels or intestine. The most common of these is the fibroid tumor that develops in many women. It is really a leiomyoma of the uterus.

Skeletal muscle sarcomas (Muscle that allows movement of arms and legs and other body parts; voluntary movement.)

Rhabdomyomas	Benign tumors of skeletal muscle (the muscle that is attached to bone and helps us to move). They are rare.

Tumors of Peripheral Nerve Tissue

Neurofibromas, schwannomas (neurilemmoma), and neuromas	Benign tumors of nerves. These tumors can occur almost anywhere in the body. An inherited condition called neurofibromatosis or von Recklinghausen disease causes people to develop many neurofibromas throughout their body. Some of these, if they formed from very large nerves such as those in the upper arms, neck, pelvis, or thigh can become malignant.

Tumors of Joint Tissue

Joints are surrounded by tough tissue called synovium, which produces the fluid that lubricates the joint surfaces so that they move smoothly. Tumors of joints start in the synovium.

Nodular tenosynovitis	Benign tumor of joint tissue. It is most common in the hands and is more common in women than in men.

Tumors of Blood Vessels and Lymph Vessels

Hemangiomas	Benign tumors of blood vessels. They are rather common, are often present at birth, and can affect the skin or internal organs. They sometimes disappear without treatment, but when located in muscles and other deep tissues, can be quite problematic and require surgical treatment.
Glomus tumors	Benign perivascular (around blood vessels) tumors. They usually are found under the skin and often under fingernails.
Hemangiopericytoma	A tumor of perivascular tissue. It most often develops in the legs, pelvis, and retroperitoneum (the back of the abdominal cavity). It is most common in adults. These can be either benign or malignant. They don't often spread to distant sites, but tend to come back where they started, even after surgery, unless very widely excised.
Lymphangiomas	Benign lymph vessel tumors that are usually present at birth. Lymph is a type of fluid that circulates in every tissue of the body, ending up in the venous system. It contains waste products from tissues and immune system cells. Lymphangiosarcomas are the malignant lymph vessel form of angiosarcomas.

Tumors of Fibrous Tissue

Fibrous tissue forms tendons and ligaments and covers bones as well as other organs in the body.

Fibromas, elastofibromas, superficial fibromatosis, and fibrous histiocytomas	All are benign tumors.

Tumors of Uncertain Tissue Type

Through microscopic examination and other laboratory tests, doctors can usually find similarities between most sarcomas and certain types of normal soft tissues. However, some sarcomas have not been linked to a specific type of normal soft tissue.

Myxoma	A benign tumor that usually is located in muscles but does not develop from muscle cells. The cells of a myxoma produce mucus-like material, a feature that distinguishes this tumor. It almost always occurs in adults.
Granular cell	Tumors are usually benign tumors of adults that occur often in the tongue but can be found almost anywhere in the body.

Tumor-like Conditions of Soft Tissue

Some conditions of soft tissues are caused by inflammation or injury and can form a mass that looks like a soft tissue tumor. Unlike a true tumor, they do not come from a single abnormal cell, they have limited capacity to grow or spread to nearby tissues, and never spread through the bloodstream or lymph system. Examples include nodular fasciitis and myositis ossificans, which involve tissues under the skin and muscle tissues, respectively.

Source: American Cancer Society: What is a soft tissue sarcoma? 2006. Available at:
.http://www.cancer.org/docroot/cri/content/cri_2_4_1x_what_is_sarcoma_38.asp?sitearea=cri. Accessed October 10, 2007

Table 8.11: Relative Incidence of Benign Bone Tumors

Benign Bone Tumor	Column 1 Mayo [1]	Column 2 UFLA [2]	Column 3 Mirra [3]	Column 4 Ward [4]	Column 5 Prevalence Relative to Osteosarcoma [5]	Column 6 National Annual Prevalence [6, 7]
Osteochrondroma	727	98	1,937	124	1.65	1,511
Unicameral Bone Cyst	NA	56	583	102	1.36	1,246 [7]
Giant Cell Tumor	425	107	1,182	63	0.84	769
Enchondroma	245	37	829	60	0.80	733
Aneurysmal Bone Cysts	208	80	492	52	0.69	632
Metaphyseal Fibrous Defect	99	30	537	47	0.63	577 [8]
Osteoid Osteoma	245	56	635	25	0.33	302 [7]
Chondroblastoma	79	43	229	14	0.19	174
Chondromyxoid Fibromas	39	27	101	6	0.08	73
Osteoblastoma	63	37	142	2	0.03	27 [7]
Malignant Bone Tumors						
Osteosarcoma [9]	1,330	324	2,525	75	1.00	916
Chondrosarcoma	732	173	746	47	0.63	987
Ewing's Sarcoma	402	141	871	33	0.44	339

[1] Source: Dahlin DC, Unni KK: *Introduction and Scope of Study in Bone Tumors: General Aspects and Data on 8,542 Cases.* Springfield, IL: Charles C. Thomas, 1986, p 8, Table 1-1.

[2] Source: Enneking WF: *Musculoskeletal Tumor Surgery,* vol II. New York, NY: Churchill Livingstone, 1983.

[3] Source: Mirra JM, Picci P, Gold RH (eds): *Bone Tumors: Clinical, Radiologic and Pathologic Correlations.* Philadelphia, PA: Lea & Febiger, 1989.

[4] Ward WG. Surgical case files, 1991-2004

[5] Ward WG. Computation of relative prevalence based on n=75 cases of osteosarcoma (i.e., (column 4)/(75)).

[6] Calculated as annual prevalence of cases relative to osteosarcoma (i.e., column 5 * national cases of osteosarcoma (n=916)).

[7] Gross underestimate due to high frequency of treatments rendered by orthopaedic surgeons other than orthopaedic oncologists.

[8] Gross underestimate of prevalence since prior studies have indicated 1%-3% of children have these at some point in their childhood. Of the symptomatic ones requiring surgery, many are managed by orthopaedists other than orthopaedic oncologists, so true incidence is vastly higher than that depicted by this conservative estimate.

[9] The national prevalence of osteosarcoma between 2000 and 2003 was 916 cases. (Table 8.7) This value is used as the base for computing the estimated national prevalence of benign bone tumors.

Table 8.12: Surgically Treated Benign Soft Tissue Tumor Incidence

Tumor	Number [1]	Incidence Relative to Osteosarcoma [2]	Minimal Estimated National Incidence [3]
Lipoma	182	2.43	2,226
Ganglion	95	1.27	1,163
Hemangioma	51	0.68	623
Pigmented Villonodular Synovitis/Giant Cell Tumor of Tendon Sheath	45	0.60	550
Myxoma	38	0.51	467
Desmoid/Fibromatosis	39	0.52	476
Neurilemmoma	30	0.40	366
Neurofibroma	19	0.25	229
Myositis Ossificans	14	0.19	174
Fibroma	14	0.19	174
Other	293	3.91	3,582

[1] Ward WG, case series 1991-2004 by patients

[2] Ward WG: Computation of relative prevalence based on n=75 cases of osteosarcoma (i.e., (number/75).

[3] Calculated as annual prevalence of cases relative to osteosarcoma (i.e., column 2 * national cases of osteosarcoma (n=916)). This provides a gross underestimate of the U.S. national burden of these tumors, as many (perhaps most) are treated by other physicians, including family physicians, general surgeons, and general orthopaedic surgeons.

Table 8.13: Neoplasms of the Bones and Joints and Soft Tissues, 20-Year Cumulative Case Counts, 1985-2004, National Cancer Data Base of the American College of Surgeons Commission on Cancer

Bone & Joint Tumors	Number	Soft Tissue Tumors by Type (continued)	Number
Total Bone Chondrosarcomas	11,585	Clear Cell Sarcoma	809
Total Bone & Joint Osteosarcomas	14,191	Dermatofibrosarcoma, NOS	2,956
		Desmoplastic Small Round Cell Tumor	162
Bone & Joint Tumors by Type		Epithelioid Sarcoma	1,271
Adamantinoma of Long Bones	196	Ewing's Sarcoma	1,113
Chondrosarcoma Dedifferentiated	238	Fibromyxosarcoma	1,523
Chondrosarcoma Juxtacortical	103	Fibrosarcoma Infantile	193
Chondrosarcoma Mesenchymal	251	Fibrosarcoma, NOS	3,421
Chondrosarcoma Myxoid	874	Giant Cell Sarcoma	1,660
Chondrosarcoma, NOS	10,119	Giant Cell Tumor of Soft Parts Malignant	132
Chordoma	2,339	Granular Cell Tumor Malignant	106
Ewing's Sarcoma	5,882	Hemangioendothelioma Malignant	162
Fibrosarcoma, NOS	405	Hemangioendothelioma Malignant Epithelioid	171
Giant Cell Tumor of Bone Malignant	606	Hemangiopericytoma Malignant	986
Hemangioendothelioma Malignant	141	Hemangiosarcoma	3,345
Hemangiosarcoma	322	Kaposi's Sarcoma	2,914
Leiomyosarcoma	161	Leiomyosarcoma*	13,719
Malignant Fibrous Histiocytoma	1,266	Leiomyosarcoma Epithelioid*	629
Osteosarcoma Chondroblastic	1,564	Leiomyosarcoma Myxoid*	274
Osteosarcoma Fibroblastic	676	Liposarcoma Mixed	627
Osteosarcoma in Pagets Disease of Bone	285	Liposarcoma Myxoid	6,026
Osteosarcoma Parosteal	756	Liposarcoma Pleomorphic	2,288
Osteosarcoma Small Cell	120	Liposarcoma Round Cell	612
Osteosarcoma Telangiectatic	354	Liposarcoma Well Differentiated	3,989
Osteosarcoma, NOS	10,436	Liposarcoma, NOS	3,551
Primitive Neuroectodermal Tumor	213	Lipsosarcoma Dedifferentiated	1,013
Sarcoma, NOS	668	Malignant Fibrous Histiocytoma	25,559
Spindle Cell Sarcoma	338	Mesenchymoma Malignant	253
All Bone and Joint Tumors	38,313	Myxosarcoma	363
		Neurilemmoma Malignant	1,343
Soft Tissue Tumors	**Number**	Neurofibrosarcoma	1,583
Soft Tissue Malignant Hemangioendothelioma	333	Osteosarcoma, NOS	571
Soft Tissue Chondrosarcomas	1,711	Peripheral Neuroectodermal Tumor	386
Soft Tissue Rhabdomyosarcomas	5,092	Primitive Neuroectodermal Tumor	581
Soft Tissue Synovial Sarcomas	5,689	Rhabdomyosarcoma Alveolar	1,419
Soft Tissue Leiomyosarcomas*	14,622	Rhabdomyosarcoma Embryonal	1,801
Soft Tissue Liposarcomas	18,106	Rhabdomyosarcoma, NOS	1,316
		Rhabdomysarcoma Pleomorphic	556
Soft Tissue Tumors (by Type)		Sarcoma Rhabdoid	140
Alveolar Soft Part Sarcoma	517	Sarcoma, NOS	9,007
Carcinosarcoma, NOS	187	Small Cell Sarcoma	501
Chondrosarcoma Mesenchymal	227	Spindle Cell Sarcoma	4,181
Chondrosarcoma Myxoid	750	Synovial Sarcoma Biphasic	1,116
Chondrosarcoma, NOS	734	Synovial Sarcoma Spindle Cell	1,168
Chordoma	303	Synovial Sarcoma, NOS	3,405

* Totals include Gynecologic Leiomyosarcomas of the Uterus

Source: American College of Surgeons National Cancer Data Base

Chapter 9

Health Care Utilization and Economic Cost of Musculoskeletal Diseases

The annual average proportion of the United States population with a musculoskeletal disease requiring medical care has increased by more than two percentage points over the past decade and now includes more than 30% of the population. The increasing prevalence of musculoskeletal diseases in a growing and aging population has resulted in a more than 41% increase in total aggregate direct cost to treat persons with a musculoskeletal disease. For the years 2002-2004, the annual average direct cost, in 2004 dollars, for musculoskeletal health care, both as a direct result of a musculoskeletal disease and for patients with a musculoskeletal disease in addition to other health issues, is estimated to be $510 billion, the equivalent of 4.6% of the national gross domestic product (GDP). Incremental medical cost, that proportion of total direct cost associated with treatment incurred beyond that of persons of similar demographic and health characteristics but who do not have one or more musculoskeletal diseases (i.e., most likely attributable to a musculoskeletal disease), is estimated to be $156.7 billion.

Indirect cost, expressed primarily as wage losses for persons aged 18 to 64 with a work history, add another $339 billion, or 3.1% of the GDP, to the cost for all persons with a musculoskeletal disease, either treated as a primary condition or in addition to another condition. The 2002-2004 annual indirect cost estimated to be associated with persons treated only for a musculoskeletal disease (incremental cost) is $110.5 billion.

Hence, the annual estimated direct and indirect cost associated with persons with a

musculoskeletal disease, but not treated for other conditions, is $267.2 billion. Taking into account all persons with a musculoskeletal disease in addition to other medical conditions, the cost for treatment in the 2002-2004 time period was estimated to be $849 billion per year.

Treatments that mitigate the long-term impact of musculoskeletal diseases and return persons to full and active lives are needed. The following chapter explores the details of cost associated with musculoskeletal diseases and establishes a baseline against which to assess future needs.

Section 9.1: Musculoskeletal Disease Prevalence

Over the period 2002-2004, an estimated 87.6 million persons reported a musculoskeletal disease in the Medical Expenditures Panel Survey (MEPS) as a primary health concern (Table 9.1 and Graph 9.1.1), a substantially lower number than the 107.7 million musculoskeletal diseases self-reported by adults aged 18 and over in the

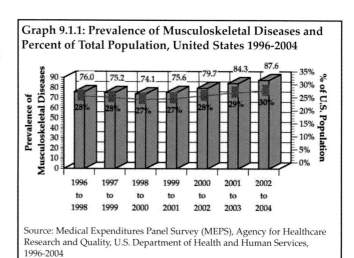

Graph 9.1.1: Prevalence of Musculoskeletal Diseases and Percent of Total Population, United States 1996-2004

Source: Medical Expenditures Panel Survey (MEPS), Agency for Healthcare Research and Quality, U.S. Department of Health and Human Services, 1996-2004

National Health Interview Survey (NHIS) in 2005 and reported in Chapter 1 (Burden of Musculoskeletal Disease Overview.) A more expansive definition of musculoskeletal diseases includes persons in whom the musculoskeletal disease is a byproduct of another condition and, therefore, is often not the primary (1ˢᵗ) diagnosis (e.g., bone metastases from cancer), as well as musculoskeletal diseases as a primary health concern. Using this more expansive definition of musculoskeletal diseases (discussed in Section 9.5 and Table 9.15), an average of 135.6 million persons, or 46.6% of the population, reported a musculoskeletal disease annually for the years 2002 to 2004. Assuming the proportion of musculoskeletal diseases among persons under the age of 18 is at least 10%, the incidence of musculoskeletal diseases in the NHIS and MEPS are similar.

Between 1996-1998 and 2002-2004, the number of persons reporting a musculoskeletal disease increased nearly 12 million from the 76 million reported in 1996. During this same time period, the prevalence of musculoskeletal diseases in the total U.S. population increased by about 2%, from 28% to 30%. (Table 9.1 and Graph 9.1.1)

Approximately 10% of all persons reporting musculoskeletal diseases in MEPS are under the age of 18, primarily due to the higher prevalence of musculoskeletal injuries (21%) in this age group. (Table 9.1 and Graph 9.1.2) Roughly one in four (23%) musculoskeletal diseases occur in persons aged 65 and over. A relatively high proportion (54%) of the category that includes osteoporosis, "Other Disorders of Bone and Cartilage," occurs in this age group. In contrast, the proportion of injuries and spine conditions are significantly lower in in persons aged 65 and over (14% and 17%, respectively). Approximately one-third (34%) of musculoskeletal diseases occur among persons aged 45 to 64, yet this group accounts for 42% of the arthritis and joint pain

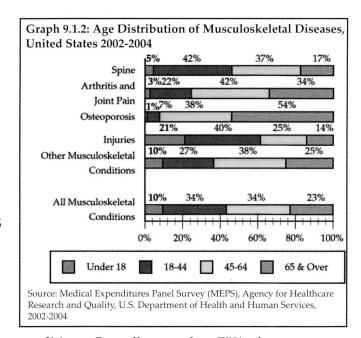

Graph 9.1.2: Age Distribution of Musculoskeletal Diseases, United States 2002-2004

Source: Medical Expenditures Panel Survey (MEPS), Agency for Healthcare Research and Quality, U.S. Department of Health and Human Services, 2002-2004

conditions. Overall, more than 75% of musculoskeletal diseases are reported by persons under the age of 65.

Among the major subgroups of musculoskeletal diseases, arthritis and joint pain have the highest prevalence, reflecting the overall aging population. In 1996-1998, just under 30 million persons (11.0%) reported one or more conditions related to arthritis and joint pain; by 2002-2004, 37.6 million persons (12.9%) reported one or more such conditions. The effect of the baby boom generation aging has been an increase in the proportion of arthritis cases among those aged 45 to 64 as they reach the typical age of onset of arthritis. As this wave ages, the proportion of persons with arthritis in the 65 and older group will increase as well. In 1996-1998, 24.8% of persons reporting arthritis were aged 18 to 44; 36.4% were aged 45 to 64. By 2002-2004, the proportions had changed to 21.7% and 41.6%, respectively. In the next decade, a higher prevalence of arthritis and joint pain is expected to occur in persons aged 65 and over.

The number of persons reporting a spine condition increased by just under 5 million, from 27.4 million in 1996-1998 to 32.7 million in 2002-

2004, while the prevalence rate increased by more than one percentage point, from 10.1% to 11.3% of the population. The majority of spine conditions occur in working age people, with 42% among persons aged 18 to 44 and another 37% among those aged 45 to 64. The higher prevalence rate among working age persons is reflected in the prominence of spine conditions in workers' compensation and disability claims. Nevertheless, about one in six spine conditions (17%) occurs among persons 65 and older.

Population aging has also led to a dramatic increase in the prevalence of the category that includes osteoporosis. In the period 1996-1998, 3.2 million people (1.2%) indicated they had these conditions, but by 2002-2004, 6.8 million (2.3%) reported having them. These numbers are substantially lower than the 8.9 million persons with self-reported osteoporosis presented in Chapter 5 (Osteoporosis and Bone Health), even though the category in this chapter is not limited to osteoporosis-related conditions, and by the National Osteoporosis Foundation, which projected 44 million persons with osteoporosis in 2002. Almost two-fifths of persons in the MEPS with these conditions are aged 45 to 64, increasing the likelihood that the more than two and a half million individuals in this age group will suffer from falls and fractures for the relatively long future they can expect to live.

In contrast to spine conditions, arthritis, and joint pain, and the category including osteoporosis, the prevalence of musculoskeletal injuries has remained steady. In 1996-1998, 23.4 million persons reported a musculoskeletal injury, while 24.7 million reported such an injury in 2002-2004. The prevalence of musculoskeletal injuries remained relatively constant at 7.7% and 8.6% of the population. Age distribution of injuries may explain why the prevalence hasn't increased. In excess of 60% of injuries occur among persons

younger than 45, a population segment growing more slowly than those who are older. It is possible improvements in the safety of automobiles and other public health prevention activities have also played a role. However, although the MEPS reporting of musculoskeletal injury trends supports trend data previously reported, the overall prevalence is substantially lower than the 57.2 million injury treatment incidents reported in Chapter 6 (Musculoskeletal Injuries) reported previously included total cases treated in doctors' offices, outpatient clinics, emergency rooms, and inpatient admissions.

The percentage of the population reporting other musculoskeletal diseases, which include a broad range of conditions of less frequent prevalence, increased from 4.4% to 5.0% between 1996-1998 and 2002-2004. The total number of persons reporting one or more such conditions increased from 12 million to 14.5 million.

Over the period 1996-2004, the proportion of persons with one or more of the major subgroups of musculoskeletal diseases, with the exception of injuries, has risen. Throughout the period under

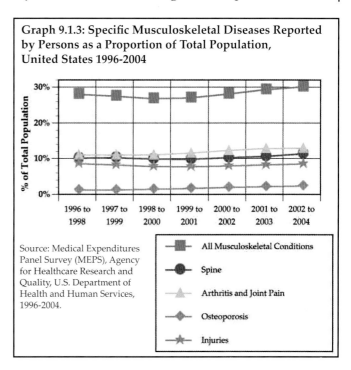

Graph 9.1.3: Specific Musculoskeletal Diseases Reported by Persons as a Proportion of Total Population, United States 1996-2004

Source: Medical Expenditures Panel Survey (MEPS), Agency for Healthcare Research and Quality, U.S. Department of Health and Human Services, 1996-2004.

All Musculoskeletal Conditions
Spine
Arthritis and Joint Pain
Osteoporosis
Injuries

study, arthritis and joint pain has been the major condition subgroup with the highest prevalence rate, followed by spine conditions (Table 9.1 and Graph 9.1.3).

Using the more expansive definition of musculoskeletal diseases (Table 9.15), in the period 2002-2004, 83.0 million persons (vs. 32.7 million using the more conservative definition) reported one or more spine conditions and 41.7 million (vs. 37.6 million) reported arthritis and joint pain. The number reporting a condition within the category that includes osteoporosis was identical in the base and expansive cases, but substantially lower than reported in Chapter 5, as noted above. The number reporting musculoskeletal injuries was slightly higher than in the more conservative definition (27.8 vs. 24.7 million). The increased prevalence in the "other" musculoskeletal diseases category was also substantial, with 45.1 million in the expansive definition versus 14.5 million, as discussed above.

Section 9.2: Musculoskeletal Health Care Utilization

Persons with musculoskeletal diseases account for a large and growing share of health care utilization. (Table 9.2 and Graph 9.2.1) In any given year, abut 85% of persons with musculoskeletal diseases have at least one ambulatory care visit to a physician's office, averaging just under six such visits per year. Between 1996-1998 and 2002-2004, ambulatory physician visits increased from 425.5 million to 507.9 million. Growth in the number of persons with musculoskeletal diseases, rather than an increase in the number of visits by individuals, is primarily responsible for this increase.

In contrast to the relatively stable number of physician office visits, there was an increase in the proportion of the U.S. population with visits to ambulatory providers other than medical physicians; the average number of visits to non-physician providers by persons with musculoskeletal diseases also increased. Non-physician ambulatory health care providers include physical therapists, occupational therapists, chiropractors, social workers, physician assistants, nurse practitioners, and other related health care workers. In 1996-1998, approximately 40% of persons with musculoskeletal diseases visited an ambulatory health care resource at least once; by 2002-2004 the proportion had jumped to nearly 52%. At the same time, the average number of such visits increased from 2.6 per person to 3.8. The result was a 69% increase, from 197.5 million to 332.8 million, in total non-physician ambulatory care visits between 1996-1998 and 2002-2004. The aggregate total for all ambulatory care visits, including those to physicians and non-physicians, thus increased over the 8 year period by 35%, from 623.0 million visits to 840.7 million visits.

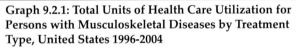
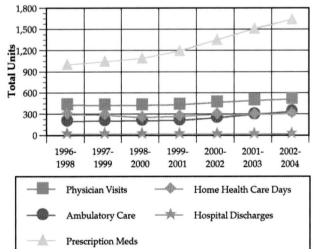

Graph 9.2.1: Total Units of Health Care Utilization for Persons with Musculoskeletal Diseases by Treatment Type, United States 1996-2004

Source: Medical Expenditures Panel Survey (MEPS), Agency for Healthcare Research and Quality, U.S. Department of Health and Human Services, 1996-2004

During this same time frame, the use of prescription medications among persons with musculoskeletal diseases rose substantially. While the proportion of persons with a musculoskeletal disease who filled at least one prescription changed only slightly, from 81.3% to 83.5%, the mean number of prescriptions filled per person increased from 13.1 to 18.6. The result was a 64% increase, from 995.3 million in 1996-1998 to more than 1.6 billion in 2002-2004, in the number of prescription medications filled by persons with a musculoskeletal disease.

Despite widespread concerns that an aging population would use an increasing amount of home health care, there is no evidence that this is occurring. Both the proportion of persons with a musculoskeletal disease using home health care and the average number of home health care visits declined slightly in the past 8 years. Only 4.7% of persons reported any home health care visits in 2002-2004, with an average of 3.5 visits incurred. The total number of home health care visits to persons with a musculoskeletal disease rose slightly, from 296.3 million to 306.5 million, and is due to population increase.

A slight increase of 15%, from 15.2 to 17.5 million, in the number of hospital discharges for persons with a musculoskeletal disease occurred in the periods 1996-1998 to 2002-2004. This may be due to the aging population. The percentage of persons with a musculoskeletal disease who were hospitalized one or more times rose by 5% in relative terms, from 11.1% to 11.7%. The average number of hospitalizations per person, at 0.2, did not change.

Over the seven 3-year averaged periods, 1996-1998 to 2002-2004, for which the MEPS data is available, prescription medications and non-physician care visits increased more than other categories of health care percentage wise. (Table 9.3 and Graph 9.2.2) Both showed a mean rise of nearly 10% per year in total health care resource usage, with the most rapid rise occurring in the past 4 years. The greatest increase in health care resource use was for persons reporting a condition in the category including osteoporosis, increasing by 13% or more annually for each of the past 7 years for all except hospital discharges. Medications filled for such diseases rose by more than 20% per year between 1996 and 2000, more than twice the rate of all other musculoskeletal diseases. This is most likely due to greater awareness of these diseases and the impact of medications on mitigating long-term impacts.

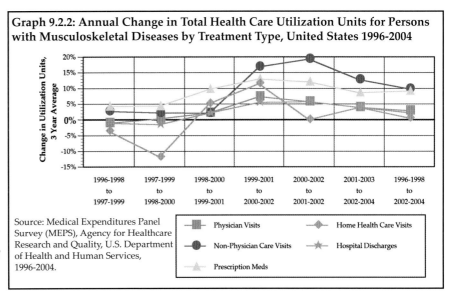

Graph 9.2.2: Annual Change in Total Health Care Utilization Units for Persons with Musculoskeletal Diseases by Treatment Type, United States 1996-2004

Source: Medical Expenditures Panel Survey (MEPS), Agency for Healthcare Research and Quality, U.S. Department of Health and Human Services, 1996-2004.

Using the more expansive definition of musculoskeletal diseases, in 2002-2004 there were an estimated 705 million visits to physicians among persons with these diseases, as well as 420 million ambulatory visits to providers other than physicians, 2.3 billion prescriptions filled, 420 million home care visits, and 27.1 million hospital discharges.

Section 9.3: Musculoskeletal Medical Care Expenditures

Musculoskeletal medical care expenditures are presented (1) for all persons with a musculoskeletal disease, regardless of whether the musculoskeletal disease was the reason for the expenditure (total cost), and (2) as a measure of the expenditures beyond those expected for persons of similar characteristics but who do not have a musculoskeletal disease (incremental cost). Incremental cost, hence, is that share estimated to be directly related to the musculoskeletal condition. Both total and incremental costs are expressed as the average cost per person with a musculoskeletal disease (Tables 9.4 and 9.4a) and the aggregate cost (total) for all persons with a musculoskeletal disease. (Table 9.5) Medical care costs are expressed in both the current year dollars (i.e., the year the data was collected) and in 2004 dollars to provide a standard of comparison across years. Throughout the following discussion, expenditures will be discussed in 2004 dollars.

Section 9.3.1: Total and Per Person Expenditures for Musculoskeletal Diseases

Overall, total average expenditures for persons with musculoskeletal diseases increased from $4,751 in 1996-1998 to $5,824 in 2002-2004, a 23%

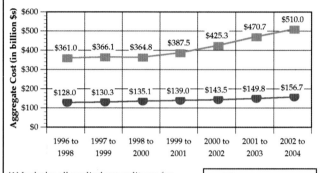

Graph 9.3.2: Aggregate Medical Care Cost for Persons with a Musculoskeletal Disease in 2004 $, United States 1996-2004

[1] Includes all medical expenditures for persons with a musculoskeletal disease regardless of whether the expenditure was to treat the musculoskeletal disease or another disease.
[2] Estimated additional medical expenditures beyond those expected for persons of similar characteristics, but without a musculoskeletal disease.

Source: Medical Expenditures Panel Survey (MEPS), Agency for Healthcare Research and Quality, U.S. Department of Health and Human Services, 2002-2004

increase. (Table 9.5, Column D and Graph 9.3.1) Aggregate total expenditures increased from $361.0 billion to $510.0 billion during this time frame (Table 9.5, Column F and Graph 9.3.2), an increase of 41%. In 1996-1998, aggregate total expenditures for persons with a musculoskeletal disease, including both primary (1st) and secondary (2nd or more) diagnoses, represented 4.4% of the GDP. By 2002-2004, the proportion had grown to 4.6% of the GDP.[1]

Incremental average expenditures for persons with musculoskeletal diseases increased from $1,685 to $1,789 between 1996-1998 and 2002-2004, or a 6% increase. (Table 9.5, Column H and Graph 9.3.1) Aggregate incremental expenditures increased from $128.0 billion to $156.7 billion (Table 9.5, Column J and Graph 9.3.2), or by about

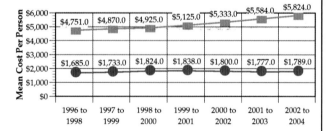

Graph 9.3.1: Mean Medical Care Cost per Person with a Musculoskeletal Disease in 2004 $, United States 1996-2000

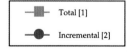

[1] Includes all medical expenditures for persons with a musculoskeletal condition regardless of whether the expenditure was to treat the musculoskeletal condition or another condition.
[2] Estimated additional medical expenditures beyond those expected for persons of similar characteristics, but without a musculoskeletal condition.

Source: Medical Expenditures Panel Survey (MEPS), Agency for Healthcare Research and Quality, U.S. Department of Health and Human Services, 1996-2004

Graph 9.3.3: Total and Incremental per Person Medical Care Expenditures for Persons with Musculoskeletal Diseases, United States 2002-2004

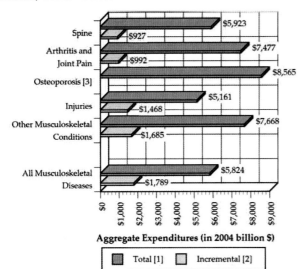

Aggregate Expenditures (in 2004 billion $)

Total [1]   Incremental [2]

[1] Includes all medical expenditures for persons with a musculoskeletal disease regardless of whether the expenditure was to treat the musculoskeletal disease or another disease.
[2] Estimated additional medical expenditures beyond those expected for persons of similar characteristics, but without a musculoskeletal disease.
[3] All individuals with osteoporosis had expenditures and total increment could not be calculated.
Source: Medical Expenditures Panel Survey (MEPS), Agency for Healthcare Research and Quality, U.S. Department of Health and Human Services, 2002-2004

Graph 9.3.4: Aggregate Total and Incremental Medical Care Expenditures for Persons with Musculoskeletal Diseases, United States 2002-2004

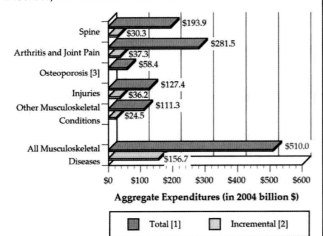

Aggregate Expenditures (in 2004 billion $)

Total [1]   Incremental [2]

[1] Includes all medical expenditures for persons with a musculoskeletal disease regardless of whether the expenditure was to treat the musculoskeletal disease or another disease.
[2] Estimated additional medical expenditures beyond those expected for persons of similar characteristics, but without a musculoskeletal disease.
[3] All individuals with osteoporosis had expenditures and total increment could not be calculated.
Source: Medical Expenditures Panel Survey (MEPS), Agency for Healthcare Research and Quality, U.S. Department of Health and Human Services, 2002-2004

22%, representing the equivalent of 1.5% and 1.4% of the GDP for the respective time frames. To provide a basis for comparison, the economy is said to be in a recession when GDP declines by at least 1% for two or more consecutive quarters. Accordingly, the aggregate economic impact of the medical expenditures on behalf of persons with musculoskeletal diseases is in excess of the amount used to define a recession and, unlike a recession, occurs in perpetuity.

Total per person medical care expenditures rose slightly for each of the major subconditions between 1996-1998 and 2002-2004 (Tables 9.4 and 9.5, Column D, and Graph 9.3.3), ranging from $5,161 per person for musculoskeletal injuries to $8,565 for conditions within the category including osteoporosis in 2002-2004. Due to the higher prevalence and relatively high level of expenditures per person, aggregate expenditures have consistently been greatest for arthritis and joint pain, accounting for $281.5 billion of musculoskeletal health care costs in 2002-2004. (Table 9.5, Column F, and Graph 9.3.4) As discussed previously, approximately one-third of the cost is for ambulatory care (33%), one-third for emergency room and inpatient care (32%), and one-third for prescriptions and other costs (36%). Spine conditions, with an estimated $193.9 billion cost in 2002-2004, have held steady as the second most expensive musculoskeletal health care condition. Spine costs also split evenly, with 34%, 32%, and 34% going to ambulatory, emergency room and inpatient, and prescriptions/other costs, respectively.

The magnitude of increase in aggregate expenditures between 1996-1998 and 2002-2004 is greatest for the diseases within the category including osteoporosis (120%), but was substantial for all musculoskeletal diseases. (Table 9.6) The aggregate cost of health care for spine conditions increased by 49%; arthritis and joint pain by 53%; musculoskeletal injuries by 37%;

and other musculoskeletal diseases by 44% over the period 1996-2004.

Sampling variability limits inference about time trends in incremental expenditures associated with the subcondition groups. However, while estimates do not have the same precision as those for all musculoskeletal diseases, it is fair to conclude that 2002-2004 aggregate incremental expenditures were between $24.5 billion for other musculoskeletal diseases and $37.3 billion for arthritis and joint pain. We were unable to estimate an increment in expenditures attributable to conditions in the category including osteoporosis. However, a "back of the envelope" estimate of the ratio of incremental to total expenditures for persons with all forms of musculoskeletal diseases for the period 2002-2004 is possible. Applying the same ratio to the category including osteoporosis yields an estimate of about $18 billion in incremental expenditures for these conditions.

Using the more expansive definition of musculoskeletal diseases, aggregate total medical care expenditures on behalf of persons with a musculoskeletal disease were $718.5 billion in 2002-2004, while the aggregate increment in expenditures was $322.2 in the same period. Total expenditures are the equivalent of 6.5% of GDP for those years, while the incremental cost is the equivalent of 2.9% of GDP.

Section 9.3.2: Medical Care Expenditures for Persons with a Musculoskeletal Disease by Demographics

Expenditures for musculoskeletal diseases are not distributed evenly across groups defined by gender, race, ethnicity, marital status, and type of insurance. (Table 9.7 and Graph 9.3.5) On an unadjusted basis, women with musculoskeletal diseases have about a 20% higher level of expenditures than men; whites have a 30% higher level than non-whites; non-Hispanics report 67% higher expenditures than Hispanics; those who are married or divorced, separated, or widowed have more than 87% higher expenditures than those who have never been married; and those with private and public health insurance have more than two and more than three times, respectively, the expenditures of those without any health insurance. Thus, lack of health insurance is associated with dramatically lower expenditure levels, inconsistent with the belief that persons who lack insurance are somehow able to obtain care. In contrast to the differences in expenditure levels found for gender, race, ethnicity, marital status, and type of health insurance, there was no discernible pattern in expenditure levels by educational attainment.

Adjustment for other characteristics reduced the magnitude of the differences in expenditures found for most demographic characteristics, but did not eliminate them. (Table 9.7 and Graph 9.3.6) Thus, whites experienced about 55% higher levels of

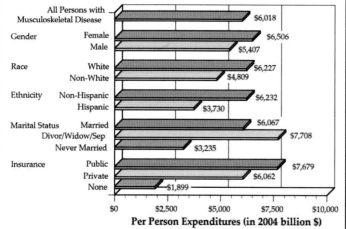

Graph 9.3.5: Per Person Total Medical Care Expenditures for Persons with Musculoskeletal Diseases by Select Demographics, United States 2002-2004

Source: Medical Expenditures Panel Survey (MEPS), Agency for Healthcare Research and Quality, U.S. Department of Health and Human Services, 2002-2004

Includes all medical expenditures for persons with a musculoskeletal disease regardless of whether the expenditure was to treat the musculoskeletal condition or another disease.

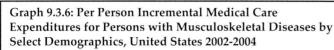

Graph 9.3.6: Per Person Incremental Medical Care Expenditures for Persons with Musculoskeletal Diseases by Select Demographics, United States 2002-2004

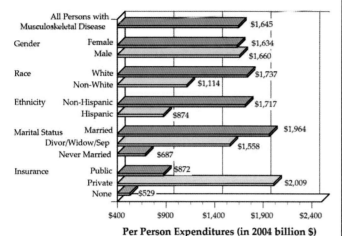

Per Person Expenditures (in 2004 billion $)

Source: Medical Expenditures Panel Survey (MEPS), Agency for Healthcare Research and Quality, U.S. Department of Health and Human Services, 2002-2004

Includes estimated additional medical expenditures beyond those expected for persons of similar characteristics, but without a musculoskeletal disease.

incremental expenditures than non-whites; non-Hispanics reported just under double the expenditures of Hispanics; and the privately insured had more than two times the expenditures of those with public insurance and almost four times the expenditures of those

without insurance. Education level presented no clear picture of differences due to an anomalous result among those who have graduated from college; in general, expenditures rose with higher levels of education. In contrast, adjustment did eliminate difference in expenditures between genders.

Section 9.3.3: Medical Care Expenditures for Persons with a Musculoskeletal Disease by Age

Total medical care expenditures for musculoskeletal diseases are disproportionately higher for persons 65 years of age or older, with a per person cost of nearly $10,000 in 2002-2004 compared to a per person cost of $5,824 for all ages. (Table 9.8 and Graph 9.3.7) Persons aged 65 and over represent more than one in five persons with a musculoskeletal disease; this age group accounted for 38%, or $195.2 billion, of total aggregate health care costs for musculoskeletal diseases in 2002-2004. (Table 9.9 and Graph 9.3.8) However, incremental aggregate

Graph 9.3.7: Total per Person Medical Care Expenditures for Persons with Musculoskeletal Diseases by Age, United States 2002-2004

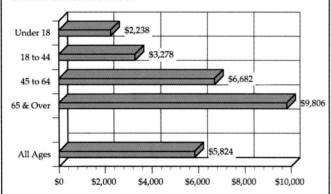

Mean per Person Cost (in 2004 billion $)

Source: Medical Expenditures Panel Survey (MEPS), Agency for Healthcare Research and Quality, U.S. Department of Health and Human Services, 2002-2004

Includes all medical expenditures for persons with a musculoskeletal disease regardless of whether the expenditure was to treat the musculoskeletal disease or another disease.

Graph 9.3.8: Aggregate Total Medical Care Expenditures for Persons with Musculoskeletal Diseases by Age, United States 2002-2004

Source: Medical Expenditures Panel Survey (MEPS), Agency for Healthcare Research and Quality, U.S. Department of Health and Human Services, 2002-2004

Includes all medical expenditures for persons with a musculoskeletal disease regardless of whether the expenditure was to treat the musculoskeletal disease or another disease.

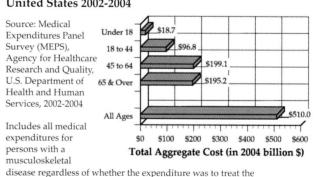

Total Aggregate Cost (in 2004 billion $)

musculoskeletal health care for the 65 and over population is estimated to comprise 25%, or $39.1 billion, of the total $156.4 billion cost. Persons aged 45 to 64 accounted for an equal or slightly higher proportion of the cost (39% of aggregate and 47% of incremental), but represent a substantially higher proportion of the population (34% aged 45 to 64; 23% aged 65 years and older).

Estimated 2002-2004 aggregate total expenditures for persons aged 18 to 64 were $295.9 billion, or 58% of total aggregate health care expenditures for musculoskeletal diseases. This share occurs disproportionately among the 45 to 64 age group, which accounted for 67% of the cost for persons aged 18 to 64, and had an 83% relative increase between 1996-1998 and 2002-2004 in total aggregate cost. This compares to a 12% to 30% relative increase in total cost for other age groups. Less than $19 billion of the total musculoskeletal health care costs went for persons under the age of 18, representing only 10% of total cost.

With a 90% relative increase in incremental cost over the two periods 1996-1998 and 2002-2004, the 45 to 64 age group also accounts for the largest share of incremental aggregate health care cost for musculoskeletal diseases. (Table 9.10) In contrast, incremental costs were relatively stable over this same time period for both persons under the age of 18 and those aged 18 to 44, while

the 65 and over population saw a 15% relative decrease in total incremental musculoskeletal health care costs.

As the population aged, both the proportion of total persons with a musculoskeletal disease and the share of cost attributed to the baby boomer generation, the majority of whom are now 45 to 64 years of age, rose steadily, while the shares attributed to other ages declined. (Table 9.8 and Graph 9.3.9) As the U.S. population aging trend continues and boomers move into the 65 and over age group, the combination of a larger patient population with potentially higher cost of care is likely to reflect increased cost associated with musculoskeletal diseases in the years to come. These increases are likely to surpass even the rapid increases seen in the past decade.

Section 9.4: Impact of Musculoskeletal Diseases on the U.S. Economy

Section 9.4.1: Overall Change in Musculoskeletal Diseases Health Care Cost

Over the period 1996-2004, slight changes in the proportion of total medical care expenditures devoted to ambulatory physicians visits (from 31% to 33% of total) and to emergency room and inpatient care (from 36% to 32%) occurred. However, the share of musculoskeletal health care costs devoted to prescription medications increased the most, growing by 50%, from 14% to 21% of total cost. Computed in 2004 dollars, the mean annual prescription cost per person increased 83%, from $653 to $1,196. During this time, development of biologic agents for several inflammatory conditions, particularly rheumatoid arthritis, occurred, as well as the widespread use of the coxibs for musculoskeletal pain,[i] and may have accounted for some of the rapid increase.

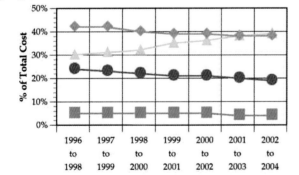

Graph 9.3.9: Proportion of Total Medical Care Expenditures for Persons with Musculoskeletal Diseases by Age, United States 1996-2004

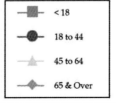

Source: Medical Expenditures Panel Survey (MEPS), Agency for Healthcare Research and Quality, U.S. Department of Health and Human Services, 2002 2004

Includes all medical expenditures for persons with a musculoskeletal disease regardless of whether the expenditure was to treat the musculoskeletal disease or another disease.

i Rofecoxib [Vioxx©] was removed from the market in September 2004; valdecoxib [Bextra©] was taken off the market in 2005; the use of celecoxib [Celebrex©] was curtailed starting in 2005.

The increment in ambulatory care expenditures for musculoskeletal diseases grew by 31% between 1996 and 2004, from $702 to $923 in 2004 dollars. Meanwhile, the increment in emergency room and inpatient care declined slightly, from $304 in the earlier years to $263 in 2002-2004, or by about 13% overall. It is noteworthy that almost no change in the increment in prescription expenditures was seen between 1996-1998 and 2002-2004, an indication that the growth in prescription medications overall did not affect those with musculoskeletal diseases disproportionately. Ambulatory care represents the largest component of the increment in expenditures, indicative of the importance of ambulatory care in musculoskeletal diseases relative to other condition groups.

The eroding share of total expenditures for emergency room and inpatient care between 1996 and 2004 is consistent across the major sub-conditions, while in each of the same subconditions, prescriptions are responsible for a growing share of total expenditures. For spine conditions, the increase in the share was from 13% to 20% of all expenditures, or an increase of 54% in relative terms. The analogous growth in the share of medical care expenditures for arthritis and joint pain was 53%. For the category including osteoporosis, it was 41%, while for injuries, it was 55%. As was the case with respect to the components of total expenditures, the increment in expenditures for prescription medications was neither large nor consistent, another indication that the growth of such expenditures did not occur disproportionately among musculoskeletal diseases relative to other condition groups.

Section 9.4.2: Indirect Cost Related to Musculoskeletal Diseases

In the studies conducted by Rice and colleagues starting in the early 1960s, indirect cost associated

with earnings losses due to musculoskeletal diseases constituted between 38% and 59% of the total cost of these diseases.[7-6] (Table 9.11 and Graph 9.4.1) The percentage shifted because in

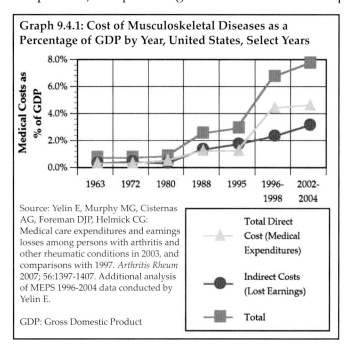

Graph 9.4.1: Cost of Musculoskeletal Diseases as a Percentage of GDP by Year, United States, Select Years

Source: Yelin E, Murphy MG, Cisternas AG, Foreman DJP, Helmick CG: Medical care expenditures and earnings losses among persons with arthritis and other rheumatic conditions in 2003, and comparisons with 1997. *Arthritis Rheum* 2007; 56:1397-1407. Additional analysis of MEPS 1996-2004 data conducted by Yelin E.

GDP: Gross Domestic Product

various eras, medical costs were rapidly escalating while earnings stagnated (1970s); in others times, wage growth exceeded the increase in medical costs (1960s and late 1990s).

Trends in earnings losses associated with musculoskeletal diseases for the period 1996-2004 show a steady increase. (Table 9.12 and Graph 9.4.2) Estimates of earnings losses are limited to persons aged 64 or younger, both because the number of workers over 65 in MEPS is too small to permit statistically reliable estimates in this age group and because in the U.S. most workers retire by that age. However, it is probable that some individuals with musculoskeletal diseases would continue working past the age of 65 in the absence of the condition. Similarly, the tabulation of earnings losses is limited to those who have established a work history either prior to or after the onset of disease. There may be some among those without a work history who would have

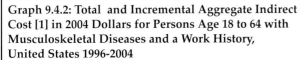

Graph 9.4.2: Total and Incremental Aggregate Indirect Cost [1] in 2004 Dollars for Persons Age 18 to 64 with Musculoskeletal Diseases and a Work History, United States 1996-2004

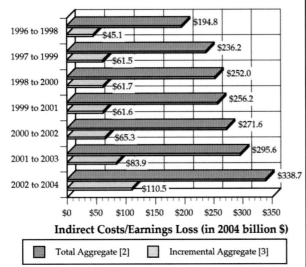

Indirect Costs/Earnings Loss (in 2004 billion $)

■ Total Aggregate [2]   □ Incremental Aggregate [3]

[1] Indirect cost calculated as estimated earnings loss per wage earner due to a musculoskeletal disease.
[2] Includes all medical expenditures for persons with a musculoskeletal disease regardless of whether the expenditure was to treat the musculoskeletal disease or another disease.
[3] Estimated additional medical expenditures beyond those expected for persons of similar characteristics, but without a musculoskeletal disease.

Source: Medical Expenditures Panel Survey (MEPS), Agency for Healthcare Research and Quality, U.S. Department of Health and Human Services, 2002-2004

begun to work in the absence of a musculoskeletal disease, but who never had the opportunity to do so. Thus, the magnitude of earnings losses shown should be considered a conservative estimate.

As of 1996-1998, slightly fewer than 64 million persons with a musculoskeletal disease had established a work history. On average, these individuals sustained $3,052 in earnings losses in 2004 terms; their earnings losses aggregated to $194.8 billion, or the equivalent of 2.4% of GDP for that period. By 2002-2004, the number of persons with musculoskeletal diseases and a work history had grown to over 73 million. On average, these 73 million workers sustained earnings losses of $4,618 each, an increase of 51% compared to 1996-1998, while aggregate earnings losses grew to $338.7 billion, an increase of 74%.

Aggregate losses in 2002-2004 were the equivalent of 3.1% of GDP for that period. Wage growth in the late 1990s played a large role in the increase in the estimate of earnings losses. Average earnings losses grew by more than one-third between 1996-1998 and 1998-2000 (from $3,052 to $4,097); they stagnated through the next two 3-year periods due to the recession, before resuming their growth.

Some of the estimated earnings losses of persons with musculoskeletal diseases might have occurred in the absence of these conditions due to other factors. For example, older workers and women, two groups with high rates of musculoskeletal diseases, have lower employment rates and earnings than the average U.S. worker. The incremental earnings loss measure takes into consideration many of the factors that might cause persons to have lower earnings even without the presence of the musculoskeletal disease. However, earnings losses using the incremental measure also grew substantially between 1996-1998 and 2002-2004. In the earlier triad of years, the 64 million persons with musculoskeletal diseases and a work history sustained average incremental earnings losses of $706, or $45.1 billion overall, the equivalent of 0.5% of GDP for 1996-1998. Average incremental earnings losses approximately doubled by 2002-2004, to $1,506; aggregate incremental earnings losses increased by 2.5 times to $110.5 billion, or 1.0% of GDP for 2002-2004.

Using the more expansive definition of musculoskeletal diseases, average earnings losses increased from $3,226 in 1996-1998 to $3,972 in 2002-2004, or by just under one-fourth in real terms. At the same time, aggregate total earnings losses rose by almost 40%, from $306.0 billion in 1996-1998 to $426.0 billion in 2002 2004. Over the same time period, the average increment in earnings losses increased from $411 to $948, while aggregate incremental earnings losses surged from $39.0 billion to $101.7 billion. Interestingly, the aggregate incremental earnings losses are smaller, however, for the more expansive definition than the more conservative definition, presumably because many persons with conditions of lesser severity are included. (Note: data on earnings losses of persons meeting the expansive definition of musculoskeletal diseases not included in the tables.)

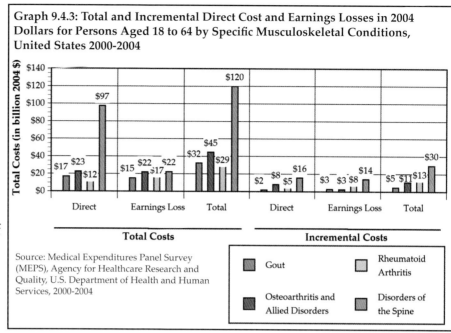

Graph 9.4.3: Total and Incremental Direct Cost and Earnings Losses in 2004 Dollars for Persons Aged 18 to 64 by Specific Musculoskeletal Conditions, United States 2000-2004

Source: Medical Expenditures Panel Survey (MEPS), Agency for Healthcare Research and Quality, U.S. Department of Health and Human Services, 2000-2004

Section 9.4.3: Medical Care Expenditures and Earnings Losses for Select Musculoskeletal Diseases

Medical conditions in MEPS are self-reported and may result in misreporting of some conditions. With respect to musculoskeletal diseases, under-reporting might occur when physicians do not provide patients with a discrete diagnosis for mild osteoarthritis, for example, because it may be too mild to be recognized or treatment is included with other conditions and not distinct. Over-reporting of a condition could occur when the respondent indicates they have a specific form of arthritis, e.g., rheumatoid arthritis, even though their physician did not so indicate. It should be noted that self-reporting of discrete medical conditions is lower than would be expected on the basis of epidemiological studies,[7] a conclusion that is supported by the higher prevalence numbers reported in the previous chapters of *The Burden of Musculoskeletal Diseases*. As a result of potential misreporting, the measures of the aggregate economic impacts of discrete conditions summarized in Table 9.13 and Graph 9.4.3 may not be as reliable as the measures previously presented that are based on larger samples, such as all musculoskeletal disease, or major subcategories, such as all forms of arthritis. Nevertheless, they do indicate in broad stroke the average economic impact for self-recognized disease and for conditions such as osteoarthritis, which are likely to be under-reported, a conservative estimate of aggregate economic impact. Estimates for discrete musculoskeletal diseases merged 5 years of MEPS data (2000-2004) to provide more stable estimates given the relatively few cases of each condition reported in individual years.

Average total direct cost for all four conditions studied—disorders of the spine, rheumatoid arthritis, osteoarthritis and allied disorders, and gout—are relatively large. In the case of gout and spinal disorders, much of the health care expenditures would not occur in the absence of the condition, as evidenced by the much smaller average incremental direct cost. Such is not the case with rheumatoid arthritis and osteoarthritis and allied disorders, where the differences between total and incremental cost are much smaller. Aggregate total cost for the persons with

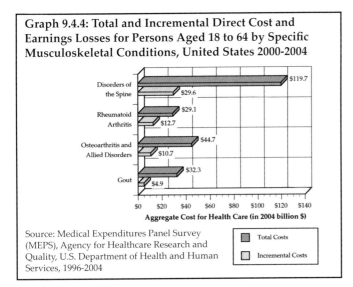

Graph 9.4.4: Total and Incremental Direct Cost and Earnings Losses for Persons Aged 18 to 64 by Specific Musculoskeletal Conditions, United States 2000-2004

Source: Medical Expenditures Panel Survey (MEPS), Agency for Healthcare Research and Quality, U.S. Department of Health and Human Services, 1996-2004

they have an aggregate impact of from $4.9 billion for gout to $29.6 billion for spine disorders. The incremental aggregate figure for rheumatoid arthritis, $12.7 billion, is particularly striking given the relatively low prevalence of this condition and no doubt reflects the growing use of biological agents to treat this condition, along with high work disability rates.

Section 9.4.4: Summary and Conclusions

The economic impact of musculoskeletal diseases is increasing due to a combination of factors that include the aging of the U.S. population with the concomitant increase in the prevalence of musculoskeletal diseases, the growth in average total expenditures to treat musculoskeletal diseases, and the average total and incremental earnings losses that result from these conditions.

Between 1996 and 2004, the number of persons with one or more musculoskeletal diseases grew from 76.0 million, or 28.0% of the population, to 87.6 million, or 30.1% of the population. Over the time period, average total expenditures for health care for persons with a musculoskeletal disease grew from $4,751 to $5,824 in 2004 dollars, while aggregate total expenditures grew from $361.0 billion to $510.0 billion. Average incremental expenditures for persons of similar characteristics but without a musculoskeletal disease grew slower from $1,685 to $1,789, but due to population growth and increased prevalence of the conditions, aggregate incremental expenditures grew from $128.0 to $156.7 billion.

one of the four musculoskeletal diseases ranged from $12.0 billion for rheumatoid arthritis to $97.4 billion for spine disorders, while aggregate incremental cost ranged from $1.9 billion for gout to $15.6 billion for back disorders.

Average total earnings losses were highest for rheumatoid arthritis, $14,175 per year, followed by osteoarthritis at $10,369 per year. They were lowest for back disorders at only $1,231 per year. As evidenced by the ratio of average total to average incremental earnings losses, a much higher proportion of earnings losses are attributable to rheumatoid arthritis and spine disorders (45% and 63%, respectively) than to osteoarthritis or gout.

On an unadjusted basis for total cost, the conditions have an aggregate economic impact ranging from $29.1 billion for rheumatoid arthritis to $119.7 billion for spine disorders. (Table 9.13 and Graph 9.4.4) The greater aggregate impact of spine disorders over average earnings losses is likely due to demographics, with spine disorders occurring more frequently in persons aged 18 to 64, prime working years, while rheumatoid arthritis has been shown to affect persons 65 and older in greater numbers. After adjustment, or the incremental cost impact,

Average per person earnings losses between 1996 and 2004 due to musculoskeletal diseases increased from $3,052 to $4,616, while total earnings losses grew from $194.8 billion to $338.7 billion in constant 2004 dollars. Incremental earnings losses also increased dramatically, from $706 to $1,506 per person and from $45.1 to $110.5 billion on an aggregate basis.

Comparing the cost of musculoskeletal diseases to the national gross domestic product (GDP) provides a perspective on these total costs (Table 9.11). Earlier estimates summarize the evidence from the studies conducted by Dorothy Rice and colleagues, the last two of which were from prior editions of the present volume,[ii] while more recent comparisons for 1996-2004 summarize the data from the present analysis. As discussed in the methodology section, the estimates of incremental medical care expenditures and earnings losses are roughly comparable to the estimates from Rice and colleagues in which costs are allocated on the basis of the primary diagnosis.

Notwithstanding the different methods of the studies by Rice and colleagues and the analysis of MEPS from the present volume, there is no question that the cost of musculoskeletal diseases has a profound economic impact on the nation, now considerably in excess of 2% of GDP. The impact has grown by at least 0.4% of GDP since the 1996-1998 period, and is likely to continue to grow more severe due to population aging, more intensive treatment—particularly with respect to prescription medications, and growing displacement of older workers from industries in decline, a phenomenon that has been shown to affect those with musculoskeletal diseases disproportionately.[9]

Society has the option of passively accepting the increasing economic impact of musculoskeletal diseases, or it can seek to alleviate this impact by the use of primary, secondary, and tertiary preventive measures with strong evidence of effectiveness. Such measures run the gamut from weight loss and exercise programs designed to reduce the prevalence of arthritic conditions, to

self-management classes designed to reduce the impact of existing conditions, to surgical and medical interventions that return the individual to higher levels of functioning and quality of life.[10-12] In the discussion of demographic variations, disparities in medical care expenditures were identified. This suggests the need for equal access to effective interventions and treatment modalities to keep individuals participating in society through work and other meaningful activities

Section 9.5: Background and Methodology

Economic cost for musculoskeletal-related health care diseases presented in this book are based on data from the Medical Expenditures Panel Survey (MEPS) using a methodology developed by the principal author and colleagues at the U.S. Centers for Disease Control (CDC).[13-16] The MEPS is a comprehensive data source designed for cost of illness studies.[17-20] The MEPS uses a random sample of the U.S. population and annually queries this sample three times about their medical conditions, health care utilization, and employment status. Two estimates are produced. The first, *total cost*, is an indication of all medical care costs and earnings losses incurred by persons with a musculoskeletal disease, regardless of the condition for which the cost was incurred. The second, *incremental cost*, is an estimate of the magnitude of cost that would be incurred beyond those experienced by persons of similar demographic and health characteristics but who do not have one or more musculoskeletal disease. Cost estimates are produced as the mean per person medical care cost and as the aggregate, or total cost, associated with all persons with musculoskeletal diseases.

Previous editions of this book based economic impact and cost of musculoskeletal diseases on

ii The National Arthritis Data Task Force concluded that about half of the increase between the 1972 and 1980 studies by Rice and colleagues was due to improvements in the data sources available to Rice and colleagues, but the remainder represented a real increase.[8]

the Rice cost of illness methodology.[5,6] The Rice model utilized the National Hospital Discharge Survey (NHDS) and other available national health care data sources. All costs associated with hospitalizations or treatments for persons with a musculoskeletal disease listed as the primary, or 1st, diagnosis were included in the model. The Rice model defines direct cost as those associated with all components of medical care (i.e., inpatient and outpatient care, medications, devices, and costs associated with procuring medical care), and indirect cost as those associated with wage loss due to morbidity or mortality, plus an estimate of intangible costs.

In the Rice model, mortality accounted for 7% of total indirect medical cost for all conditions. The MEPS data do not provide a comparable method for calculating wage loss associated with mortality. Hence, total cost presented here represents an undercount by a similar percentage. Because musculoskeletal diseases have a smaller impact on mortality than most other major categories of illness, the undercount will be an unknown, but smaller, percentage.

Comparing total cost for 1995,[6] updated to 1996 terms, the first year for which MEPS data is available, and omitting cost associated with mortality, the current analysis results in $207 billion in total cost associated with musculoskeletal diseases using the Rice method and about $173 billion using the MEPS database. This suggests the two methods yield estimates of similar magnitude, although the estimates based on MEPS may be more conservative. A series of papers provide a detailed description of the methods of estimating total and incremental direct and indirect cost of conditions, and outline the regression model used to adjust for differences of persons with and without musculoskeletal diseases due to demographic characteristics and health status.[13,15]

Conditions included in the musculoskeletal disease rubric include spine conditions, arthritis and joint pain, the category that includes osteoporosis (other diseases of bone and cartilage), injuries, and an inclusive "other" category for the remaining conditions. Conditions selected for the cost analysis presented above are based on preceding chapters in the book. Data are reported primarily for base case ICD-9-CM codes, or those codes for which musculoskeletal disease is the principal etiology rather than a consequence of a condition for which the principal etiology is another major health condition (e.g., cancer). (Table 9.14) Estimates are also provided for a more expansive list of codes of musculoskeletal-related diseases that includes the conditions for which the musculoskeletal diseases are the primary and secondary etiologies. (Table 9.15) Although this more expansive list of conditions yields a vastly larger prevalence estimate than the base case list, it is reasonable to assume the cost of musculoskeletal diseases probably exceeds the conservative estimates presented here. For example, a person with bone metastases would incur costs to treat the bone manifestation, even though the cancer, not the bone condition, is the primary etiology. ICD-9-CM codes included in each subcategory for the base and expansive conditions are listed in Tables 9.14 and 9.15.

Although generally prevalence and cost associated with musculoskeletal diseases increase over time, sampling variability in the MEPS does not reflect this in each successive year. The impact of sampling variability is partially mitigated by smoothing, or averaging, data across 3-year periods.

1. US Bureau of the Census: *Statistical Abstract of the US*, 2007. Available at: http://www.census.gov/prod/2006pubs/07statab/income.pdf. Accessed July 6, 2007

2. Rice D: *Estimating the Cost of Illness*. Hyattsville, MD: National Center for Health Statistics, Health Economic Series, 1966, No. 6.

3. Cooper B, Rice D: The economic cost of illness revisited. Health Economics Series No. 6. *Social Security Bulletin* 1979;39:21-35.

4. Rice D, Hodgson T, Kopstein A: The economic costs of illness: A replication and update. *Health Care Fin Rev* 1985;7:61-80.

5. Rice D: Cost of musculoskeletal conditions, in Praemer A, Furner S, Rice D (eds): *Musculoskeletal Conditions in the US*, ed 1. Rosemont, IL: American Academy of Orthopaedic Surgeons, 1992.

6. Rice D: Cost of musculoskeletal conditions, in Praemer A, Furner S, Rice D (eds): *Musculoskeletal Conditions in the US*, ed 2. Rosemont, IL: American Academy of Orthopaedic Surgeons, 1999.

7. Lawrence R, Helmick C, Arnett F, et al: Estimates of the prevalence of arthritis and selected musculoskeletal disorders in the United States. *Arthritis Rheum* 1998;41:788-799.

8. Yelin E, Callahan L: The economic cost and social and psychological impact of musculoskeletal conditions. *Arthritis Rheum* 1995;38:1351-1362.

9. Yelin E, Katz P: Labor force participation among persons with musculoskeletal conditions, 1970-1987: National estimates derived from a series of cross sections. *Arthritis Rheum* 1991;34:136-170.

10. Kruger J, Helmick C, Callahan L, Haddix A: Cost-effectiveness of the arthritis self-help course. *Arch Int Med* 1998;158:1245-1249.

11. Minor M: 2002 Exercise and Physical Activity Conference, St. Louis, Missouri: Exercise and arthritis "We know a little bit about a lot of things." *Arth Rheum* 2003;49:1-2.

12. Redelmeier D, Lorig K: Assessing the clinical importance of symptomatic improvements: An illustration in rheumatology. *Arch Int Med* 1993;153:1337-1342.

13. Yelin E, Cisternas M, Pasta D, et al: Medical care expenditures and earnings losses of persons with arthritis and other rheumatic conditions in the United States in 1997: Total and incremental estimates. *Arthritis Rheum* 2004;50(7):2317-2326.

14. Yelin E, Herrndorf A, Trupin L, Sonneborn D: A national study of medical care expenditures for musculoskeletal conditions: The impact of health insurance and managed care. *Arthritis Rheum* 2001;44:1160-1169.

15. Yelin E, Murphy L, Cisternas MG, et al: Medical care expenditures and earnings losses among persons with arthritis and other rheumatic conditions in 2003 and comparisons with 1997. *Arthritis Rheum* 2007;56(5):1397-1407.

16. Yelin E, Trupin L, Cisternas M: *Direct and Indirect Costs of Musculoskeletal Conditions in 1997: Absolute and Incremental Estimates*. Atlanta, GA: Centers for Disease Control, 2002.

17. Cohen J, Monheit A, Beauregard K. The medical expenditures panel survey: A national information resource. *Inquiry* 1996/1997;33:373-389.

18. Cohen S: *Sample Design of the 1996 Medical Expenditure Panel Survey Household Component*. Agency for Health Care Policy and Research: U.S. Department of Health and Human Services, 1997.

19. Cohen S: *Sample Design of the 1997 Medical Expenditure Panel Survey Household Component*. Agency for Health Care Policy and Research: U.S. Department of Health and Human Services, 2000.

20. Cohen S, DiGaetano R, Goksel H: *Estimation Procedures in the 1996 Medical Expenditure Panel Survey Household Component*. Agency for Health Care Policy and Research: U.S. Department of Health and Human Services, 1999.

Section 9.6: Health Care Utilization and Economic Cost of Musculoskeletal Diseases Data Tables

Table 9.1: Number and Percent of Population with Musculoskeletal Diseases by Age, United States, 1996-2004

		Total Population (in millions)	Persons with Condition			Age Distribution			
			# Individuals (in millions)	% Total Population	Under 18	18-44	45-64	65 & Over
All Musculoskeletal Diseases	1996-1998	6,964	271.2	76.0	28.0%	11.6%	38.0%	28.7%	21.7%
	1997-1999	7,004	273.7	75.2	27.5%	11.4%	36.7%	29.5%	22.4%
	1998-2000	6,025	276.1	74.1	26.8%	11.2%	35.7%	30.5%	22.6%
	1999-2001	6,814	279.7	75.6	27.0%	10.5%	35.0%	31.6%	22.9%
	2000-2002	8,252	283.6	79.7	28.1%	9.8%	34.8%	32.5%	22.8%
	2001-2003	9,166	287.7	84.3	29.3%	9.5%	34.3%	33.4%	22.7%
	2002-2004	9,337	290.8	87.6	30.1%	9.5%	33.7%	34.0%	22.7%
Spine	1996-1998	2,510	271.2	27.4	10.1%	5.4%	47.5%	31.0%	16.1%
	1997-1999	2,580	273.7	27.9	10.2%	5.4%	45.8%	32.0%	16.8%
	1998-2000	2,199	276.1	27.2	9.9%	5.6%	44.6%	33.0%	16.9%
	1999-2001	2,411	279.7	27.3	9.8%	5.6%	44.4%	33.6%	16.4%
	2000-2002	2,927	283.6	28.8	10.2%	5.2%	44.1%	34.0%	16.7%
	2001-2003	3,258	287.7	30.6	10.6%	4.7%	42.8%	35.5%	17.0%
	2002-2004	3,408	290.8	32.7	11.3%	4.5%	41.5%	36.7%	17.3%
Arthritis and Joint Pain	1996-1998	2,804	271.2	29.9	11.0%	3.1%	24.8%	36.4%	35.7%
	1997-1999	2,853	273.7	30.0	11.0%	3.1%	23.3%	37.4%	36.3%
	1998-2000	2,498	276.1	30.3	11.0%	3.3%	22.0%	38.5%	36.2%
	1999-2001	2,936	279.7	32.2	11.5%	3.3%	21.4%	39.0%	36.2%
	2000-2002	3,632	283.6	34.7	12.2%	3.1%	21.6%	39.9%	35.4%
	2001-2003	4,058	287.7	36.9	12.8%	2.8%	22.1%	40.8%	34.3%
	2002-2004	4,103	290.8	37.6	12.9%	2.7%	21.7%	41.6%	34.0%
Osteoporosis	1996-1998	299	271.2	3.2	1.2%	4.3%	10.7%	34.8%	50.1%
	1997-1999	321	273.7	3.4	1.2%	3.1%	8.6%	32.8%	55.5%
	1998-2000	308	276.1	3.8	1.4%	2.3%	7.3%	31.5%	58.9%
	1999-2001	395	279.7	4.4	1.6%	2.2%	6.5%	32.1%	59.2%
	2000-2002	537	283.6	5.3	1.9%	1.9%	6.5%	34.7%	56.9%
	2001-2003	645	287.7	6.1	2.1%	1.7%	6.3%	37.5%	54.5%
	2002-2004	705	290.8	6.8	2.3%	1.3%	6.5%	38.2%	54.0%
Injuries	1996-1998	2,093	271.2	23.4	8.6%	24.2%	43.4%	19.4%	13.0%
	1997-1999	2,047	273.7	22.5	8.2%	24.8%	41.8%	20.0%	13.3%
	1998-2000	1,698	276.1	21.6	7.8%	24.5%	41.8%	21.0%	12.7%
	1999-2001	1,869	279.7	21.4	7.7%	23.0%	41.8%	22.4%	12.8%
	2000-2002	2,235	283.6	22.3	7.9%	21.4%	41.8%	23.4%	13.4%
	2001-2003	2,492	287.7	23.6	8.2%	21.0%	41.1%	24.1%	13.8%
	2002-2004	2,545	290.8	24.7	8.5%	21.2%	40.2%	24.6%	14.0%
Other Musculoskeletal Conditions	1996-1998	1,173	271.2	12.0	4.4%	11.8%	30.6%	31.5%	26.1%
	1997-1999	1,174	273.7	11.8	4.3%	10.4%	30.4%	32.9%	26.3%
	1998-2000	983	276.1	11.3	4.1%	9.7%	29.7%	34.2%	26.4%
	1999-2001	1,098	279.7	11.5	4.1%	9.7%	28.6%	35.5%	26.2%
	2000-2002	1,345	283.6	12.4	4.4%	9.6%	28.3%	36.4%	25.7%
	2001-2003	1,546	287.7	13.6	4.7%	9.8%	27.8%	37.1%	25.3%
	2002-2004	1,618	290.8	14.5	5.0%	9.5%	27.0%	38.4%	25.1%

Note: Totals may differ by orders of magnitude, e.g. prescriptions filled vs. hospital discharges

Source: Medical Expenditures Panel Survey (MEPS), Agency for Healthcare Research and Quality, U.S. Department of Health and Human Services, 1996-2004

Table 9.2: Health Care Utilization by Type for Persons with Musculoskeletal Diseases, United States 1996-2004

Condition	Year	Ambulatory Physician Visits			Non-physician Care Visits			Prescription Medications Filled			Home Health Care Visits			Hospital Discharges		
		% With Any	Mean Visits	Total Visits (in millions)	% With Any	Mean Visits	Total Visits (in millions)	% With Any	Mean Meds Filled	Total Meds (in millions)	% With Any	Mean Visits	Total Visits (in millions)	% With Any	Mean Visits	Total (in millions)
All Musculo-skeletal Diseases	1996-1998	84.8%	5.6	428.5	39.7%	2.6	197.5	81.3%	13.1	995.3	5.1%	3.9	296.3	11.1%	0.2	15.2
	1997-1999	84.9%	5.6	421.0	40.9%	2.7	203.0	81.3%	13.8	1,037.4	5.0%	3.8	285.7	11.6%	0.2	15.0
	1998-2000	85.3%	5.7	422.2	41.0%	2.8	207.4	82.5%	14.6	1,081.5	4.6%	3.4	251.9	11.6%	0.2	14.8
	1999-2001	85.9%	5.7	430.9	42.0%	2.8	211.7	83.8%	15.7	1,186.9	4.6%	3.5	264.6	11.8%	0.2	15.1
	2000-2002	86.0%	5.8	462.5	45.1%	3.1	247.2	84.5%	16.8	1,339.8	4.7%	3.7	295.1	11.7%	0.2	15.9
	2001-2003	85.8%	5.8	488.9	49.2%	3.5	295.0	84.5%	17.8	1,500.5	4.8%	3.5	295.1	11.8%	0.2	16.9
	2002-2004	85.1%	5.8	507.9	51.5%	3.8	332.8	83.5%	18.6	1,628.9	4.7%	3.5	306.5	11.7%	0.2	17.5
Spine	1996-1998	83.2%	6.2	169.7	46.7%	3.7	101.3	80.3%	12.9	353.2	4.1%	2.7	73.9	10.7%	0.2	5.5
	1997-1999	83.0%	6.1	170.2	48.4%	3.9	108.8	80.3%	13.3	371.0	3.9%	3.0	83.7	11.0%	0.2	5.6
	1998-2000	84.0%	6.2	168.7	49.1%	4.1	111.5	81.5%	14.2	386.3	3.6%	2.8	76.2	11.1%	0.2	5.4
	1999-2001	84.6%	6.2	169.0	49.5%	4.2	114.5	82.9%	15.4	419.9	3.5%	2.5	68.2	11.5%	0.2	5.5
	2000-2002	84.7%	6.2	178.7	52.4%	4.5	129.7	83.5%	16.7	481.4	3.7%	2.2	63.4	11.4%	0.2	5.8
	2001-2003	84.3%	6.1	186.7	56.1%	4.9	150.0	83.6%	17.8	544.8	3.9%	2.2	67.3	11.5%	0.2	6.1
	2002-2004	83.6%	6.1	199.7	58.6%	5.3	173.5	82.6%	18.6	609.0	4.0%	2.3	75.3	11.6%	0.2	6.5
Arthritis and Joint Pain	1996-1998	90.1%	6.8	203.3	42.4%	2.6	77.7	89.4%	18.9	565.0	7.9%	6.3	188.3	13.5%	0.2	5.0
	1997-1999	90.4%	6.8	204.0	43.4%	2.6	78.0	89.1%	20.1	603.0	7.7%	6.3	189.0	14.2%	0.2	5.0
	1998-2000	90.1%	6.8	205.7	43.2%	2.6	78.7	89.6%	21.0	635.3	7.0%	5.6	169.4	14.0%	0.2	6.1
	1999-2001	90.3%	6.8	218.8	44.7%	2.8	90.1	90.5%	22.3	717.6	6.8%	5.4	173.8	14.4%	0.2	6.4
	2000-2002	90.5%	6.9	239.2	47.8%	3.3	114.4	91.3%	23.5	814.6	6.9%	5.3	183.7	14.4%	0.2	6.9
	2001-2003	90.8%	7.0	258.6	52.2%	3.8	140.4	91.3%	24.8	916.1	7.1%	5.1	188.4	14.6%	0.2	7.4
	2002-2004	90.3%	7.1	267.3	55.0%	4.1	154.3	90.7%	26.0	978.7	6.9%	5.2	195.7	14.5%	0.2	7.5
Osteopor-osis	1996-1998	96.4%	9.5	30.0	54.1%	3.4	30.3	95.6%	27.8	87.8	10.3%	7.7	24.3	19.2%	0.3	0.9
	1997-1999	97.3%	9.5	32.4	54.7%	4.0	32.4	95.5%	28.0	95.4	10.4%	8.5	28.9	18.5%	0.3	1.0
	1998-2000	97.2%	9.2	34.8	54.6%	4.0	34.8	95.5%	27.9	105.7	8.7%	7.4	28.0	17.8%	0.3	1.1
	1999-2001	96.6%	8.9	39.6	56.3%	3.6	39.6	95.9%	29.3	130.2	8.9%	7.8	34.7	17.2%	0.2	0.9
	2000-2002	95.9%	8.8	46.3	58.9%	3.7	46.3	96.6%	31.4	165.3	9.4%	8.2	43.2	17.1%	0.2	1.1
	2001-2003	95.2%	8.7	53.4	63.5%	4.2	53.4	97.2%	32.2	197.6	10.3%	8.6	52.8	17.1%	0.3	1.8
	2002-2004	95.6%	8.4	57.3	64.8%	4.4	57.3	97.1%	31.3	213.5	9.7%	7.6	51.8	15.4%	0.2	1.4
Injuries	1996-1998	83.0%	4.8	112.1	36.2%	2.3	53.7	76.3%	8.6	200.9	4.2%	2.7	63.1	10.3%	0.1	2.3
	1997-1999	83.9%	4.9	110.2	37.4%	2.6	58.5	76.4%	9.3	209.2	4.1%	3.1	69.7	10.8%	0.1	2.2
	1998-2000	83.5%	5.0	108.0	37.3%	2.8	60.5	77.6%	10.0	215.9	4.1%	3.2	69.1	11.1%	0.1	2.2
	1999-2001	84.0%	5.2	111.5	37.9%	2.8	60.0	78.7%	11.0	235.9	4.0%	3.3	70.8	11.4%	0.2	4.3
	2000-2002	83.8%	5.3	118.1	40.3%	3.0	66.9	79.1%	12.1	269.7	4.2%	3.6	80.2	11.4%	0.2	4.5
	2001-2003	83.6%	5.3	124.9	44.2%	3.3	77.8	78.5%	13.2	311.1	4.4%	3.4	80.1	11.3%	0.2	4.7
	2002-2004	82.7%	5.2	128.3	46.3%	3.7	91.3	77.8%	13.8	340.6	4.3%	3.2	79.0	10.7%	0.2	4.9
Other Musculo-skeletal Conditions	1996-1998	89.8%	7.5	90.3	44.4%	3.4	41.0	86.6%	18.8	226.5	8.3%	6.7	80.7	14.0%	0.2	2.4
	1997-1999	90.6%	7.6	89.8	45.5%	3.6	42.5	87.7%	19.9	235.0	8.1%	6.5	76.8	14.9%	0.2	2.4
	1998-2000	90.8%	7.5	84.9	44.8%	3.4	38.5	88.4%	21.2	240.0	7.4%	6.0	67.9	16.2%	0.3	3.4
	1999-2001	90.8%	7.5	86.4	46.7%	3.4	39.2	89.6%	22.5	259.3	7.4%	6.5	74.9	16.3%	0.3	3.5
	2000-2002	90.6%	7.6	93.9	49.4%	3.7	45.7	89.8%	24.1	297.6	7.0%	6.8	84.0	16.0%	0.2	2.5
	2001-2003	89.9%	7.7	105.1	54.4%	4.5	61.4	90.0%	25.4	346.5	6.7%	6.0	81.9	15.0%	0.2	2.7
	2002-2004	90.2%	7.8	113.2	56.4%	4.9	71.1	89.5%	26.4	383.3	6.6%	5.8	84.2	15.3%	0.2	2.9

Note: Totals may differ by orders of magnitude, e.g. prescriptions filled vs. hospital discharges.
Source: Medical Expenditures Panel Survey (MEPS), Agency for Healthcare Research and Quality, U.S. Department of Health and Human Services, 1996-2004

Table 9.3: Annual Average Change in Total Units of Health Utilization by Type of Care for Persons with Musculoskeletal Diseases, United States 1996-2004

MEPS Data Years Averaged	Ambulatory Physician Visits	Ambulatory Non-physician Visits (Ambulatory Care)	Prescription Medication Filled (Meds)	Home Health Care Days	Hospital Discharges
1996-1998 to 1997-1999	-1.1%	2.7%	4.2%	-3.6%	-1.1%
1997-1999 to 1998-2000	0.3%	2.2%	4.3%	-11.8%	-1.5%
1998-2000 to 1999-2001	2.1%	2.1%	9.7%	5.1%	2.1%
1999-2001 to 2000-2002	7.3%	16.8%	12.9%	11.5%	5.5%
2000-2002 to 2001-2003	5.7%	19.3%	12.0%	0.0%	5.7%
2001-2003 to 2002-2004	3.9%	12.8%	8.6%	3.9%	3.9%
1996-1998 to 2002-2004	2.8%	9.8%	9.1%	0.5%	2.2%
Annual Average Change for Select Musculoskeletal Diseases, 1996-1998 to 2002-2004					
Spine	2.5%	10.2%	10.3%	0.3%	2.8%
Arthritis and Joint Pain	4.5%	14.1%	10.5%	0.6%	3.7%
Osteoporosis	13.0%	13.0%	20.4%	16.2%	6.3%
Musculoskeletal Injuries	2.1%	10.0%	9.9%	3.6%	15.9%
Other Musculoskeletal Conditions	3.6%	10.5%	9.9%	0.6%	2.9%

Source: Medical Expenditures Panel Survey (MEPS), Agency for Healthcare Research and Quality, U.S. Department of Health and Human Services, 1996-2004

Table 9.4: Per Person Components of Total Direct Cost in 2004 Dollars for Musculoskeletal Diseases, United States 1996-2004

Condition	Year	Total Mean and % of All Costs								
		Ambulatory Care		ER and Inpatient		Prescription		Residual		All
All Musculoskeletal Diseases	1996-1998	$1,496	31%	$1,728	36%	$653	14%	$874	18%	$4,751
	1997-1999	$1,493	31%	$1,791	37%	$728	15%	$858	18%	$4,870
	1998-2000	$1,525	31%	$1,795	36%	$798	16%	$808	16%	$4,925
	1999-2001	$1,600	31%	$1,762	34%	$908	18%	$853	17%	$5,125
	2000-2002	$1,734	33%	$1,742	33%	$998	19%	$858	16%	$5,333
	2001-2003	$1,823	33%	$1,771	32%	$1,119	20%	$871	16%	$5,584
	2002-2004	$1,898	33%	$1,865	32%	$1,196	21%	$864	15%	$5,824
Spine	1996-1998	$1,675	35%	$1,728	36%	$638	13%	$714	15%	$4,756
	1997-1999	$1,618	34%	$1,692	35%	$700	15%	$782	16%	$4,791
	1998-2000	$1,697	34%	$1,738	35%	$767	15%	$766	15%	$4,967
	1999-2001	$1,757	34%	$1,786	34%	$871	17%	$775	15%	$5,190
	2000-2002	$1,895	36%	$1,652	31%	$973	19%	$729	14%	$5,249
	2001-2003	$1,905	35%	$1,724	31%	$1,108	20%	$738	13%	$5,475
	2002-2004	$2,022	34%	$1,900	32%	$1,200	20%	$801	14%	$5,923
Arthritis and Joint Pain	1996-1998	$1,849	30%	$2,272	37%	$945	15%	$1,100	18%	$6,166
	1997-1999	$1,831	29%	$2,405	38%	$1,065	17%	$1,100	17%	$6,400
	1998-2000	$1,762	29%	$2,233	36%	$1,160	19%	$1,004	16%	$6,160
	1999-2001	$1,865	29%	$2,168	34%	$1,308	20%	$1,044	16%	$6,384
	2000-2002	$2,072	31%	$2,247	34%	$1,397	21%	$981	15%	$6,697
	2001-2003	$2,281	32%	$2,299	32%	$1,573	22%	$993	14%	$7,145
	2002-2004	$2,393	32%	$2,425	32%	$1,684	23%	$976	13%	$7,477
Osteoporosis	1996-1998	$2,586	31%	$3,040	36%	$1,451	17%	$1,344	16%	$8,422
	1997-1999	$2,603	31%	$2,914	35%	$1,570	19%	$1,269	15%	$8,357
	1998-2000	$2,511	31%	$2,857	35%	$1,615	20%	$1,168	14%	$8,151
	1999-2001	$2,689	33%	$2,498	31%	$1,769	22%	$1,224	15%	$8,179
	2000-2002	$2,779	32%	$2,588	30%	$1,939	23%	$1,310	15%	$8,616
	2001-2003	$2,776	31%	$2,630	30%	$2,092	24%	$1,348	15%	$8,845
	2002-2004	$2,781	32%	$2,488	29%	$2,089	24%	$1,207	14%	$8,565
Musculoskeletal Injuries	1996-1998	$1,332	33%	$1,342	34%	$420	11%	$889	22%	$3,983
	1997-1999	$1,416	33%	$1,485	35%	$485	11%	$868	20%	$4,254
	1998-2000	$1,451	33%	$1,571	36%	$542	12%	$821	19%	$4,384
	1999-2001	$1,563	34%	$1,540	33%	$631	14%	$902	19%	$4,636
	2000-2002	$1,618	33%	$1,565	32%	$718	15%	$969	20%	$4,869
	2001-2003	$1,718	33%	$1,635	32%	$835	16%	$983	19%	$5,171
	2002-2004	$1,721	33%	$1,588	31%	$898	17%	$953	18%	$5,161
Other Musculoskeletal Conditions	1996-1998	$1,918	30%	$2,435	38%	$914	14%	$1,168	18%	$6,435
	1997-1999	$2,040	30%	$2,639	39%	$1,033	15%	$1,140	17%	$6,852
	1998-2000	$2,076	29%	$2,915	41%	$1,127	16%	$1,039	15%	$7,156
	1999-2001	$2,181	30%	$2,793	38%	$1,283	17%	$1,125	15%	$7,382
	2000-2002	$2,229	30%	$2,603	35%	$1,421	19%	$1,187	16%	$7,440
	2001-2003	$2,388	32%	$2,261	30%	$1,603	22%	$1,188	16%	$7,440
	2002-2004	$2,447	32%	$2,390	31%	$1,712	22%	$1,120	15%	$7,668

[1] Due to the sample size, increment not calculated for this subcondition.

Note: Due to estimation errors, increment components do not always equal the total; percentages were not calculated due to this unknown error.

Source: Medical Expenditures Panel Survey (MEPS), Agency for Healthcare Research and Quality, U.S. Department of Health and Human Services, 1996-2004

Table 9.4a: Per Person Components of Incremental Direct Cost in 2004 Dollars for Musculoskeletal Diseases, United States 1996-2004

Condition	Year	Ambulatory Care	ER and Inpatient	Prescription	Residual
			Mean Increment		
All Musculoskeletal Diseases	1996-1998	$702	$304	$210	$280
	1997-1999	$714	$370	$196	$255
	1998-2000	$783	$357	$206	$247
	1999-2001	$798	$353	$188	$239
	2000-2002	$849	$281	$179	$245
	2001-2003	$874	$275	$219	$247
	2002-2004	$923	$263	$212	$258
Spine	1996-1998	$690	$209	$99	$111
	1997-1999	$641	$253	$76	$100
	1998-2000	$780	$364	$60	$108
	1999-2001	$752	$473	$43	$101
	2000-2002	$767	$282	$55	$105
	2001-2003	$660	$155	$52	$90
	2002-2004	$737	$176	$1	$101
Arthritis and Joint Pain	1996-1998	$578	$26	$138	$137
	1997-1999	$529	$125	$77	$135
	1998-2000	$511	$4	$56	$139
	1999-2001	$478	$97	$69	$118
	2000-2002	$508	$112	$59	$103
	2001-2003	$548	$189	$145	$89
	2002-2004	$560	$283	$88	$104
Osteoporosis	1996-1998	[1]	[1]	[1]	[1]
	1997-1999	[1]	[1]	[1]	[1]
	1998-2000	[1]	[1]	[1]	[1]
	1999-2001	[1]	[1]	[1]	[1]
	2000-2002	[1]	[1]	[1]	[1]
	2001-2003	[1]	[1]	[1]	[1]
	2002-2004	[1]	[1]	[1]	[1]
Musculoskeletal Injuries	1996-1998	$486	$485	$36	$400
	1997-1999	$547	$581	$19	$413
	1998-2000	$587	$655	$52	$426
	1999-2001	$624	$627	-$18	$455
	2000-2002	$581	$654	-$19	$442
	2001-2003	$569	$644	$12	$417
	2002-2004	$545	$593	$53	$411
Other Musculoskeletal Conditions	1996-1998	$647	$742	$194	$247
	1997-1999	$845	$744	$260	$252
	1998-2000	$845	$1,186	$293	$249
	1999-2001	$843	$1,052	$245	$226
	2000-2002	$679	$840	$191	$253
	2001-2003	$744	$412	$249	$245
	2002-2004	$755	$532	$205	$225

[1] Due to the sample size, increment not calculated for this subcondition.

Note: Due to estimation errors, increment components do not always equal the total; percentages were not calculated due to this unknown error.

Source: Medical Expenditures Panel Survey (MEPS), Agency for Healthcare Research and Quality, U.S. Department of Health and Human Services, 1996-2004

Table 9.5: Total and Incremental Direct Costs for Musculoskeletal Diseases in Current and 2004 Dollars, United States 1996-2004

Condition	Year	Persons with Condition		Total				Incremental			
		Mean		Aggregate [1]				Mean		Aggregate [1]	
		Sample N	Total Population	Current $ [2]	2004 $ [2]	Current $ (in billions)	2004 $ (in billions)	Current $s [2]	2004 $ [2]	Current $s (in billions)	2004 $ (in billions)
		Column A	Column B	Column C	Column D	Column E	Column F	Column G	Column H	Column I	Column J
All Musculo-skeletal Diseases	1996-1998	6,964	75,978,133	3,600	4,751	273.5	360.0	1,276	1,685	96.9	128.0
	1997-1999	7,004	75,173,840	3,808	4,870	286.3	366.1	1,356	1,733	101.9	130.3
	1998-2000	6,025	74,077,194	3,993	4,925	295.8	364.8	1,482	1,824	109.8	135.1
	1999-2001	6,814	75,600,394	4,323	5,125	326.8	387.5	1,546	1,838	116.9	139.0
	2000-2002	8,252	79,748,298	4,704	5,333	375.1	425.3	1,582	1,800	126.2	143.5
	2001-2003	9,166	84,297,419	5,142	5,584	433.5	470.7	1,638	1,777	138.1	149.8
	2002-2004	9,337	87,575,871	5,594	5,824	489.9	510.0	1,715	1,789	150.2	156.7
Spine	1996-1998	2,510	27,376,436	3,600	4,756	98.6	130.2	759	1,006	20.8	27.5
	1997-1999	2,580	27,893,654	3,749	4,791	104.6	133.6	812	1,033	22.6	28.8
	1998-2000	2,199	27,203,474	4,030	4,967	109.6	135.1	1,050	1,286	28.6	34.0
	1999-2001	2,411	27,263,245	4,376	5,190	119.3	141.5	1,151	1,370	31.4	37.4
	2000-2002	2,927	28,825,976	4,623	5,249	133.3	151.3	998	1,148	28.8	33.1
	2001-2003	3,258	30,607,329	5,044	5,475	154.4	167.6	754	826	23.1	25.3
	2002-2004	3,408	32,740,018	5,700	5,923	186.6	193.9	898	927	29.4	30.3
Arthritis and Joint Pain	1996-1998	2,804	29,893,915	4,675	6,166	139.8	184.3	799	1,057	23.9	31.6
	1997-1999	2,853	29,998,123	5,000	6,400	149.0	191.0	783	1,007	23.5	30.2
	1998-2000	2,498	30,254,301	4,989	6,160	150.9	186.4	666	823	20.1	24.9
	1999-2001	2,936	32,177,862	5,387	6,384	173.3	205.4	723	857	23.3	27.6
	2000-2002	3,632	34,664,846	5,914	6,697	205.0	232.2	757	858	26.2	29.7
	2001-2003	4,058	36,938,769	6,580	7,145	243.1	263.9	916	992	33.8	36.6
	2002-2004	4,103	37,643,137	7,181	7,477	270.3	281.5	951	992	35.8	37.3
Osteoporosis	1996-1998	299	3,158,916	6,391	8,422	20.2	26.6	[3]	[3]	[3]	[3]
	1997-1999	321	3,405,501	6,529	8,357	22.2	28.5	[3]	[3]	[3]	[3]
	1998-2000	308	3,787,044	6,587	8,151	24.9	30.9	[3]	[3]	[3]	[3]
	1999-2001	395	4,444,849	6,914	8,179	30.7	36.4	[3]	[3]	[3]	[3]
	2000-2002	537	5,264,938	7,605	8,616	40.0	45.4	[3]	[3]	[3]	[3]
	2001-2003	645	6,136,560	8,121	8,845	49.8	54.3	[3]	[3]	[3]	[3]
	2002-2004	705	6,819,738	8,212	8,565	56.0	58.4	[3]	[3]	[3]	[3]
Injuries	1996-1998	2,093	23,358,073	3,021	3,983	70.6	93.0	1,051	1,386	24.5	32.4
	1997-1999	2,047	22,495,891	3,329	4,254	74.9	95.7	1,258	1,604	28.3	36.1
	1998-2000	1,698	21,590,412	3,555	4,384	76.8	94.7	1,423	1,751	30.7	37.8
	1999-2001	1,869	21,442,353	3,912	4,636	83.9	99.4	1,438	1,715	30.8	36.8
	2000-2002	2,235	22,285,775	4,297	4,869	95.8	108.5	1,378	1,571	30.7	35.0
	2001-2003	2,492	23,570,429	4,763	5,171	112.3	121.9	1,392	1,508	32.8	35.5
	2002-2004	2,545	24,680,193	4,947	5,161	122.1	127.4	1,404	1,468	34.7	36.2
Residual	1996-1998	1,173	12,046,200	4,876	6,435	58.7	77.5	1,426	1,885	17.2	22.7
	1997-1999	1,174	11,809,322	5,362	6,852	63.3	80.9	1,727	2,191	20.4	25.9
	1998-2000	983	11,322,533	5,811	7,156	65.8	81.0	2,142	2,633	24.3	29.8
	1999-2001	1,098	11,524,129	6,217	7,382	71.6	85.1	2,049	2,456	23.6	28.3
	2000-2002	1,345	12,350,398	6,550	7,440	80.9	91.9	1,719	1,971	21.2	24.3
	2001-2003	1,546	13,643,094	6,853	7,440	93.5	101.5	1,500	1,624	20.5	22.2
	2002-2004	1,618	14,518,291	7,359	7,668	106.8	111.3	1,615	1,685	23.4	24.5

[1] All aggregates (including total) are created by multiplying smoothed means by smoothed population in year.

[2] 2004 and current $ for year are no longer equal due to smoothing.

[3] All individuals with osteoporosis had expenditures and total increment could not be calculated

Source: Medical Expenditures Panel Survey (MEPS), Agency for Healthcare Research and Quality, U.S. Department of Health and Human Services, 1996-2004

Table 9.6: Annual Average and Total Change in Health Care Cost for Persons with Musculoskeletal Diseases, United States 1996-2004

| MEPS Data Years Averaged | Average Annual Increase | | | |
| | Total | | Incremental | |
	Mean	Aggregate [1]	Mean	Aggregate [1]
1996-1998 to 1997-1999	2.5%	1.4%	2.8%	1.8%
1997-1999 to 1998-2000	1.1%	-0.3%	5.3%	3.7%
1998-2000 to 1999-2001	4.1%	6.2%	0.8%	2.8%
1999-2001 to 2000-2002	4.1%	9.8%	-2.1%	3.3%
2000-2002 to 2001-2003	4.7%	10.7%	-1.3%	4.4%
2001-2003 to 2002-2004	4.3%	8.4%	0.7%	4.6%
1996-1998 to 2002-2004	3.2%	5.9%	0.9%	3.2%
Total Increase 1996-1998 to 2002-2004	22.6%	41.3%	6.2%	22.4%
Annual Average Change for Select Musculoskeletal Diseases, 1996-1998 to 2002-2004				
Spine	3.5%	7.0%	-1.1%	1.5%
Arthritis and Joint Pain	3.0%	7.5%	-0.9%	2.6%
Osteoporosis	0.2%	17.1%	[2]	[2]
Musculoskeletal Injuries	4.2%	5.3%	0.8%	1.7%
Other Musculoskeletal Conditions	2.7%	6.2%	-1.5%	1.1%
Total Increase in Health Care Cost for Select Musculoskeletal Diseases, 1996-1998 to 2002-2004				
Spine	24.5%	48.9%	-7.9%	10.2%
Arthritis and Joint Pain	21.3%	52.7%	-6.1%	18.2%
Osteoporosis	1.7%	119.6%	[2]	[2]
Musculoskeletal Injuries	29.6%	36.9%	5.9%	11.9%
Other Musculoskeletal Conditions	19.2%	43.6%	-10.6%	7.7%

[1] All aggregates (including total) are created by multiplying smoothed means by smoothed population in year.

[2] All individuals with the conditions within the category including osteoporosis had expenditures and total increment could not be calculated.

Source: Medical Expenditures Panel Survey (MEPS), Agency for Healthcare Research and Quality, U.S. Department of Health and Human Services, 1996-2004

Table 9.7: Total and Incremental Expenditures for Musculoskeletal Diseases by Demographic Characteristics, United States 2004

Demographic Characteristics	Number of Respondents		Estimated Population (in 1000s)		Total Expenditures			Incremental Expenditures	
	Total	With Musculo-skeletal Diseases	Total	With Musculo-skeletal Diseases	Mean	Standard Error (±)	Aggregate (in millions)	Mean	Aggregate (in millions)
Total Population	32,737	9,027	293,527	89,740	$6,018	$213	$540.16	$1,645	$147.6
Gender									
Female	17,298	5,264	149,658	49,916	$6,506	$225	$324.8	$1,634	$81.6
Male	15,439	3,763	143,869	39,824	$5,407	$371	$215.3	$1,660	$66.1
Race									
White	25,210	7,301	236,409	76,489	$6,227	$244	$476.3	$1,737	$132.9
Non-White	7,527	1,726	57,118	13,252	$4,809	$261	$63.7	$1,114	$14.8
Ethnicity									
Hispanic	9,022	1,523	42,212	7,668	$3,730	$323	$28.6	$874	$6.7
Non-Hispanic	23,715	7,504	251,315	82,072	$6,232	$229	$511.5	$1,717	$140.9
Education [1]									
	8,359	2,299	49,087	16,141	$6,509	$402	$105.1	$1,056	$17.0
High School	10,422	2,876	91,613	28,947	$6,165	$297	$178.5	$1,731	$50.1
Some College	6,935	1,956	70,070	21,377	$5,847	$384	$125.0	$2,070	$44.3
College Graduate	4,071	1,103	48,284	13,596	$4,762	$334	$64.7	$730	$9.9
Graduate School	2,681	737	32,730	9,256	$6,974	$1,195	$64.6	$2,770	$25.6
Marital status [2]									
Never Married	7,012	1,469	62,411	14,975	$3,235	$194	$48.4	$687	$10.3
Married or w/Partner	19,205	5,043	175,791	51,417	$6,067	$298	$311.9	$1,964	$101.0
Divorced-Widowed-Separated	6,457	2,507	55,005	23,289	$7,708	$426	$179.5	$1,558	$36.3
Insurance									
Any Private	18,364	5,530	200,787	63,323	$6,062	$284	$383.9	$2,009	$127.2
Public	9,180	2,535	56,530	18,347	$7,679	$313	$140.9	$872	$15.0
None	5,193	962	36,211	8,071	$1,899	$192	$15.3	$529	$4.3

[1] Education status for individuals < 18 was set to the highest level in the household.   *Education status for individuals < 18 was set to the highest level in the household; marital status for individuals < 18 were set hierarchically by household to married, div/wid/sep, and never married.

[2] Marital status for individuals < 18 was set hierarchically by household to married, div/wid/sep, and never married.

Source: Medical Expenditures Panel Survey (MEPS), Agency for Healthcare Research and Quality, U.S. Department of Health and Human Services, 2004

Table 9.8: Age Distribution of Total and Incremental Direct Costs [1] of Musculoskeletal Diseases, United States 1996-2004

| | Age | **Years Averaged** | | | | | | |
		1996-1998	1997-1999	1998-2000	1999-2001	2000-2002	2001-2003	2002-2004
TOTAL COST								
	<18	858	849	715	762	893	989	1,002
Persons with Condition	18-44	2,481	2,419	2,020	2,252	2,715	3,012	3,030
(Sample N)	45-64	2,118	2,171	1,922	2,243	2,765	3,102	3,179
	65+	1,506	1,564	1,368	1,557	1,879	2,063	2,127
	<18	8,837,738	8,587,926	8,270,671	7,909,778	7,812,654	8,015,131	8,339,766
Persons with Condition	18-44	28,857,105	27,582,172	26,465,903	26,434,506	27,764,847	28,914,760	29,523,069
(Total Population)	45-64	21,794,220	22,136,282	22,574,221	23,930,631	25,951,528	28,209,432	29,802,135
	65+	16,489,070	16,867,460	16,766,399	17,325,479	18,219,269	19,158,096	19,910,901
	<18	$1,880	$2,034	$2,271	$2,586	$2,535	$2,359	$2,238
Total Mean	18-44	$2,945	$3,019	$3,036	$3,101	$3,148	$3,221	$3,278
in 2004 $	45-64	$4,993	$5,062	$5,237	$5,598	$5,934	$6,401	$6,682
	65+	$9,132	$9,092	$8,792	$8,712	$9,009	$9,283	$9,806
	<18	$16.6	$17.5	$18.8	$20.5	$19.8	$18.9	$18.7
Total Aggregate	18-44	$85.0	$83.3	$80.4	$82.0	$87.4	$93.1	$96.8
in 2004 $ (in billions)	45-64	$108.8	$112.1	$118.2	$134.0	$154.0	$180.6	$199.1
	65+	$150.6	$153.4	$147.4	$150.9	$164.1	$177.8	$195.2
INCREMENTALAL COST								
	<18	858	849	715	762	893	989	1,002
Persons with Condition	18-44	2,481	2,419	2,020	2,252	2,715	3,012	3,030
(Sample N)	45-64	2,118	2,171	1,922	2,243	2,765	3,102	3,179
	65+	1,506	1,564	1,368	1,557	1,879	2,063	2,127
	<18	8,837,738	8,587,926	8,270,671	7,909,778	7,812,654	8,015,131	8,339,766
Persons with Condition	18-44	28,857,105	27,582,172	26,465,903	26,434,506	27,764,847	28,914,760	29,523,069
(Total Population)	45-64	21,794,220	22,136,282	22,574,221	23,930,631	25,951,528	28,209,432	29,802,135
	65+	16,489,070	16,867,460	16,766,399	17,325,479	18,219,269	19,158,096	19,910,901
	<18	$1,145	$1,191	$1,365	$1,445	$1,355	$1,261	$1,250
Increment Mean	18-44	$1,140	$1,251	$1,185	$1,208	$1,175	$1,156	$1,105
in 2004 $	45-64	$1,794	$1,884	$2,186	$2,336	$2,364	$2,577	$2,492
	65+	$2,797	$2,598	$2,569	$2,289	$2,156	$1,735	$1,965
	<18	$10.1	$10.2	$11.3	$11.4	$10.6	$10.1	$10.4
Increment Aggregate	18-44	$32.9	$34.5	$31.4	$31.9	$32.6	$33.4	$32.6
in 2004 $ (in billions)	45-64	$39.1	$41.7	$49.3	$55.9	$61.3	$72.7	$74.3
	65+	$46.1	$43.8	$43.1	$39.7	$39.3	$33.2	$39.1

[1] In 2004 $.

Source: Medical Expenditures Panel Survey (MEPS), Agency for Healthcare Research and Quality, U.S. Department of Health and Human Services, 1996-2004

Table 9.9: Distribution of Total Direct Cost for Musculoskeletal Diseases by Age, United States 1996-2004

	Total Aggregate Cost Based on 2004 $			
	≤18	18-44	45-64	65+
1996-1998	5%	24%	30%	42%
1997-1999	5%	23%	31%	42%
1998-2000	5%	22%	32%	40%
1999-2001	5%	21%	35%	39%
2000-2002	5%	21%	36%	39%
2001-2003	4%	20%	38%	38%
2002-2004	4%	19%	39%	38%

	Increment Aggregate Cost Based on 2004 $			
	≤18	18-44	45-64	65+
1996-1998	8%	26%	30%	36%
1997-1999	8%	26%	32%	34%
1998-2000	8%	23%	37%	32%
1999-2001	8%	23%	40%	29%
2000-2002	7%	23%	43%	27%
2001-2003	7%	22%	49%	22%
2002-2004	7%	21%	47%	25%

Source: Medical Expenditures Panel Survey (MEPS), Agency for Healthcare Research and Quality, U.S. Department of Health and Human Services, 1996-2004

Table 9.10: Annual Change in Total and Incremental Health Care Cost for Persons with Musculoskeletal Diseases by Age, United States 1996-2004

MEPS Data Years Averaged	Total Aggregate Cost			
	≤18	18 to 44	45 to 64	65 & Over
1996-1998 to 1997-1999	5.1%	-2.0%	3.0%	1.8%
1997-1999 to 1998-2000	7.5%	-3.5%	5.5%	-3.9%
1998-2000 to 1999-2001	8.9%	2.0%	13.3%	2.4%
1999-2001 to 2000-2002	-3.2%	6.6%	15.0%	8.7%
2000-2002 to 2001-2003	-4.5%	6.6%	17.3%	8.4%
2001-2003 to 2002-2004	-1.3%	3.9%	10.3%	9.8%
Annual Average Increase	1.8%	2.0%	11.9%	4.2%
Total Increase	12.3%	13.9%	83.0%	29.7%

MEPS Data Years Averaged	Incremental Aggregate Cost			
	≤18	18 to 44	45 to 64	65 & Over
1996-1998 to 1997-1999	1.1%	4.9%	6.7%	-5.0%
1997-1999 to 1998-2000	10.4%	-9.1%	18.3%	-1.7%
1998-2000 to 1999-2001	1.2%	1.8%	13.3%	-7.9%
1999-2001 to 2000-2002	-7.4%	2.2%	9.7%	-1.0%
2000-2002 to 2001-2003	-4.5%	2.5%	18.5%	-154%
2001-2003 to 2002-2004	3.1%	-2.4%	2.2%	17.7%
Annual Average Increase	0.4%	-0.1%	12.8%	-2.2%
Total Increase	3.0%	-0.8%	89.9%	-15.2%

Source: Medical Expenditures Panel Survey (MEPS), Agency for Healthcare Research and Quality, U.S. Department of Health and Human Services, 1996-2004

Table 9.11: Cost of Musculoskeletal Diseases as a Percentage of GDP by Year, United States, Select Years

Year	Direct Cost	Indirect Cost	Total
1963	0.3%	0.3%	0.7%
1972	0.3%	0.4%	0.7%
1980	0.5%	0.3%	0.8%
1988	1.2%	1.3%	2.5%
1995	1.2%	1.7%	2.9%
1996-1998			
Total	4.4%	2.3%	6.7%
Incremental	1.5%	0.5%	2.0%
2002-2004			
Total	4.6%	3.1%	7.7%
Incremental	1.4%	1.0%	2.4%

Source: Yelin E, Murphy MG, Cisternas AG, Foreman DJP, Helmick CG: Medical care expenditures and earnings losses among persons with arthritis and other rheumatic conditions in 2003, and comparisons with 1997. *Arthritis Rheum* 2007;56:1397-1407. Additional analysis of MEPS 1996-2004 data conducted by Yelin E.

Table 9.12: Total and Incremental Indirect Cost [1] for Persons Aged 18 to 64 with Musculoskeletal Diseases and a Work History, United States 1996-2004

Year	Population with Musculoskeletal Disease Who Ever Worked	Indirect Cost (Earnings Loss)			
		Raw		**Increment**	
		Mean	Aggregate (in billion $s)	Mean	Aggregate (in billion $s)
1996-1998	63,840,865	$3,052	$194.8	$706	$45.1
1997-1999	62,603,143	$3,773	$236.2	$983	$61.5
1998-2000	61,508,942	$4,097	$252.0	$1003	$61.7
1999-2001	63,182,182	$4,055	$256.2	$975	$61.6
2000-2002	66,886,534	$4,061	$271.6	$977	$65.3
2001-2003	70,931,602	$4,167	$295.6	$1183	$83.9
2002-2004	73,343,698	$4,618	$338.7	$1506	$110.5

[1] Calculated as estimated earnings loss per wage earner due to a musculoskeletal condition in 2004 $.

Source: Medical Expenditures Panel Survey (MEPS), Agency for Healthcare Research and Quality, U.S. Department of Health and Human Services, 1996-2004

Table 9.13: Average Annual Total and Incremental Direct Costs and Total and Incremental Earnings Losses of Persons Aged 18 to 64 for Select Musculoskeletal Diseases, United States 2000-2004

			Gout [1]	Osteoarthritis and Allied Disorders [2]	Rheumatoid Arthritis [3]	Other and Unspecified Disorders of the Back [4]
	Sample N		227	206	128	1,860
	# Individuals		2,309,103	2,120,057	1,205328	18,160,441
	% Total Population		0.8%	0.7%	0.4%	6.3%
Direct Cost	Total	Mean	$7,389	$10,730	$9,938	$5,361
		Aggregate (in billions)	$17.1	$22.7	$12.0	$97.4
	Incremental	Mean	$834	$3,883	$4,116	$857
		Aggregate (in billions)	$1.9	$8.2	$5.0	$15.6
Earnings Losses	Total	Mean	$6,594	$10,369	$14,175	$1,231
		Aggregate (in billions)	$15.2	$22.0	$17.1	$22.4
	Incremental	Mean	$1,296	$1,175	$6,414	$771
		Aggregate (in billions)	$3.0	$2.5	$7.7	$14.0
Total	Total	Aggregate (in billions)	$32.3	$44.7	$29.1	$119.7
	Incremental	Aggregate (in billions)	$4.9	$10.7	$12.7	$29.6

Musculoskeletal Disease

[1] ICD-9-CM Codes: Gout=274

[2] ICD-9-CM Codes: Osteoarthritis and Allied Disorders=715

[3] ICD-9-CM Codes: Rheumatoid Arthritis=714

[4] ICD-9-CM Codes: Other and Unspecified Disorders of the Back=724

Source: Medical Expenditures Panel Survey (MEPS), Agency for Healthcare Research and Quality, U.S. Department of Health and Human Services, 2000-2004

Table 9.14: Base Case ICD-9-CM Codes by Musculoskeletal Disease Included in Economic Impact Analysis

ICD-9-CM Code	Condition Name	ICD-9-CM Code	Condition Name
Spine		**Musculoskeletal Injuries** (continued)	
720	Ankylosing Spondylitis and Other Inflammatory Spondylopathies	810	Fracture of Clavicle
721	Spondylosis and Allied Disorders	811	Fracture of Scapula
722	Intervertebral Disc Disorders	812	Fracture of Humerus
723	Other Disorders of Cervical Region	813	Fracture of Radius and Ulna
724	Other and Unspecified Disorders of Back	814	Fracture of Carpal Bone(s)
737	Curvature of Spine	815	Fracture of Metacarpal Bone(s)
781	Symptoms Involving Nervous and Musculoskeletal Systems	816	Fracture of One or More Phalanges of Hand
805	Fracture of Vertebral Column without Mention of Spinal Cord Injury	817	Multiple Fractures of Hand Bones
		818	Ill-defined Fractures of Upper Limb
806	Fracture of Vertebral Column with Spinal Cord Injury	819	Multiple Fractures Involving Both Upper Limbs, and Upper Limb with Rib(s) and Sternum
830	Dislocation of Jaw	820	Fracture of Neck of Femur
846	Sprains And Strains of Sacroiliac Region	821	Fracture of Other and Unspecified Parts of Femur
847	Sprains And Strains of Other and Unspecified Parts Of Back	822	Fracture of Patella
Arthritis and Joint Pain		823	Fracture of Tibia and Fibula
274	Gout	824	Fracture of Ankle
390	Rheumatic Fever without Mention of Heart Involvement (arthritis, rheumatic, acute or subacute)	825	Fracture of One or More Tarsal and Metatarsal Bones
		826	Fracture of One or More Phalanges of Foot
391	Rheumatic Fever with Heart Involvement	827	Other, Multiple, and Ill-defined Fractures of Lower Limb
710	Diffuse Diseases of Connective Tissue	828	Multiple Fractures Involving Both Lower Limbs, Lower with Upper Limb, and Lower Limb(s) with Rib(s)*
711	Arthropathy Associated with Infections		
712	Crystal Arthropathies	829	Fracture of Unspecified Bones
713	Arthropathy Associated w/Disorders Classified Elsewhere	831	Dislocation of Shoulder
714	Rheumatoid Arthritis and Other Inflammatory Polyarthropathies	832	Dislocation of Elbow
715	Osteoarthrosis and Allied Disorders	833	Dislocation of Wrist
716	Other and Unspecified Arthropathies	834	Dislocation of Finger
719	Other and Unspecified Disorders of Joint	835	Dislocation of Hip
725	Polymyalgia Rheumatica	836	Dislocation of Knee
726	Peripheral Enthesopathies and Allied Syndromes	837	Dislocation of Ankle
727	Other Disorders of Synovium, Tendon, and Bursa	838	Dislocation of Foot
Osteoporosis		839	Other, Multiple, and Ill-defined Dislocations
733	Other Disorders of Bone and Cartilage	840	Sprains and Strains of Shoulder and Upper Arm
Other Musculoskeletal Conditions		841	Sprains and Strains of Elbow and Forearm
015	Tuberculosis of Bones and Joints	842	Sprains and Strains of Wrist and Hand
135	Sarcoidosis: Lupoid of Boeck;Lupus Pernio	843	Sprains and Strains of Hip and Thigh
170	Malignant Neoplasm of Bone and Articular Cartilage	844	Sprains and Strains of Knee and Leg
171	Malignant Neoplasm of Connective and Other Soft Tissue	845	Sprains and Strains of Ankle and Foot
213	Benign Neoplasm of Bone and Articular Cartilage	848	Other and Ill-defined Sprains and Strains
268	Vitamin D Deficiency	875	Open Wound of Chest (wall)
728	Disorders of Muscle, Ligament, And Fascia	876	Open Wound of Back
729	Other Disorders of Soft Tissues	877	Open Wound of Buttock
730	Osteomyelitis, Periostitis, and Other Infections Involving Bone	880	Open Wound of Shoulder and Upper Arm
731	Osteitis Deformans & Osteopathies Assoc w/Disorders Classified Elsewhere	881	Open Wound of Elbow, Forearm, and Wrist
		882	Open Wound of Hand Except Finger(s) Alone
732	Osteochondropathies	883	Open Wound of Finger(s)
734	Flat Foot: Pes planus (acquired); Talipes planus (acquired)	884	Multiple and Unspecified Open Wound of Upper Limb
735	Acquired Deformities of Toe	885	Traumatic Amputation of Thumb (complete) (partial)
736	Other Acquired Deformities of Limbs	886	Traumatic Amputation of Other Finger(s) (complete) (partial)
738	Other Acquired Musculoskeletal Deformity	887	Traumatic Amputation of Arm and Hand (complete) (partial)
739	Nonallopathic Lesions, NEC	890	Open Wound of Hip and Thigh
741	Spina Bifida	891	Open Wound of Knee, Leg (except Thigh), and Ankle
754	Certain Congenital Musculoskeletal Deformities	892	Open Wound of Foot Except Toe(s) Alone
755	Other Congenital Anomalies of Limbs	893	Open Wound of Toe(s)
756	Other Congenital Musculoskeletal Anomalies	894	Multiple and Unspecified Open Wound of Lower Limb
V49	Other Conditions Influencing Health Status	895	Traumatic Amputation of Toe(s) (complete) (partial)
V54	Other Orthopedic Aftercare	896	Traumatic Amputation of Foot (complete) (partial)
Musculoskeletal Injuries		897	Traumatic Amputation of Leg(s) (complete) (partial)
717	Internal Derangement of Knee	905	Late Effects of Musculoskeletal and Connective Tissue Injuries
718	Other Derangement of Joint	927	Crushing Injury of Upper Limb
807	Fracture of Rib(s), Sternum, Larynx, and Trachea	928	Crushing Injury of Lower Limb
808	Fracture of Pelvis	929	Crushing Injury of Multiple and Unspecified Sites
809	Ill-defined Fractures of Bones of Trunk		

Table 9.15: Expansive List ICD-9-CM Codes by Musculoskeletal Disease Included in Economic Impact Analysis

ICD-9-CM Code	Condition Name	ICD-9-CM Code	Condition Name
Spine		**Other Musculoskeletal Conditions**	
307	Special Symptoms or Syndromes, NEC	3	Other Salmonella Infections
346	Migraine	26	Rat-bite Fever
350	Trigeminal Nerve Disorders	36	Meningococcal Infection
353	Nerve Root and Plexus Disorders	56	Rubella
524	Dentofacial Anomalies, Including Malocclusion	88	Other Arthropod-borne Diseases
625	Pain and Other Symptoms Associated w/Female Genital Organs	91	Early Syphilis, Symptomatic
627	Menopausal and Postmenopausal Disorders	95	Other Forms of Late Syphilis, with Symptoms
780	General Symptoms	102	Yaws
782	Symptoms Involving Skin and Other Integumentary Tissue	137	Late Effects of Tuberculosis
784	Symptoms Involving Head and Neck	195	Malignant Neoplasm of Other and Ill-defined Sites
786	Symptoms Involving Respiratory System and Other Chest Symptoms	198	Secondary Malignant Neoplasm of Other Specified Sites
		202	Other Malignant Neoplasms of Lymphoid and Histiocytic Tissue
787	Symptoms Involving Digestive System	203	Multiple Myeloma and Immunoproliferative Neoplasms
789	Other Symptoms Involving Abdomen and Pelvis	215	Other Benign Neoplasm of Connective and Other Soft Tissue
951	Injury to Other Cranial Nerve(s)	238	
953	Injury to Nerve Roots and Spinal Plexus		Neoplasm of Uncertain Behavior of Other and Unspecified Sites and Tissues
Arthritis and Joint Pain		239	Neoplasms of Unspecified Nature
98	Gonococcal Infections	252	Disorders of Parathyroid Gland
99	Other Venereal Diseases	272	Disorders of Lipoid Metabolism
136	Other and Unspecified Infectious and Parasitic Diseases	275	Disorders of Mineral Metabolism
277	Other and Unspecified Disorders of Metabolism	282	Hereditary Hemolytic Anemias
287	Purpura and Other Hemorrhagic Conditions	327	Organic Sleep Disorders
344	Other Paralytic Syndromes	355	Mononeuritis of Lower Limb and Unspecified Site
354	Mononeuritis of Upper Limb and Mononeuritis Multiplex	567	Peritonitis and Retroperitoneal Infections
357	Inflammatory and Toxic Neuropathy	682	Other Cellulitis aAnd Abscess
437	Other and Ill-defined Cerebrovascular Disease	759	Other and Unspecified Congenital Anomalies
443	Other Peripheral Vascular Disease	906	Late Effects of Injuries to Skin and Subcutaneous Tissues
446	Polyarteritis Nodosa and Allied Conditions	958	Certain Early Complications of Trauma
447	Other Disorders of Arteries and Arterioles	996	Complications Peculiar to Certain Specified Procedures
696	Psoriasis and Similar Disorders	V13	Personal History of Other Diseases
Musculoskeletal Injuries		V42	Organ or Tissue Replaced by Transplant
874	Open Wound of Neck	V43	Organ or Tissue Replaced by Other Means
879	Open Wound of Other and Unspecified Sites, Except Limbs	V45	Other Postprocedural States
922	Contusion of Trunk	V48	Problems with Head, Neck, and Trunk
923	Contusion of Upper Limb	V53	Fitting and Adjustment of Other Device
924	Contusion of Lower Limb and Of Other and Unspecified Sites	V66	Convalescence and Palliative Care
926	Crushing Injury of Trunk	V67	Follow-up Examination
		V74	Special Screening Examination for Bacterial and Spirochetal Diseases

Appendices

Appendix A - Musculoskeletal Diseases Diagnosis Codes

ICD-9-CM Diagnosis Codes for Specific Musculoskeletal Diseases

Condition	ICD-9-CM Code	Description
Chapter 2: Spinal Deformity and Related Conditions		
	737	Curvature of the spine
Chapter 3: Spine: Low Back and Neck Pain		
Back Pain (Lumbar and Low Back)		
Back Disorders	720*	Ankylosing spondylitis and other inflammatory spondylopathies
	721.2-.721.9	Spondylosis and allied disorders
	724	Other and unspecified disorders of back
Disc Disorders	722.10, 722.11	Displacement of intervertebral disc
	722.30-722.39	Schmorl's nodes
	722.51, 722.52, 722.60	Degeneration of intervertebral disc
	722.72, 722.73	Intervertebral disc disorder with myelopathy
	722.80, 722.82, 722.83	Postlaminectomy syndrome
	722.90, 722.92, 722.93	Other and unspecified disc disorder
Back Injury	805.20-805.80	Closed fracture of vertebra without mention of spinal cord injury
	806.20-806.90	Closed fracture of vertebra with spinal cord injury
	839.20-839.49	Closed dislocation, vertebra
	846	Sprains and strains of sacroiliac region
	847.10-749.90	Other sprains and strains of back
Cervical (Neck) Pain		
Neck Disorders	721.00, 721.11	Cervical spondylosis
	723.00-723.90	Disorders of cervical region
Disc Disorders	722.00	Displacement of cervical intervertebral disc
	722.40	Degeneration of cervical intervertebral disc
	722.71	Intervertebral disc disorder, with myelopathy
	722.81	Postlaminectomy syndrome of cervical region
	722.91	Other and unspecified disc disorders of cervical region
Neck Injury	805	Closed fracture of cervical vertebra without mention of spinal cord injury
	806	Closed fracture of cervical vertebra with spinal cord injury
	839	Closed dislocation, cervical vertebra
	847.00	Neck sprain
Spine Procedures (ICD-9-CM Procedure Codes)	81.02, 81.03	Cervical fusion
	81.04, 81.05	Thoracic fusion
	81.06-81.08	Lumbar fusion
	81.00, 81.01	Other fusion
	81.62-81.64	Fusion/refusion multiple vertebrae
	81.30-81.39	Spine refusion
	03.09	Spinal decompression
	80.50, 80.51	Spinal diskectomy

ICD-9-CM Diagnosis Codes for Specific Musculoskeletal Diseases (continued)

Condition	ICD-9-CM Code	Description

Chapter 4: Arthritis and Joint Pain

Condition	ICD-9-CM Code	Description
Arthritis and Other Rheumatic Conditions	715	Osteoarthritis
	714	Rheumatoid arthritis
	274, 712	Gout and other crystal arthropathies
	710.00	Systemic lupus erythematosus (Lupus)
	710.01	Systemic sclerosis
	710.20	Sjogren's syndrome
	729.10	Fibromyalgia
	446.50, 725.00	Polymyalgia rheumatica and giant cell arteritis
	099.30, 696.00, 720, 721	Spondylarthropathies
	716, 719	Joint pain
	354, 711, 726, 727, 728, 729.40	All other arthritis and rheumatic conditions
Joint Rreplacement (ICD-9-CM Procedure Codes)	81.54, 815.5, 00.80-00.84	Knee arthroplasty/revision arthroplasty
	81.51-81.53, 00.70-00.76	Hip arthroplasty/revision arthroplasty
	81.56, 81.57, 81.59	Ankle, foot, toe arthroplasty
	81.71, 81.72	Finger arthroplasty
	81.73-81.73, 81.79	Wrist arthroplasty
	81.80, 81.81, 81.83	Shoulder arthroplasty
	81.84, 81.85	Elbow arthroplasty
	81.97	Upper extremity unspecified

Chapter 5: Osteoporosis and Bone Health

Condition	ICD-9-CM Code	Description
Primary Osteoporosis	733	Osteoporosis
Low Energy Fractures	805.00-805.08, 805.20, 805.40, 805.60, 805.80, 808.00, 808.41-808.49, 808.80	Vertebral and pelvic fracture
	810.00-810.03, 811.00-811.03, 811.09, 812.00-812.03, 812.09, 812.20, 812.21, 812.40-812.44, 812.49	Upper limb fracture (closed)
	813.00-813.08, 813.20-813.23, 813.40-813.45, 813.80-813.83, 814.00-814.09, 815.00-815.04, 815.09	Wrist fracture (closed)
	820.00-820.03, 820.09, 820.20-820.22, 820.80	Hip fracture (closed)
	821.00-821.01, 821.20-821.23, 821.29, 822.00, 823.00-823.02, 823.20-823.22, 823.80-823.82	Lower limb fracture, excluding foot and ankle (closed)
	824.00, 824.20, 824.40, 824.60, 824.80, 825.00, 825.20-825.25, 825.29	Ankle and foot fracture (closed)
	733.10-733.16, 733.19, 733.93-733.95	Stress and pathological fractures
	E800-E807, E810-E838, E840-E848, E990-E999	Exclude cases with E-code of high energy fracture
Secondary Osteoporosis	242.90-242.91, 252.00-252.02, 252.08, 255.00, 255.30, 256.20, 256.31, 256.39, 257.10, 257.20, 259.30, 259.90, 268.20, 268.90, 588.00, 588.81, 627.20, 627.40, 627.80, 627.90	Diagnosis that may lead to osteoporosis
	806.00-806.40, 806.50, 806.60-806.62, 806.69, 807.70-706.72, 706.79, 806.80, 806.90	Vertebral fractures with spinal cord injury

ICD-9-CM Diagnosis Codes for Specific Musculoskeletal Diseases (continued)

Condition	ICD-9-CM Code	Description
Chapter 6: Musculoskeletal Injuries		
Fractures	807.00-807.4, 808, 809, 819, 828, 829	Trunk and multiple site fractures
	810, 811, 812, 813, 814, 815, 816, 817	Upper limb fractures
	820, 821, 822, 823, 824, 825, 826, 827	Lower limb fractures
Derangement	717	Knee derangement
	718	Other joint derangement
Dislocation	831, 832, 833	Upper limb dislocation
	834, 835, 836, 837, 838	Lower limb dislocation
	839	Other site dislocation
Sprains/Strains	840, 841, 842	Upper limb sprain/strain
	843, 844, 845	Lower limb sprain/strain
	848	Other site sprain/strain
Contusions	922, 923, 924	
Crushing Injury	926, 927, 928, 929	
Open Wound	874, 875, 876, 877, 879, 880, 881, 882, 883, 884, 890, 891, 892, 893, 894	
Traumatic Amputation	885, 886, 887, 895, 896, 897	
Late Effect of Injury	954, 955, 956, 957, 959	
Chapter 7: Musculoskeletal Congenital and Infantile Developmental Conditions		
	741	Spina bifida
	754.1-754.9	Certain congenital musculoskeletal deformities
	755	Other congenital anomalies of limbs
	756	Other congenital musculoskeletal anomalies
Chapter 8: Neoplasm of Bone and Connective Tissue		
	Data based on National Cancer Institute Classifications	

Appendix B - Musculoskeletal Data Summaries

Table B1: Hospitalizations by First Listed Diagnosis, All Musculoskeletal Diseases, by Age Category and Diagnosis Code, United States 2004

ICD-9-CM	Description	≤18	18-44	45-64	64+	Total
88.8	Other arthropod-borne disease; Other specified arthropod-borne diseases	*	*	*	*	2,271
135	Sarcoidosis	*	2,816	32,966	*	6,900
170.7	Malignant neoplasm of bone and articular cartilage; Long bones of lower limb	890	*	*	*	1,606
171.2	Malignant neoplasm of connective and other soft tissue; Upper limb, including shoulder	*	*	*	*	869
171.3	Malignant neoplasm of connective and other soft tissue; Lower limb, including hip	*	*	867	*	2,207
171.4	Malignant neoplasm of connective and other soft tissue; Thorax	*	*	*	*	853
171.5	Malignant neoplasm of connective and other soft tissue; Abdomen	*	*	*	*	1,286
171.6	Malignant neoplasm of connective and other soft tissue; Pelvis	*	*	*	*	1,059
198.5	Secondary malignant neoplasm of other specified sites; Bone and bone marrow	*	2,761	13,015	19,779	35,682
203	Multiple myeloma ad immunoproliferative neoplasm	*	*	7,179	11,663	19,324
213.7	Benign neoplasm of bone and articular cartilage; Long bones of lower limb	*	*	*	*	861
214.1	Lipoma; Other skin and subcutaneous tissue	*	*	*	*	1,030
238.1	Neoplasm of uncertain behavior of other and unspecified sites and tissues; Connective and other soft tissue	*	*	*	*	1,028
239.2	Neoplasm of unspecified nature; Bone soft tissue and skin	*	*	*	*	949
252	Disorders of parathyroid gland; Hyperthyroidism	*	1,404	372	3,569	8,751
252.1	Disorders of parathyroid gland; Hypoparathyroidism	*	*	*	*	1,172
274	Gout; Gouty arthropathy	*	1,049	2,993	7,075	11,117
275.4	Disorders of mineral metabolism; Disorders of calcium metabolism	*	2,163	4,780	7,864	14,943
282.6	Hereditary hemolytic anemia; Sickle-cell disease	18,597	47,744	6,515	*	72,910
343	Infantile cerebral palsy	1,449	*	*	*	2,097
344	Other paralytic syndromes	*	1,396	10,206	904	3,880
354	Mononeuritis of upper limb and mononeuritis multiplex	*	928	1,851	1,530	4,359
355	Mononeuritis of lower limb and unspecified site	*	1,597	2,370	2,492	6,600
356.90	Hereditary and idiopathic peripheral neuropathy; Unspecified	*	*	*	1,549	2,716
682.20	Other cellulitis and abscess; Trunk	4,859	14,386	16,776	7,087	43,108
682.30	Other cellulitis and abscess; Upper arm and forearm	3,959	20,414	15,686	13,361	53,421
682.40	Other cellulitis and abscess; Hand, except fingers and thumb	2,341	12,390	9,173	6,770	30,674
682.60	Other cellulitis and abscess; Leg, except foot	11,577	52,038	74,888	92,290	230,793
682.70	Other cellulitis and abscess; Foot, except toes	3,635	8,829	15,380	16,893	44,737
696.00	Psoriasis and similar disorders; Psoriatic arthropathy	*	*	*	*	811
710	Diffuse diseases of connective tissue	2,634	10,716	5,722	2,865	21,937
711	Arthropathy associated with infections	2,515	6,259	7,627	7,910	2,431
714	Rheumatoid arthritis and other inflammatory polyarthropathies	*	2,864	7,200	8,982	19,832

* Estimate does not meet standard of reliability or precision.
Source: National Center for Health Statistics, National Inpatient Survey, 2004
Table B1 continued next page.

Table B1: Hospitalizations by First Listed Diagnosis, All Musculoskeletal Diseases, by Age Category and Diagnosis Code, United States 2004 (continued)

ICD-9-CM	Description	≤18	18-44	45-64	64+	Total
715	Osteoarthrosis and allied disorders	*	19,347	236,387	406,485	662,357
716	Other and unspecified arthroplasties	*	4,404	7,891	7,583	20,133
717	Internal derangement of knee	891	3,567	2,538	931	7,927
718	Other derangement of joint	2,399	6,444	4,074	3,116	16,033
719	Other and unspecified disorders of joint	1,442	4,855	7,794	14,723	28,814
720	Ankylosing spondylitis and other inflammatory spondylopathies	*	*	*	*	1,854
721	Spondylosis and allied disorders	*	13,290	43,215	40,516	97,104
722	Intervertebral disc disorders	*	121,008	143,816	70,139	335,619
723	Other disorder of cervical region	*	5,603	13,572	7,858	27,461
724	Other and unspecified disorders of back	*	18,634	46,448	82,387	148,266
725	Polymyalgia rheumatica	*	*	*	2,147	2,397
726	Peripheral enthesopathies and allied syndromes	*	7,862	14,997	14,128	37,633
727	Synovitis & tenosynovitis	2,656	4,645	9,321	7,795	24,417
728	Disorders of muscle, ligament, and fascia	1,604	9,027	9,463	12,411	32,504
729	Other disorders of soft tissue	1,892	8,998	12,507	11,628	35,025
730	Acute osteomyelitis	3,968	11,866	20,069	22,188	58,091
732	Osteochondropathies	3,135	*	*	*	4,046
733	Osteoporosis	4,993	24,706	40,572	89,527	159,797
734	Flat foot	*	*	*	*	975
735	Acquired deformities of toe	*	*	1,044	1,148	2,564
736	Acquired deformities of forearm	2,189	1,695	2,760	2,604	9,249
737	Curvature of spine	6,637	1,820	2,130	1,776	12,364
738.1	Other acquired deformity of head, other specified deformity	*	1,888	1,198	*	3,874
738.4	Other acquired deformity (acquired spondylolisthesis)	*	4,401	11,008	10,493	26,181
741	Spina bifida	1,261	*	*	*	2,043
754.3	Congenital musculoskeletal deformities (congenital dislocation of hip), unilateral dislocation	1,368	*	*	*	1,514
754.5	Congenital musculoskeletal deformities (varus deformities of feet)	1,097	*	*	*	1,422
754.8	Congenital musculoskeletal deformities (other specified nonteratogenic anomalies), pectus excavatum	1,697	*	*	*	1,887
755	Other congenital anomalies of limbs (polydactyly)	2,813	1,101	*	*	4,743
756.1	Other congenital musculoskeletal anomalies (spine)	*	1,787	3,557	2,762	8,877
756.6	Other congenital musculoskeletal anomalies (anomalies of diaphragm)	852	*	*	*	902
756.7	Other congenital musculoskeletal anomalies (anomalies of abdominal wall)	1,123	*	*	*	1,123
781.00	Symptoms involving nervous & musculoskeletal systems (Abnormal involuntary movements)	982	1,217	827	906	3,932

* Estimate does not meet standard of reliability or precision.
Source: National Center for Health Statistics, National Inpatient Survey, 2004
Table B1 continued next page.

Table B1: Hospitalizations by First Listed Diagnosis, All Musculoskeletal Diseases, by Age Category and Diagnosis Code, United States 2004 (continued)

ICD-9-CM	Description	<18	18-44	45-64	64+	Total
781.20	Symptoms involving nervous & musculoskeletal systems (Abnormality of gait)	*	*	1,947	10,884	13,691
781.30	Symptoms involving nervous & musculoskeletal system (lack of coordination)	*	966	2,238	3,550	7,068
781.9	Symptoms involving nervous & musculoskeletal systems (other symptoms)	*	*	1,252	*	2,534
805	Fracture of vertebral column without mention of spinal cord injury	3,523	20,394	15,436	46,025	85,379
806	Fracture of vertebral column with mention of spinal cord injury	*	5,347	3,207	2,415	11,502
807	Fracture of vertebral column with mention of spinal cord injury	919	7,832	12,255	20,178	41,184
808	Fracture of pelvis (acetabulum, closed)	2,577	12,013	9,590	34,950	59,130
810	Fracture of clavicle (closed)	*	2,364	1,304	1,352	5,581
811	Fracture of scapula (closed)	*	1,325	*	*	2,549
812	Fracture of humerus (upper end, closed)	16,000	8,607	12,414	35,858	72,879
813	Fracture of radius and ulna (upper end, closed)	11,633	17,762	14,859	18,220	62,473
814	Fracture of carpal bone(s) (closed)	*	845	*	*	1,659
815	Fracture of metacarpal bone(s) (closed)	*	2,776	951	*	4,906
816	Fracture of one or more phalanges of hand (closed)	821	4,253	2,520	1,136	8,730
820	Fracture of neck of femur (transcervical fracture, closed)	2,500	7,988	27,812	263,244	301,545
821	Fracture of other and unspecified parts of femur (shaft or unspecified part, closed)	14,140	16,619	9,643	21,646	62,047
822	Fracture of patella	*	2,763	3,751	6,072	12,907
823	Fracture of tibia & fibula, upper end (closed)	8,601	30,748	22,136	14,314	75,799
824	Fracture of ankle	7,631	33,878	35,469	29,586	106,564
825	Fracture of one or more tarsal and metatarsal bones	1,290	11,257	5,784	2,607	20,938
826	Fracture of one or more phalanges of foot	*	1,252	902	*	2,818
831	Dislocation of shoulder	*	810	*	1,375	3,085
835	Dislocation of hip	*	1,060	*	*	2,739
836	Dislocation of knee	*	1,744	1,001	1,096	4,027
839	Other, multiple, and ill-defined dislocations	*	1,425	*	1,103	3,677
840	Sprains and strains of shoulder and upper arm	*	1,352	6,027	6,854	14,327
843	Sprains and strains of hip and thigh	*	*	*	2,120	2,695
844	Sprains and strains of knee and leg	1,123	4,873	3,139	3,257	12,391
845	Sprains and strains of ankle and foot	*	1,844	1,158	852	4,050
846	Sprains and strains of sacroiliac region	*	911	*	814	2,348
847	Sprains and strains of other and unspecified parts of back	*	6,353	4,457	2,800	14,326
848.8	Other and ill-defined sprains and strains (other specified sites of sprains and strains)	*	*	*	*	1,121
876.00	Open wound of back	*	940	*	*	1,267

* Estimate does not meet standard of reliability or precision.
Source: National Center for Health Statistics, National Inpatient Survey, 2004
Table B1 continued next page.

Table B1: Hospitalizations by First Listed Diagnosis, All Musculoskeletal Diseases, by Age Category and Diagnosis Code, United States 2004 (continued)

ICD-9-CM	Description	<18	18-44	45-64	64+	Total
877.00	Open wound of buttock	*	*	*	*	813
880.00	Open wound of shoulder and upper arm	*	1,831	*	*	2,813
881.00	Open wound of elbow, forearm, and wrist	828	5,264	2,138	1,207	9,436
882.00	Open wound of hand except finger(s) alone	*	4,248	1,767	948	7,723
883.00	Open wound of finger(s)	*	4,667	1,879	*	7,638
885	Traumatic amputation of thumb	*	925	*	*	1,715
886	Traumatic amputation of other finger(s)	*	3,097	1,425	*	5,624
890	Open wound of hip and thigh	951	2,236	*	*	4,068
891	Open wound of knee, leg (except thigh), and ankle	1,748	5,448	2,151	2,762	12,110
892	Open wound of foot except toe(s) alone	1,243	1,610	1,049	*	4,325
893	Open wound of toe(s)	*	*	*	*	925
895	Traumatic amputation of toe(s)	*	*	*	*	1,102
897	Traumatic amputation of leg(s)	*	*	*	*	932
922	Contusion of trunk	1,036	3,638	3,205	5,420	13,300
923	Contusion of upper limb	*	986	*	1,674	3,748
924	Contusion of lower limb and of other and unspecified sites	892	2,611	3,811	14,159	21,472
927	Crushing injury of upper limb	*	1,379	*	*	23,899
928	Crushing injury of lower limb	*	1,218	899	*	2,733
955	Injury to peripheral nerve(s) of shoulder girdle and upper limb	*	1,953	*	*	2,975
958.30	Posttraumatic wound infection, not else classified	*	1,120	995	*	2,769
959.10	Injury, other & unspecified (trunk)	910	1,465	1,229	1,785	5,390
959.60	Injury, other & unspecified (hip & thigh)	*	*	*	1,174	1,416
959.70	Injury, other & unspecified (knee, leg, ankle & foot)	*	*	*	*	1,248
996.40	Mechanical complication of internal orthopaedic device, implant & graft	*	10,484	31,651	50,958	94,061
996.60	Infection & inflammatory reaction due to internal prosthetic device, implant & graft-internal joint prosthesis	10,623	35,215	67,178	74,523	187,540
996.70	Infection and inflammatory reaction (due to other internal orthopaedic device, implant, and graft)	2,316	20,266	59,662	67,863	150,107
997.60	Amputation stump complication	*	2,755	9,939	10,618	23,457
997.79	Other complication of internal prosthetic device, implant, and graft-due to internal joint prosthesis	*	*	*	*	1,004
V54.00	Other orthopaedic aftercare	860	1,424	2,934	10,229	15,447
V67.00	Follow-up examination, following surgery	*	*	1,261	1,276	3,285

* Estimate does not meet standard of reliability or precision.

Source: National Center for Health Statistics, National Inpatient Survey, 2004

Table B2: Total Hospitalizations for the 30 Most Frequently Listed Musculoskeletal Diseases, by 3-digit ICD-9-CM Code, United States 2004

3-Digit ICD-9-CM Code	Description	Hospitalizations
715	Osteoarthrosis and allied disorders	826,021
272	Disorders of lipoid metabolism	467,005
722	Intervertebral disc disorders	416,140
733	Other disorders of bone and cartilage	352,170
V45	Other post-procedural states	328,291
820	Fracture of neck of femur	305,553
996	Complications peculiar to certain specified procedures	239,841
724	Other and unspecified disorders of back	199,935
V10	Personal history of malignant neoplasm	190,378
V43	Organ or tissue replaced by other means	171,072
721	Spondylosis and allied disorders	148,515
997	Complications affecting specified body systems, not elsewhere classified	127,801
824	Fracture of ankle	117,404
682	Other cellulitis and abscess	117,052
730	Osteomyelitis, periostitis, and other infections involving bone	102,332
813	Fracture of radius and ulna	92,250
823	Fracture of tibia and fibula	83,320
726	Peripheral enthesopathies and allied syndromes	75,361
812	Fracture of humerus	74,556
716	Other and unspecified arthroplasties	72,445
714	Rheumatoid arthritis and other inflammatory polyarthropathies	66,511
821	Fracture of other and unspecified parts of femur	66,502
727	Other disorders of synovium, tendon and bursa	61,697
729	Other disorders of soft tissue	61,241
790	Nonspecific findings on examination of blood	60,881
805	Fracture of vertebral column without mention of spinal cord injury	60,866
738	Other acquired deformity	56,730
357	Inflammatory and toxic neuropathy	51,501
274	Gout	51,032
719	Other and unspecified disorders of joint	50,055

Source: National Center for Health Statistics, National Inpatient Survey, 2004

Table B3: Most Frequently Performed Operations on the Musculoskeletal System Excluding Jaw, United States 2004

ICD-9-CM	Description	Procedures
81.54	Total knee replacement	463,269
03.31	Spinal tap	378,072
80.51	Excision of intervertebral disc	336,847
03.09	Other exploration and decompression of spinal canal	268,954
81.62	Fusion or refusion of 2-3 vertebrae	243,798
03.90	Insertion of catheter into spinal canal for infusion of therapeutic or palliative substances	234,820
81.51	Total hip replacement	230,092
79.35	Open reduction of fracture with internal fixation, femur	171,027
79.36	Open reduction of fracture with internal fixation, tibia and fibula	155,035
03.91	Injection of anesthetic into spinal canal for analgesia	137,290
81.08	Lumbar lumbosacral fusion, posterior technique	126,441
81.02	Other cervical fusion, anterior technique	123,143
77.79	Excision of bone for graft, other (pelvic bones, phalanges, vertebrae)	110,962
84.51	Insertion of interbody spinal fusion device	108,576
81.52	Partial hip replacement	105,199
81.91	Arthrocentesis	69,104
03.92	Injection of other agent into spinal canal	59,587
84.11	Amputation of toe	59,485
79.15	Closed reduction of fracture with internal fixation, femur	57,453
79.32	Open reduction of fracture with internal fixation, radius and ulna	48,832
04.81	Injection of anesthetic into peripheral nerve for analgesia	43,993
84.15	Other amputations below knee	38,440
81.53	Revision of hip replacement	38,042
78.55	Internal fixation of bone without fracture reduction, femur	36,213
81.92	Injection of therapeutic substance into joint or ligament	35,874
81.55	Revision of knee replacement	35,757
79.31	Open reduction of fracture with internal fixation, humerus	35,047
78.69	Removal of implanted devices from bone, Other (pelvic bones, phalanges, vertebrae)	33,031
84.17	Amputation above knee	32,723
83.63	Rotator cuff repair	32,175

Source: National Center for Health Statistics, National Inpatient Survey, 2004

Appendix C - Data Sources

The primary sources of data used in this publication were the National Health Care Surveys (NHCS) family of provider-based surveys conducted by the National Center for Health Statistics (NHCS). NHCS surveys are designed to meet the need for objective, reliable information about the organizations and providers that supply health care, the services rendered, and the patients they serve. The National Health Care Surveys are designed to answer key questions of interest to health care policy makers, public health professionals, and researchers. These can include the factors that influence the use of health care resources, the quality of health care, including safety, and disparities in health care services provided to population subgroups in the United States.

Collectively, NCHS surveys have a combination of design features that make them unique. The surveys are nationally representative, provider-based, and cover a broad spectrum of health care settings. Within each setting, data are collected from a sample of organizations that provide care (such as home health care agencies, inpatient hospital units, or physician offices) and from samples of patient (or discharge) encounters within the sampled organizations.

Each of the National Health Care Surveys collects core information which remains stable over time. Consequently, trends in the types of care delivered in each setting can be monitored in an objective and reliable manner and can be examined in relation to characteristics of providers, patients, and clinical management of patients' care. In addition, the surveys are flexible enough to accommodate special data collection modules and to sample new provider organizations as new information is needed. For most databases, the most current year of data available at the time of analysis was for the year 2004.

Timeliness of data releases and the time required for thorough analysis of multiple databases limits the time span for data presented in the book. In recent years, the release of NCHS databases has shortened. Currently data for 2005 is available. However, at the time work began on this project, 2004 data was the most current year available for most databases.

NHCS surveys used in the *Burden of Musculoskeletal Diseases in the United States* include:

[1] The National Health Interview Survey (NHIS), a nationwide cross-sectional survey of the non-institutional population conducted by household interview, designed to monitor the health of the United States population through the collection and analysis of data on a broad range of health topics. 2005 survey data used; sample size 98,649.

[1a] The National Health Interview Survey Injury Database (NHIS-Injury).

[2] The National Hospital Discharge Survey (NHDS), is a national probability survey designed to meet the need for information on characteristics of inpatients discharged from non-Federal short-stay hospitals in the United States. The NHDS collects data from a sample of approximately 270,000 inpatient records acquired from a national sample of about 500 hospitals. Only hospitals with an average length of stay of fewer than 30 days for all patients, general hospitals, or children's general hospitals are included in the survey. Federal, military, and Department of Veterans Affairs hospitals, as well as hospital units of institutions (such as prison hospitals), and hospitals with fewer than six beds staffed for patient use, are excluded. 2004 survey data used; sample size 370,785.

[3] The National Ambulatory Medical Care Survey (NAMCS), based on a sample of visits to

nonfederally employed office-based physicians who are primarily engaged in direct patient care (physicians in the specialties of anesthesiology, pathology, and radiology are excluded from the survey). 2004 survey data used; sample size 25,286.

[4]&[5] The National Hospital Ambulatory Medical Care Survey (NHAMCS), which collects data on the utilization and provision of ambulatory care services in hospital emergency (ER) and outpatient departments (OP). Findings are based on a national sample of visits to the emergency departments and outpatient departments of noninstitutional general and short-stay hospitals, exclusive of Federal, military, and Veterans Administration hospitals, located in the 50 States and the District of Columbia. 2004 survey data used; sample size 36,589 (ER) and 31,783 (OP).

[6] The National Health and Nutrition Examination Survey (NHANES), the only national survey that collects extensive health information from both face-to-face interviews and medical examinations, providing unique opportunities to study major nutrition, infection, environmental, and chronic health conditions in the U.S. 2004 survey data used; sample size 10,122.

[7] The National Nursing Home Survey (NNHS), one in a continuing series of nationally representative sample surveys of United States nursing homes, their services, their staff, and their residents. 2004 survey data used; sample size 13,507.

The following surveys were also used:

[8] The Healthcare Cost and Utilization Project Nationwide Inpatient Sample (HCUP-NIS), conducted by the Agency for Healthcare Research and Quality (AHRQ), a family of health care databases that brings together the data collection efforts of state data organizations, hospital

associations, private data organizations, and the Federal government to create a national information resource of patient-level health care data. 2004 survey data used; sample size 800,457.

[9] The Medical Expenditures Panel Survey (MEPS) , conducted by the Agency for Healthcare Research and Quality, a set of large-scale surveys of families and individuals, their medical providers, and employers across the United States, and the most complete source of data on the cost and use of health care and health insurance coverage. Data averaged for seven 3-year periods from 1996 to 2004.

[10] The Survey of Occupational Injuries and Illnesses, conducted by the Bureau of Labor Statistics, U.S. Department of Labor, that provides data on illnesses and injuries on the job and data on worker fatalities. Published summary data from 2005.

[11] The National Birth Defects Prevention Network (NBDPN), from which estimates of prevalence for selected defects are drawn based on state birth defects surveillance programs.

[12] The Centers for Disease Control and Prevention (CDC) Metropolitan Atlanta Congenital Defects Program (MACDP), which collects data on birth defects.

[13] The CDC Metropolitan Atlanta Developmental Disabilities Surveillance Program (MADDSP), which monitors the occurrence of selected developmental disabilities in school-age children.

[14] The Surveillance, Epidemiology, and End Results (SEER) Program of the National Cancer Institute, DCCPS, Surveillance Research Program, Cancer Statistics Branch, an authoritative source of information on cancer incidence and survival in

the United States, including cancer incidence and survival data from population-based cancer registries covering approximately 26% of the U.S. population. Published summary data from 2005 data submission.

[15] National Cancer Data Base (NCDB), maintained by the American College of Surgeons Commission on Cancer.

The small size of some databases precludes analysis at a detailed level. In general, ICD-9-CM codes were combined into major musculoskeletal disease classifications to provide sufficient sample size for reliable estimates.

Extensive use was also made of published studies in scientific and epidemiologic journals as secondary sources of data.

it is important to recognize that any one source of data provides an incomplete view of the frequency and impact of a disease or condition. Interview surveys, for instance, generally underestimate the frequency of most musculoskeletal diseases. However, information obtained through the use of interviews is essential to assess an individual's symptoms or how that individual indicates he or she has been affected by a disease. In addition, for some conditions, this may be the only possible means of diagnosis and collection of data.

In contrast, the use of objective methods such as physical examination, laboratory measurements, and radiographs for the detection and diagnosis of disease and injury is not dependent on the subjective reporting of symptoms. However, the objective evidence used to establish the presence or absence of a condition does not always correlate with reported symptoms. It is clear that numerous individuals who report symptoms do not have evidence of disease upon examination and, conversely, some individuals who have objective evidence of disease do not experience symptoms. Thus, although objective measures are valuable tools, they may yield an incomplete picture of the impact of a given disease. They are also more expensive, involve a smaller number of individuals, and may underrepresent less frequently occurring disorders.

Data obtained from medical records are also subject to certain limitations. Many persons affected with certain musculoskeletal diseases do not seek medical care. Although records of visits to physicians and hospitals provide estimates of the volume of visits, these records do not include those who do not seek medical care. Therefore, data based on existing records, will yield only a partial representation of how various musculoskeletal diseases affect the population.

Medical records do not necessarily indicate the underlying musculoskeletal condition. For instance, fractures at various sites, especially hip fractures, are a major consequence of osteoporosis. when admitted to the hospital; however, a fracture diagnosis is usually listed rather than osteoporosis. Medical records may also be subject to "upcoding" to maximize reimbursement and may overstate the frequency of more severe conditions.

By analyzing and including data from a wide range of sources, each with its own strength and weaknesses, it is hoped that the results presented have been integrated into a comprehensive and reasonable understanding of the impact of musculoskeletal diseases on the United States population.

Index

A

Activities of daily living, 1. *See also* Bed days, Lost work days
    Related to arthritis, 82
    Related to injury, 128, 129
    Related to medical conditions, 4, 5
    Related to osteoporosis, 97
    Related to spine problems, 29
Activity restrictions, 28. *See also* Activities of daily living; Impairment; Limitations
Adolescent idiopathic scoliosis. *See* Scoliosis
Aging, 6, 22, 29, 62, 64, 97, 104, 195, 196, 197, 199, 204, 208, 209
Allergies, 21
Ambulatory care, 198, 19, 201, 204, 205. *See also* Outpatient care
    Arthritis, 72, 74, 75, 76, 77, 78, 83
    Injuries, 137
    Spine, 33
American College of Surgeons, 173, 179, 184
Amputation. *See* Injuries
Ankylosing spondylitis, 78
Arthritis, 3, 4, 6, 8, 71-96, 97, 129, 173, 196, 197, 198, 201, 202, 204, 205, 207, 208, 210. *See also* Fibromyalgia; Giant cell arteritis; Gout; Juvenile Arthritis; Lupus; Osteoarthritis; Polymyalgia rheumatica; Rheumatoid; Sclerosis; Sjögren's syndrome
Arthroplasty, 73, 79-83

B

Back pain, 3, 6, 21-53, 61, 62, 130, 131. *See also* Low back pain; Neck pain
    Age, 23, 24, 26
    Bed days, 6, 28-29, 47
    Burden, 27
    Cervical (neck), 3, 21, 25-26, 27, 28, 31, 33
    Gender, 25, 26-27
    Length of stay (inpatient), 24, 26
    Limitations, 27-29
    Lost work, 27-28, 47
    Lumbar (low back), 3, 6, 21-24, 25, 26, 27, 28, 29, 31, 57
    Procedures (spine), 29-32
    Prevalence, 3, 6

    Radiating leg pain, 6, 21, 29
    Site, 22
    Treatment episodes, 22
    Treatment location, 23, 25

Bed days, due to
    Chronic conditions, 5-6
    Musculoskeletal injuries, 129
    Spine conditions, 28-29
Biological agent, 78
Blacks/African Americans, 5, 61, 71, 99
Bone and Joint Decade, 1
Bone mass, 97, 98, 99
Bracing, 55, 57, 58, 59, 60, 61, 64
Burden, 1, 2, 6
    Arthritis, 71, 72, 73, 78, 82
    Back pain, 27
    Congenital conditions, 163
    Musculoskeletal injury, 123, 134
    Neoplasms, 175, 178, 179, 181, 184
    Osteoporosis, 97, 104, 107

C

Carpal tunnel syndrome, 130, 131, 132, 133
Centers for Disease Control and Prevention (CDC), 163, 209
Cerebral palsy, 60, 163, 164-165, 168-169
Cervical pain. *See* Neck pain
Chondrosarcoma. *See* Neoplasms
Chronic conditions
    Chronic circulatory conditions, 2-6
    Chronic joint pain, 3-4, 6, 78
    Chronic musculoskeletal conditions, 3-4
    Chronic respiratory conditions, 2-6
Clubfoot, 163, 164, 166-167
Cobb angle, 55, 56, 58
Congenital
    Cerebral palsy, 60, 163, 164-165, 168-169
    Clubfoot, 163, 164, 166-167
    Dysplasia of the hip, 163, 164, 166, 169
    Limb deficiencies, 163, 164, 167
    Metropolitan Atlanta Congenital Defects Program (MACDP), 163, 164, 168, 169, 170
    National Birth Defects Prevention Network (NBDPN), 163, 164, 169
    Polydactyly, 163, 164, 168
    Prevalence, 163-165, 166, 167, 168, 169, 170